C
CONTEXT

Nancy Roper trained at the General Infirmary, Leeds, UK and later spent 15 years at the Cumberland Infirmary School of Nursing as Principal Tutor. In 1970 she was awarded a fellowship from the Commonwealth Nurses' War Memorial Fund and in 1975 she received an MPhil degree for the thesis based on the research project; she also wrote the monograph *Clinical Experience in Nurse Education* (1976). From 1975–1978 she was Nursing Officer (Research) at the Scottish Home and Health Department. In 1964 she became a self-employed writer and since 1978 she has been a full-time author.

She is the editor of the Churchill Livingstone Pocket Medical Dictionary, Churchill Livingstone Nurses' Dictionary, and New American Pocket Medical Dictionary; and the author of *Man's Anatomy, Physiology, Health and Environment.* In 1976 Winifred Logan and Alison Tierney joined her to work on the first edition of *The Elements of Nursing* which was published in 1980. This was followed by *Learning to Use The Process of Nursing* in 1981 and in 1983 they edited *Using a Model for Nursing*. The second edition of *The Elements of Nursing* appeared in 1985.

PRINCIPLES OF NURSING IN PROCESS CONTEXT

NANCY ROPER MPhil RGN RSCN RNT

FOURTH EDITION

Churchill Livingstone
EDINBURGH LONDON MELBOURNE AND NEW YORK 1988

CHURCHILL LIVINGSTONE
Medical Division of Longman Group UK Limited

Distributed in the United States of America by Churchill Livingstone Inc., 1560 Broadway, New York, N.Y. 10036, and by associated companies, branches and representatives throughout the world.

First edition 1967
Second edition 1973
Third edition 1982
Fourth edition 1988

ISBN 0-443-03576-8

British Library Cataloguing in Publication Data
Roper, Nancy
Principles of nursing in a process context.
4th ed.
1. Nursing
I. Title II. Roper, Nancy. Principles of nursing
610.73 RT41

Library of Congress Cataloging in Publication Data,
Roper, Nancy.
Principles of nursing in a process context.
Rev. ed. of: Principles of nursing. 3rd ed. 1982.
Includes bibliographies and index.
1. Nursing. I. Roper, Nancy. Principles of nursing. II. Title. [DNLM: 1. Nursing Care. 2. Nursing Process. WY 100 R784p]
RT41.R726 1988 610.73 87–34122

Produced by Longman Singapore Publishers Pte Ltd
Printed in Singapore.

Preface

I have to confess to an initial unwillingness to write a fourth edition of *Principles of Nursing*! I started by re-reading the prefaces of the previous three editions and realised that each was considerably different from its predecessors. And this is no less true of the fourth, because the language of nursing has changed and this has necessitated a major re-write.

There is an introductory chapter — Nursing in process context. The process of nursing is currently widely incorporated into nurse education and practice, consequently only a broad overview is given of this problem-oriented process, or method of implementing nursing. However there is an innovation; an economical documentation system comprising a patient assessment form, a patient's nursing plan and a patient's nursing notes is discussed before proceeding to the four phases of the process. To remind readers that a three document recording system is used throughout the book, a 'logo' has been prepared and is placed at the beginning of each chapter. The three documents (or they could be called three parts of one nursing document) are those advocated by Roper, Logan & Tierney (1985) and here I acknowledge my indebtedness to Win and Alison for the many hours we have spent together in our 'trio' work, refining our ideas about nursing, the result of which must inevitably influence 'solo' authorship, however much one tries to wear a 'solo' hat! Beginning with a description of the 'three' documents means that the four phases can then be discussed in relation to them, and this pattern has been adopted in each of the ensuing chapters. Unfortunately in introducing the process of nursing to the wards, the time, which might have been better spent in developing the skills which are necessary to think in process context, was spent in trying to 'fit' each patient into the 'nursing process documents' which appeared on the wards. Understandably, 'documentation' of nursing in process format is still the most common complaint about using the process. There is another innovation in the introductory chapter. This is an attempt to convey the difference between a medical diagnosis and a nursing diagnosis; a nursing diagnosis is a clear statement of those problems which are amenable to nurse-initiated intervention, written in the words the patient uses to describe them. At appropriate places in the text this exercise is repeated.

The headings of the ensuing 24 chapters have been re-worded where necessary, so that each enunciates a principle of nursing. Such an interpretation of 'nursing' cannot be exhaustive; furthermore the principles are not congruent, in that some are concerned with helping patients to carry out a particular everyday living activity; others are concerned with helping patients who are experiencing particular symptoms; some are associated with helping patients to avoid hazards of treatment, and yet others helping patients to avoid the hazards associated with admission to hospital. The common denominator is 'Helping patients ...'. Stating principles of nursing is a much less vigorous exercise than developing a theory of nursing.

The chapters can be used in any order, for example, preventing nosocomial infection, medications, and operations are found towards the end of the book, but these subjects need to be introduced in the first year of a nursing programme. To achieve an additional objective for this fourth edition, which is to help nurses to develop skills for, and confidence in, using their interpretation of 'nursing' in a process context, a format which involves considerable repetition in each chapter has been necessary. To avoid other repetitions, in some chapters objective and subjective information is emphasised, yet it is applicable in all chapters. The same can be said for disabled people being admitted for a reason other than their disablement; for the decision-making inherent in using the process; for the recording of second choice nursing interventions due to lack of equipment or human resources, thus providing factual evidence of these deficiencies; for the personal ethical dilemmas about, for example, medical prescription, or the constraints on the standard of nursing because of, for example, lack of clean linen for changing an incontinent patient; for the increasing emphasis on the nurse's accountability regarding the standard of nursing implemented.

New words are not always explained as it is hoped that students will have a nursing dictionary to hand while reading. Many of the new words are in fact medical diagnoses; the student will learn much more about them throughout a 3 year programme, and a sound base of biological knowledge will facilitate learning, but the important point is that students are being introduced to them in a nursing context.

Account has been taken of the increasing emphasis on 'health' as portrayed by the World Health Organization's project 'Health for all by the year 2000', the UK Government publication 'Health is everybody's business' and the United Kingdom Central Council for Nursing Midwifery and Health Visiting's publication 'Project 2000 : a new preparation for practice'. This last publication is currently being considered by the Government and in the lifetime of readers of this fourth edition it is likely to have considerable influence on nursing education and practice.

The idea of health being incorporated into a concept of nursing emphasises another complex concept, that of habilitation/rehabilitation which is discussed in Chapter 2. However, it is only for the purpose of description that nursing knowledge can be divided into chapters, for in reality each nursing activity is so complex that it requires a synthesis of knowledge from several chapters. This synthesising process, together with clinical experience and response to clinical intuition, contributes to the concept of professional judgement.

The other objectives of the book are unchanged; they are to provide updated references in the Reading Assignments at the beginning of each chapter so that students become aware of the extent of literature available to them; learn to scan it and accept this as a professional responsibility. Many of the references are annotated for two reasons: firstly to help students locate those items which could be read in preparation for class discussion/demonstration. Members of the group can decide who is going to read which references as class preparation, and each member could accept the responsibility of making a précis and presenting it to the others, thus facilitating participative learning. Secondly the annotation will help students to locate items of particular interest when they need them, for instance during their individual clinical allocations. It is hoped that students will develop library skills in locating references, and literary skills in relation to writing references, together with the habit of reading journals, which is one important means of continually updating professional knowledge. Many of the articles also have references so that in following them students can learn the rudiments of literature search.

Stating a principle of nursing explicitly in the heading of each of the chapters has necessitated change at the end of each chapter. There is a new heading 'Applying the principle' and under it, a registered nurse's responsibilities are stated in breadth as before; they are intended as a goal towards which the student of nursing is progressing. Under a new heading 'Working assignment' the subheading 'Topics for discussion' has been retained; they are meant to 'air' problems which can arise in the wards and departments, some of which are of an ethical or moral nature. The subheading 'Writing assignment' has also been retained but re-worded to convey its active nature; the required definitions are of dictionary type; the students will learn more about them as they advance in the educational programme, but, as already mentioned, it is advantageous to introduce them in a nursing context.

Having completed the text, I realise that my current anxiety about what I sincerely believe to be a highly complex answer to an apparently simple question 'What is nursing?' has resulted in a text suitable for a diverse readership. This may be currently appropriate, but it is not good authorship as one should write for a specific readership! Students of nursing may therefore need to draw on the experience of qualified staff regarding some of the discussions.

I have learned a lot from preparing this text, but I do not have all the answers! If it helps nurses to gain satisfaction from implementing individualised nursing, then the enormous task will have been worth while. Feedback from readers' reaction to this fourth edition will provide impetus for further thinking!

I cannot conclude this Preface without saying a big 'thank you' to my publishers, Churchill Livingstone. They coped admirably with my change of mind half-way through the revision to rewrite the text so that it would help readers to practise thinking about the selected principles of nursing in process context. Extra time was needed for me to accomplish this, and staff co-operated in a positive way by adjusting work schedules to facilitate this.

Edinburgh 1988 N.R.

Contents

Introduction: Nursing in process context

READING ASSIGNMENT: PROCESS OF NURSING

Aggleton P, Chalmers H 1984 Models and theories.
1. Defining the terms. Nursing Times 80 (36) September 5: 24–28
2. The Roy adaptation model. Nursing Times 80 (40) October 3:45–48
3. The Riehl interaction model. Nursing Times 80 (45) November 7: 58–61
4. Roger's unitary field model. Nursing Times 80 (50)December 12: 35–39
5. Orem's self-care model. Nursing Times 81 (1) January 2: 36–39
6. Roper's activities of living model. Nursing Times 81 (7) February 13: 59–61
7. Henderson's model. Nursing Times 81 (10) March 6: 33–35

Aggleton P, Chalmers H 1986 Model choice. Senior Nurse 5 (5/6) November/December: 18–20
Offers some guidelines to help nurses to evaluate and choose between different nursing models.

Alibhai Y 1986 Can't they see I'm me? Nursing Times 82 (1) January 1: 56
'If nursing is to do with individual care' then the broad generalisations acquired in studying ethnic minorities can be counter productive.

Barker P 1986 Mechanical faults. Nursing Times 82 (39) September 24: 55–56

'Assessment is about releasing information held within the patient. Much of it is contained in his actions and interactions and needs decoding into the language we all know.'

Barnett D 1985 Making your plans work. Nursing Times 81 (2) January 9: 24–27
Setting realistic goals is a common difficulty in using a problem-solving approach. Suggests some ways to avoid the pitfalls.

Barnett D 1985 The information exchange. Nursing Times 81 (9) February 27: 27–29
Describes an experiment to increase the flow of information from hospital to the community nurse.

Behi R 1986 Look after yourself. Nursing Times 82 (37) September 10: 35–37
Outlines some of the limitations to implementing Orem's self-care model, but concludes it could be introduced in general wards in the UK.

Bond S 1984 The Open University pack: a systematic approach to nursing care.

Buckenham M 1986 Patient's points of view. Senior Nurse 4 (3) March: 26–27
Patients' answers more often concerned attitudes and interpersonal relationships than the practical activities of the nurses.

Carter D 1986 Part of the process. Senior Nurse 5 (5/6) November/December: 20–21
Describes how the Riehl interaction model and the Health belief model can provide a framework for patient education.

Castledine G 1985 Guidelines for success. Nursing Times 81 (34) August 21: 22
Is there enough evidence to prove the worth of 'the nursing process'. Suggests ways in which success can be measured.

Chiarella M 1985 Monitoring the nursing process. Nursing Mirror 160 (20) May 15: 40–42
Describes the work of a nursing process working party.

Clark J 1985 Putting the patient first. Nursing Times 81 (7) February 13: 22
Are you for or against the nursing process? Gives a glowing reference for the process — from a patient.

Clark J 1985 Delivering the goods. Community Outlook January: 23–24, 26–28
Explains why she has become increasingly convinced of the usefulness of the nursing process in health visiting.

Claxton J 1984 The rewarding world of the micro. Nursing Mirror 158 (23) June 13: 8–10
Microcomputers can be integrated successfully with more traditional methods of implement-ing the process of nursing. They are also used in the field of mental handicap as aids for teaching and assessing residents' skills.

Clayton J 1981 Just call me Mrs Begum. Health and Social Service Journal XCI (4736) March 27: 360
Describes the training materials to help health workers in their contacts with Asian people.

Cooper I 1986 The nursing process at work. Nursing Times 82 (1) January 1: 32–35
Occupational health nurses advocate use of the process to provide holistic nursing care.

Cruttenden L 1987 The right to reject care. Nursing Times 83 (5) February 4: 33–35
Do the professionals always know best what the patient requires?

Devlin R 1981 If you've named one you've named them all! Nursing Mirror 152 (22) May 27: 8
Looks at a training kit for health workers — on Asian names.

Dimond B 1987 Doing the right thing. Nursing Times 83 (5) February 4: 61
If there is conflict between a nurse's professional code and a doctor's orders, what should the nurse do?

Draper P 1986 Any use for an American import? Nursing Times 82 (2) January 8: 37–39
Nursing care plans often reveal confusion as to what is and is not a problem amenable to nursing intervention (nursing diagnosis).

Dunn C 1986 An holistic approach to intensive care. Nursing Times 82 (33) August 13: 36–38
Describes the development of plans which have proved successful.

Dyer J 1985 A model of care. Nursing Mirror 160 (17) April 24: 28– 30
Describes use of the Roper, Logan, Tierney model for nursing to care for a patient who had an abdominoperineal resection of colon.

Ellis B 1985 Making it work. Community Outlook January: 22–23

Describes how the process of nursing was implemented in a district.

Evans M 1985 Handled with care. Nursing Times 81 (37) September 11: 32–36
A patient study using Roy's model as a conceptual framework for the nursing process.

Ewles L, Simnett I 1985 Promoting health. Senior Nurse 3 (2) July: 40–42
Discusses the integration of health education into the nursing curriculum.

Faulkner A 1984 Infection control: an integral part of the nursing process. Nursing: The Add-On Journal of Clinical Nursing 3 (3) March: 84–86
Assessment of infection risks. Role modelling.

Filkins J 1986 Introducing change. Nursing Times 82 (7) February 12: 26, 29–30
Describes how a model ward resulted from implementation of individualised patient care.

Fitton J 1985 For the record. Community Outlook June: 19–20, 22
Describes an audit of nursing process records which were designed for action by health visitors.

Fleming I, Tosh M 1985 Going for goals. Nursing Mirror 160 (20) May 15: 42–45
The concept of goal planning and its use with mentally handicapped people are clearly described, and compared to the process of nursing. Goal planning entails a clear and detailed assessment of the client, and the clear identification of goals which the intervention will be attempting to achieve. An assessment is made of the individual's strengths or abilities, and needs or deficits. By doing this, the client is viewed in a positive manner and emphasis on 'problems' is avoided.

Flood N, Saunders M 1984 The process of recording. Nursing Mirror 158 (22). May 30: 34–37
A study of record-keeping by nurses resulted in improved care plans and a more appropriate form for history taking.

Fox C 1985 What's in a name? Nursing Mirror 161 (15) October 9: 44– 45
Describes some of the backlashes from using patients' first names.

Fraser R 1985 The nursing process — a core concept for mental handicap nursing. Nursing: The Add-On Journal of Clinical Nursing 2 (37) May: 1096–1097

Glasper A, Stonehouse J, Martin L 1987 Core care plans. Nursing Times 83 (10) March 11: 55–57
Contains an illustration of a core plan for patient with chronic obstructive airways disease using the Henderson model of nursing.

Gould D 1985 Measuring recovery. Nursing Mirror 160 (13) March 27: 17–18
Useful references. Discusses the problems of measuring patients' recovery and the weaknesses in so many current methods of assessment.

Grahame C 1985 Mutton dressed as lamb? Nursing Times 81 (40) October 2: 56
Claims that some nurses were carrying out the nursing process before the term was invented.

Henley A 1981 Asian patients in hospital and at home. King's Fund, London

Holmes P 1985 Celebrating the process. Nursing Times 8 (14) January 23: 20
Reports a one-day seminar. Does the process encourage patients to participate in their own care?

Howie C 1986 On the record. Nursing Times 82 (50) December 10: 29– 30
Discusses the debate on patients' rights to see their medical and nursing records.

Jackson A 1985 Follow the charts. Nursing Times 81 (6) February 6: 24–25
Application of knowledge is essential to the process of nursing. Considers the use of flow charts in problem solving.

Jayram R 1984 Radical treatment indicated. Nursing Mirror 159 (1) July 18: 21
Despair and confusion about the process of nursing.

Kilgour D, Logan W 1985 A model for health: its use in an undergraduate nursing programme. Nurse Education Today 5: 215–220
Discusses use of the Roper, Logan, Tierney model for nursing based on a model of living.

Miller A 1985 Are you using the nursing process? Nursing Times 81 (50) December 11: 36–39

Mitchell J R A 1984.Is nursing any business of doctors? A simple guide to the 'nursing

process'. Nursing Times 80 (19) May 9: 28–32
Moheeputh R 1984 The light in the ward. Nursing Mirror 159 (19) November 21: 38–39
Offers advice about implementation of the process of nursing on night duty.
Roper N, Logan W, Tierney A 1985 The elements of nursing, 2nd edn. Churchill Livingstone Edinburgh, p 347–357
Ross T 1984 Opening out the process. Nursing Times 80 (17) April 25: 16–17
Discusses the Open University teaching package about the process of nursing.
Royal College of Nursing 1986 Nursing process. Royal College of Nursing, London
Report of a working party of the RCN Association of Nursing Practice.
Slack P 1985 Standards of care. Nursing Times 81 (22) May 29:
Describes the use of Monitor and Qualpacs as audit systems for measuring standards of care.
Sparrow S, Pearson A 1985 Teach yourself goal setting. Nursing Times 81 (42) October 16: 24–25
A lively self-teaching programme.
Tierney A J 1984 Defending the process. Nursing Times 80 (20) May 16: 38–41
Tutton L 1986 What is primary nursing? The Professional Nurse 2 (2) November: 39–40
Primary nurses accept full responsibility for assessing individual patients and planning their nursing until their discharge.
Waters K 1986 Cause and effect. Nursing Times 82 (5) January 29: 28, 30
Evaluation is an important part of the process of nursing but it is difficult to do. A thoughtful article about the difficulties.
Wertheimer A 1986 Information retrieval. Nursing Times 82 (50) December 10: 31–33
Why is the patient's right to see his records so hotly disputed? Outlines some of the arguments for and against right of access.
Williamson C 1984 What's in a name? Nursing Times 80 (48) November 28: 30, 32
Although nurses usually ask if they can call a patient by first name, they don't always get an honest answer; this can upset the relationship between nurse and patient.
Wilson-Barnett J 1985 Principles of patient teaching. Nursing Times 81 (8) February 20: 28–29
The golden rule is ask the patient.
Wright S 1984 In praise of patient-centred nursing. Nursing Times 80 (26) June 27: 11
Wright S 1985 Real plans for real patients. Nursing Times 81 (34) August 21: 36–38
Wright S 1985 Special assignment. Nursing Times 81 (35) August 28: 36–37
A system of patient allocation can be rewarding for both nurse and patient.
Wright S 1985 A rich experience. Nursing Times 81 (36) September 4: 38–39
Looks back at 5 years using the process in the ward.
Wright S 1985 How one nurse was converted. Nursing Times 81 (33) August 14: 24–27
The process can work even in a busy 25-bed geriatric ward.

Nursing in a very broad sense is helping people, whatever the medical diagnosis, to manage their everyday living activities so that they achieve their individual optimal status of well-being or health, which is discussed on page 34.

'People' includes those born with a congenital mental and/or physical handicap, or physical abnormality, so that health visitors, school nurses, and mental handicap nurses are involved. Occupational health departments, well women's /men's clinics are domains in which the nurse's knowledge of health is of paramount importance. And there are nurses in more recently appointed health education posts.

Use of the term 'medical model' in a nursing context implies that the main focus of nursing is the patient's medical diagnosis (whether disease or trauma) and the ensuing doctor's orders, many of which are carried out by nurses. It is an undeniable fact that even when seeking to clarify nursing's unique contribution to the total health care programme, there continues to be a number of medical prescriptions which are carried out by nurses. However, modern technology has increased the sophistication of methods for treatment and investigation available to doctors. In view of these methods, some of which are very frightening to patients, they require more than ever, nurses who will not only help them to make sense of their actual experience of the treatment and/or investigation, but will also help them to continue their everyday living activities. This cannot be done unless the nurse is aware of the individualised pattern of these activities, and one objective in using the process of nursing is to accomplish this.

THE PROCESS OF NURSING

From articles in the Reading Assignment you will be aware that there are differences of opinion about the 'nursing process'. Jayram (1984) expresses his 'despair at the confusion and uncertainty that exists about the nursing process'. One of the fundamental facts about the process of nursing is that it is merely a method/a process of carrying out nursing; it does not tell us what to assess and so on.

Use of the term 'nursing process' may well have predisposed nurses to expect that what constitutes 'nursing' is defined as well as the logical, systematic approach. The broad interpretation throughout this text is that nursing is concerned with helping people to carry out everyday living activities to their maximal potential of independence congruent with their condition and circumstances. 'Everyday' is used in the Concise Oxford Dictionary meaning of 'commonplace'.

What to assess is guided by an explicit interpretation of what constitutes nursing, and some authors have published their interpretation of what constitutes nursing as a model for nursing (p. 115). A selection of items in the Reading Assignment gives an introduction to this subject.

It cannot be stressed too strongly that the process is merely a method of carrying out nursing. The majority of items in the Reading Assignment describe the method as comprising four phases, steps or stages, and any of these words are currently acceptable. In this text the word 'phase' will be favoured, though all three words have the disadvantage of linearity, that is, they convey the idea that the phases are sequential, whereas the notion of an ongoing circular activity is nearer reality. An interesting idea and illustration — 'nursing process spiral' — is given by Barnett (1985); this could be pursued as it might help clarification of some aspects of the process of nursing.

The number of phases referred to in the previous paragraph is not set in stone and some authors use six. What is important is that you fully understand what is included in each phase in the context in which it is being used, for example, on the documents in the clinical areas to which you will be allocated in the programme, or when writing a patient study, exact details should be given.

From the Reading Assignment you will have identified a mixture of words used to describe the phases of the process of nursing, which in verb form are:

- to assess
- to plan
- to implement
- to evaluate.

The World Health Organization in its medium term programme which attempted to identify the nursing contribution to total health care programmes used the words:

- assessment
- planning
- implementation
- evaluation.

Using the nouns — assessment, implementation and evaluation — has a possibility of conveying the idea of a one-off activity and this is not the case. The four phases in this text will therefore be referred to as:

- assessing
- planning
- implementing
- evaluating.

There are two reasons for this choice:

- to emphasise the active ongoing nature of each phase
- to achieve consistency in the use of words.

It was mentioned earlier that one objective in using the process is to individualise nursing.

Other uses are:

- to be part of a monitoring programme related to the quality of nursing service
- to give greater job satisfaction to practising nurses
- to provide factual information to managers when, because of staff shortages, items in the 'planned nursing' had to be omitted
- to provide factual information to managers when a second best nursing intervention had to be planned because of lack of resources
- to provide information during investigation of patients' complaints, even in a legal setting
- to help nurses to describe nursing's contribution to other paramedicals, the public and the politicians.

From the background reading you will be aware that the process of assessing, planning, implementing and evaluating is not the sole prerogative of nursing. You will realise that you use it in your everyday activities; industrial management uses it; and in another guise the National Health Service is beginning to use it — Performance Indicators, Quality Assurance and Quality Circles are terms which appear in particular items in the Reading Assignment (Slack 1985). First-year students of nursing cannot be expected to have detailed knowledge of these concepts which are likely to assume greater significance during their 3-year programme. In an ever-increasingly competitive world and in a health service short of finance it is difficult to justify the existence of nursing if it cannot be demonstrated that it benefits the recipient in some way. Use of the process of nursing is an attempt to achieve this.

Various documents are being used in different clinical areas on which to record in process format, information related to the patient's nursing. Documenting is undoubtedly a highly complex activity, but understanding the rationale involved is more important than the actual pieces of paper on which relevant information is documented. The stance taken in this text is that taken by Roper, Logan & Tierney (1985). We believe that to make documenting manageable and minimal, three documents are necessary: the patient assessment form, the nursing plan, and the patient's nursing notes. These will be discussed briefly from the point of view of how they work.

Patient assessment form

Patient profile and nursing history are other names for this document. It is used in the initial interview between patient and nurse and is the first opportunity of establishing a nurse/patient relationship.

Most forms request biographical information to help nurses on succeeding shifts to individualise their interactions with the patient. An item included in several assessment forms, 'preferred name' seems to have resulted in nurses and patients being on first name terms, but it is beginning to have a backlash from patients as depicted by Fox (1985) and Williamson (1984). We tend to believe that the British naming system is the only one, but this is far from the truth. Help is at hand regarding the intricate Asian naming systems (Clayton 1981, Devlin 1981, Henley 1981).

Another item included in some forms, 'significant others' resulted in a negative medical response (Mitchell 1984) followed by a nursing explanation (Tierney 1984). Other information requested relates to such things as occupation and hobbies and is used by nurses to individualise their conversation with the patient, and to help prevention of boredom, a frequent complaint of patients (p. 38). Whatever biographical information is requested on an assessment form, its objective is to help nurses on succeeding shifts to individualise their interactions with patients and should be written with this in mind.

An assessment form usually requests information about everyday living activities, first of all to give a vignette of previous habits of carrying out each activity to help nurses on each shift to individualise each patient's day. The admitting nurse is also seeking to discover the person's level of independence in each activity. If any aids are used to maintain independence in one or more of the activities, this should be carefully recorded so that the person is not deprived of this way of coping by any nurse on any shift. There may be things which the person habitually cannot do and with which he will need nursing help, and the nurse will elicit what sort of help. This information should be written in such a way that all nurses will offer the same sort of help. It is not a new problem: the patient has learned to cope with it by arranging help from another person. In the interests of minimising paper work this information need not be re-written on the nursing plan as long as nurses agree to use information on the assessment form throughout the person's stay in the health care service.

If the reason for the person's entry to the health care service is a problem with one or more everyday living activity(ies) which will require a nursing intervention, it becomes an entry in the patient's nursing plan which will be discussed later. However the description of the problem on the assessment form is only applicable on the day on which it was written and therefore further information about it should not be written on the

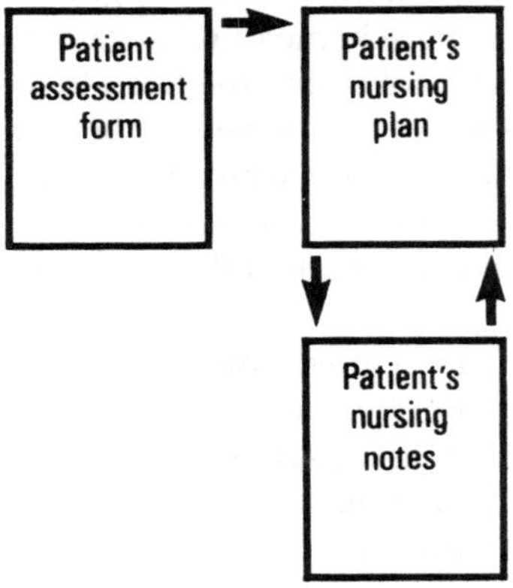

Fig. I.1

assessment form. In Figure I.1 the assessment form stands alone, yet it informs the nursing plan when particular problems, actual or potential, which require planned nursing intervention have been identified, and indeed it guides many of the nursing activities which are part and parcel of the patient's day, but which do not require to be written on the nursing plan. However one exception to this, concerns eating and drinking (p. 143) and it resulted from the discovery of malnutrition in hospital patients. The illustration also shows that the assessment form is not influenced by either the nursing plan or the nursing notes.

Nurses vary as to whether identification of the patient's problems, actual or potential, should be written on the assessment form or on the nursing plan. From published documents, writing them in the first column of the nursing plan seems to be favoured. It is probably the most difficult part — describing the problem from the patient's point of view. Barnett (1985) gives some good advice about this. To state a problem as 'At present has a urinary infection' and the goal as 'To clear up urinary infection' is not helping the development of nursing knowledge. Nursing is concerned with the problems arising in everyday living because of the medical condition. 'Urinary infection' (cystitis) is a medical diagnosis confirmed by the laboratory. Identification of the problem from the patient's perspective might read:

- passing urine x 10 day, x 3 night
- confined to house
- pain on passing scalding urine
- perineum sore
- avoiding painful sexual intercourse

Some nurses consider this cluster of patient's problems a nursing diagnosis.

The fact that there are numbers for the increased frequency of passing urine gives base data against which evaluation can take place, and will give rise to the goal statement/patient outcome — decreasing the number of times urine is passed by day and night and might be recorded as PU ↓ day/night. 'Confined to house' is the patient's way of coping with the increased frequency and urgency related to passing urine. The goal will be 'patient socialising in previous pattern'. The remaining three patient's problems will respond to the nursing intervention:

- facilitating patient's understanding about:
  - cystitis
  - perineal hygiene
  - hygiene and sexual intercourse.

These will not only aid recovery but will prevent recurrence of the condition.

Patient's nursing plan

'Nursing care plans' and 'care plans' are other terms used for this document. You might like to debate whether or not 'nursing care' is a tautology! And 'care plans' could apply to any other paramedical's plans. Because nursing is the subject of this book, the term 'nursing plans' will be strictly adhered to. There are other forms of planning which concern nurses and in, for instance, the chapter about eating and drinking the opportunity is taken to discuss generalised planning, ward planning and individualised planning.

The patient's problems related to one or more everyday living activities, actual or potential, for which nurse-initiated interventions are required, are written on the nursing plan. A goal is set related to alleviation or solution of the problem and a date by which it is to be achieved is appended. Each time the intervention is carried out it will be recorded on the patient's nursing notes, not on the nursing plan. When the goal is achieved the intervention on the nursing plan is cancelled and dated. Roper, Logan & Tierney (1985) suggest that this part of the nursing plan is kept separate from that resulting from medical or other prescription (as mentioned later) so that the nurse-initiated part of nursing can be identified.

There will be some nursing activities on the nursing plan which are not related to a patient's problem — several preoperative preparations come into this category. In the interests of economy of time and paperwork some wards find it acceptable for the nurses who carry out these activities to sign the plan. This would seem to be sensible for one-off 'activities' as opposed to regular 'interventions'.

There will also be some delegated nursing interventions arising from medical prescriptions written in the medical notes, and some resulting from physiotherapists', occupational therapists' and speech therapists' prescriptions which are usually verbal and not written. Roper, Logan & Tierney (1985) suggest that these are recorded in the nursing plan on a separate sheet from that used for nurse-initiated interventions related to problems with everyday living activities.

Patient's nursing notes

These do not have a particular design, merely a margin in which the date and time of each entry are recorded. All planned nursing interventions as they are carried out are recorded, together with any nursing activities/observations (assessments) which the nurses on the next shift need to know. If the patient develops another problem related to his everyday living activities this will be described, and an agreed nursing intervention to achieve a set goal/patient outcome/objective will be written on the nursing plan. The carrying out of this extra nursing intervention will be recorded on the patient's nursing notes.

Having discussed briefly the documents on which nursing is recorded, there follows a discussion of selected aspects of the four phases of the process of nursing — assessing, planning, implementing and evaluating.

Assessing

There is ample information about assessing in the Reading Assignment. Here, it might be useful to collect together a scheme of what can be observed about a patient, following the head to toe pattern. Written lists look formidable but the probability is that very little will need to be written! However, by learning this scheme you will be able to 'scan' patients — the hallmark of the effective nurse.

head:	large/medium/small	
bossing:	forehead/occiput	
fontanelles:	bulging/sunken	
eyes:	bulging/sunken	
	pupils:	dilated/unequal /constricted
	squint:	right/left/both
	cataract:	right/left/both
	artificial:	right/left/both
	spectacles:	all the time/ reading only/ bifocal
earlobes:	right/left/both	
	protruding:	right/left/both
	earrings:	right/left/both
		number: right/ left

hair: shiny/dull
short/long
current colour
current style
malodorous
dandruff
nits/headlice baldness

facial appearance: rash/acne/scars

mood: up
normal
down

expression:

lips: cold sores (herpes simplex)
scar of hare-lip
intertrigo at corners of mouth
upper lip: active/inactive when speaking
lower lip: active/inactive when speaking
mouth: presence of teeth
state of teeth
dentures: upper/lower/both
sordes
tongue: clean/furred
gums
breath

neck: front view: are both sides symmetrical?
side view: Adam's apple area larger/smaller than 'normal'
swelling over Adam's apple area symmetrical/left/right
pulsation of blood vessels: right/left /both

shoulders: well braced: athletic prowess/ confidence/feeling good
drooping: poor physique/ loss of confidence/ depression

spine: upright posture/noticeably curved spine

upper limbs: presence/absence of right/left/both
scars from previous operation/ trauma right/left
limitation of movement from operation/trauma right/left
length relative to age: short/long

hands: skin: chafed from immersion in water
endangered by work
suggestive of clean working conditions
nicotine stains: index fingers right/left/both
nails: bitten/state of manicure/ spoon-shaped

chest: respiratory rate: abnormalities are quickly observed with practice
symmetry of breast: male/female
pigeon chest
discharge from nipples
let-down of milk in postnatal period
size of breasts: large/medium/small
maceration under breasts

abdomen: different exaggerated shapes in obese people
upper abdominal breathing indicative of chronic heart failure
swellings
scars

lower limbs: presence/absence of right/left/both
scars from previous operation/ trauma right/left
limitation of movement from operation/trauma
length relative to age: short/long
bow legs
pigeon-toed
bunion: right/left
hammer toe: right/left, which toe?
corns
verruca
nails
hardened skin
athlete's foot

Planning

We do not yet seem to have solved the many difficulties related to use of nursing plans, the outcome of the planning phase of the process. Most published ones start with a problem column and it is here that our lack of skill is evident — in verbalising the patient's personal problems caused by the medical diagnosis. Take as an example:

medical diagnosis: gastric ulcer

patient's problem:

- experiences 'indigestion'/pain shortly after eating (epigastric pain)
- belches, passes wind per rectum, experiences discomfort from distended abdomen (flatulence)
- afraid to eat
- anxious about loss of weight because of lessened food intake
- anxious about constipation because of lessened food intake
- rumbling noises in stomach/belly/abdomen (borborygmi)

Given that a nursing diagnosis is a clear statement of the patient's problems which are amenable to nursing and related to everyday living, it would seem that we can use the term 'nursing diagnosis' when we have gained sufficient skill in stating the patient's problems as he experiences them. However, in the UK we do not have a sufficient data bank of correctly stated patients' problems to attempt a classification system of nursing diagnoses. We imported uncritically from the USA 'the nursing process' without realising that it only made sense when used with an explicit acknowledgement of what constitutes 'nursing'. My current stance in relation to nursing diagnosis classification is — make haste slowly and reliably (Draper 1986).

In our zeal to individualise nursing by using the process, we must not forget that as well as planning to individualise nursing for each patient, a great deal of ward planning is necessary to facilitate individualised nursing (p. 92), and even more generalised planning goes on in a higher echelon to provide the resources such as linen, dressings, equipment, furniture, food, non-nursing, nursing, paramedical and medical staff to facilitate individualised nursing.

Implementing

Implementing would seem to be the most straightforward phase of the process of nursing. However the planned nursing interventions relate to problems which the patient is experiencing, and to identified potential problems to prevent them becoming actual ones. Yet there will be other nursing activities required if the patient is to continue carrying out the non-problematic everyday living activities.

In going along with the four phases of the process of nursing, one positive point has emerged — it has compelled nurses to analyse and verbalise the cognitive skills which are a part of each nursing intervention/activity. Previously a first year student would be privileged to observe a registered nurse carrying out a technique; she would be baffled by the dexterity and the ability to change, for example the previous dressing to a different one. The registered nurse found it difficult to explain the cognitive skills employed in realising that change was necessary, and what the change should be. Well founded clinical judgement cannot be taken for granted and every effort should be made to analyse it, to verbalise the analysis to justify the selection of one nursing activity/intervention as opposed to other options. Of course in an emergency situation this can only be done after the event, by reflecting on what happened. In the substantiation of the 'science' of nursing, equal emphasis requires to be given to the 'art' of nursing.

Documenting the implementing phase of the process has already been referred to. Each time the planned intervention is carried out it will be recorded on the patient's nursing notes together with any observed change or untoward reaction such as the patient feeling nauseated. But there will be some nursing activities to facilitate a patient attending to the other non-problematic everyday activities, and these may not need to be documented, but should be remembered when nurse staffing levels are being discussed.

Evaluating

From articles in the Reading Assignment you will be aware that nurses feel they have been given least help with this phase of the process of nursing. In many ways this is understandable because it is so closely related to the other three. The result of vigorous discussion between Roper, Logan & Tierney about evaluating is to be found on pages 78 and 79 of the second edition of *The Elements of Nursing* and I recommend that you read them.

In view of the current staffing position and the decreasing number of 18-year-olds on the labour market, written nursing records will be the main communicating tool between nurses on different shifts. The next chapter is about communicating but here it is appropriate to say that in patient satisfaction surveys a recurrent theme is inadequate communication between staff, 'one doesn't know what the other is doing' (Buckenham 1986).

This introductory chapter has given a brief account of the process of nursing, a patient assessment form and how it informs the nursing plan, a case of one-directional information. The nursing plan must inform the patient's nursing notes and the nursing notes may inform the nursing plan. A selective discussion of the four phases of the process of nursing followed. In each of the ensuing chapters a principle of nursing (see Preface) will be considered in a process of nursing context.

APPLYING THE PRINCIPLE

A registered nurse must be capable of:

- organising work by selecting a model for nursing and using it
- teaching other staff about the process of nursing
- carrying out the code of conduct set by UKCC
- acting as a role model to other staff.

WORKING ASSIGNMENT

Topics for discussion

- task allocation
- patient allocation
- team nursing
- primary nursing
- United Kingdom Central Council (UKCC)
- Royal College of Nursing (RCN)
- the function of a model
- the process of nursing
- health
- medical model in nursing
- a model for nursing.

Writing assignment

- define the process of nursing
- state the words which can be used to describe the parts of the process of nursing
- define assessing
  planning
  implementing
  evaluating
- state the objectives in using the process of nursing
- name some of the programmes which aim to evaluate the quality of nursing
- reproduce Figure I.1
- define the following:

athlete's foot	borborygmi	bow legs
cataract	bossing	bunion
epigastric	corns	cystitis
hammer toe	flatulence	fontanelle
intertrigo	hare-lip	herpes simplex
squint	occiput	pigeon-toed
	verruca	

- 'cystitis' is erroneously written as a patient's problem in a nursing context. Work out the problems with everyday living activities which the patient might experience because of cystitis
- 'gastric ulcer' is erroneously written as a patient's problem in a nursing context. Write out some problems which the patient may be experiencing (in his words — a nursing diagnosis).

1

Helping patients to communicate

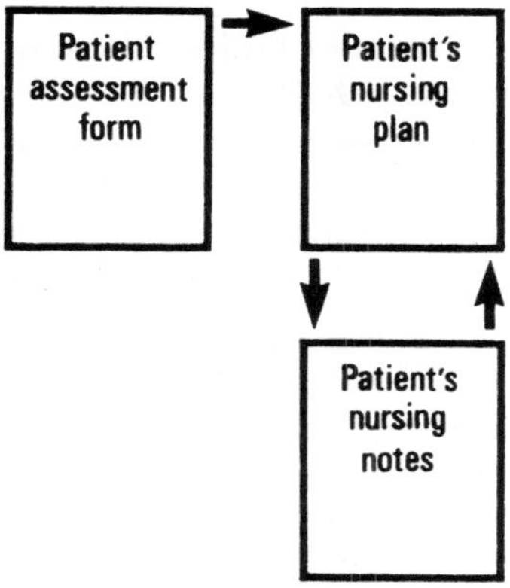

Reading assignment

Background information
- *Communicating*
  - *Listening skills*
  - *Communicating non-verbally*
  - *Communicating by name badges*
  - *Communicating with anxious patients*
  - *Communicating and displaced concern*
  - *Offering to communicate*
  - *Patients' lack of information*

Ward organisation to facilitate the process of nursing

Emotional involvement and the process of nursing

Communicating and the process of nursing
- *Assessing*
- *Planning*
- *Implementing*
- *Evaluating*

Applying the principle
- *A registered nurse must be capable of:*

Working assignment
- *Topics for discussion*
- *Writing assignment*

READING ASSIGNMENT

Argyle M 1972 The psychology of interpersonal behaviour. Penguin, Harmondsworth, p 48–49

Armstrong M 1987 Contemporary ethics. Nursing: The Add-On Journal of Clinical Nursing 3 (14) February: 518–520

Berry A 11986 Knowledge at one's fingertips. Nursing Times 82 (49) December 3: 56–57
Nurses often touch patients during nursing procedures but they could use touch as a therapeutic tool, rather than a gesture made spontaneously or haphazardly.

Bleazard R 1984 Knowing oneself. Nursing Times 80 (10) March 7: 44– 46
Describes the essential qualities for counselling, pointing out the importance of self-knowledge.

Burnard P 1986 Picking up the pieces. Nursing Times 82 (17) April 23: 37–38
How does the nurse respond to the patient who is not clinically depressed but feels an increasing sense of futility? Describes dispiritedness and methods of treatment.

Dainow S 1986 Believe in yourself. Nursing Times 82 (27) July 2: 49– 51
Highlights assertiveness techniques and shows how they can benefit every nurse.

Darbyshire P 1986 When the face doesn't fit. Nursing Times 82 (39) September 24: 28–29
Discusses why some patients are treated better than others.

Dickson N 1986 Editorial. Nursing Times 82 (27) July 2: 3
If access to records causes professionals to justify their comments, so much the better.

Dimond B 1987 Your disobedient servant. Nursing Times 83 (4) January 28: 28–31
Looks at the legal implications and questions whether nurses can any longer shelter behind the accountability of their medical colleagues.

Drane L 1986 Watch my lips. Nursing Times 82 (20) May 14: 52
To help patients who are ventilated via a tracheostomy and therefore unable to speak.

Drummond P 1986 Blind spot. Nursing Times 82 (34) August 20: 18–19
Nurses are well placed to counsel visually impaired people.

Eardley A 1986 Expectations of recovery. Nursing Times 82 (17) April 23: 53–54
Describes how patients nearing the end of a radiotherapy course felt about the treatment. Could help nurses provide the right information and support.

Eardley A 1986 What do patients need to know? Nursing Times 82 (16) April 16: 24–26
Radiotherapy is a common treatment for cancer, but patients are not clear what it entails. Increasing patient understanding can reduce stress.

Faulkner A 1986 Human interest. Nursing Times 82 (33) August 13: 33– 345.
Suggests ways of teaching nurses the necessary skills of communication.

Faulkner A 1984 (ed) Communication. Recent advances in nursing, no.7. Churchill Livingstone, Edinburgh

Fawcus M
1. How to help the dysphasic patient with writing
2. How to help the dysphasic patient with reading
3. How to help the dysphasic patient with understanding speech
4. How to help the dysphasic patient with speech and communication
5. How you can help the dysphasic patient — alternative communication systems

Action for Dysphasic Adults (ADA), Northcote House, 37a Royal Street, London SE1 7LL.

Flanagan L 1986 A question of ethics. Nursing Times 82 (35) August 27: 39–41
Many psychiatric nurses seem unaware of the ethical dilemmas which surround their work. The moral problems which they face are discussed, and the hierarchy which fuels the system is questioned.

Franklin B L 1974a Patient anxiety on admission to hospital. Royal College of Nursing, London, pp vii and 39–41

Franklin B L 1974b Patient anxiety on admission to hospital. Royal College of Nursing, London, p 16

Garrett G 1984 Caught and not taught? Nursing Times 80 (43) October 24: 48–51
The stereotyped image of the elderly is being challenged. Examines the attitudes of nurse learners in their care of the elderly.

Hills K 1985 Gaining and giving insight. Nursing Mirror 160 (6) February 6: 28–29
A course designed to develop counselling skills and self-awareness.

Holland S 1987 Teaching patients and clients. Nursing Times 83 (3) January 21: 59–62
Explains a range of ways to create learning opportunities for patients and clients.

Hoy R 1986 Setting the record straight. Nursing Times 82 (13) March 26: 58
The Data Protection Act has implications for all, whether we use information about patients or whether information about us as staff is stored by management.

Isted C R 1979 Learning to speak again after a stroke. King's Fund Book, distributed by Pitman Medical Publishing Company, London
Written by a man who suffered a stroke.

Jolly J 1986 Communicating with children. The Professional Nurse 1 (10) July: 266–267
Gives real-life situations which could form the basis for discussion groups.

Keighley T 1984 The right to know. Nursing Standard 36 (3) September 6: 6
Discusses a major re-think about confidentiality.

Kempton M 1984 Keeping in touch. Nursing Mirror 159 (18) November 14: i–iii, vi–viii
Describes reality orientation to help withdrawn patients to keep in touch with the

world around them.
King J 1984 Psychology in nursing.
1. Striking it right. Nursing Times 80 (42) October 17: 28–31
2. The health belief model. Nursing Times 80 (43) October 24: 53–55
3. Your health in your hands. Nursing Times 80 (44) October 31: 51–52
4. A question of attitude. Nursing Times 80 (45) November 7: 51–52
Le May A 1986 The human connection. Nursing Times 82 (47) November 19: 28-30
Suggests that nurses can do much to reassure anxious patients by the appropriate use of touch.
Melia K 1986 Dangerous territory. Nursing Times 82 (21) May 21: 27
Discusses informed consent as it relates to nurses and concludes that it is a responsibility which belongs strictly to doctors.
Melia K 1987 Everyday ethics for nurses. Nursing Times 83 (3) January 31: 28–29
Ethics is a severely practical business affecting every clinical nurse every day.
Melia K 1987 To lie or not to lie? Nursing Times 83 (3) January 31: 30–32
Can we really justify being less than honest with patients? Indeed are there times when we should conceal the truth?
Menzies I E P 1961 A case study in the functioning of social systems as a defence against anxiety. Report from the Tavistock Institute of Human Relations, London
McDonald N 1987 Ask the family. Nursing Times 83 (3) January 21: 46– 47
Family therapy involves all members in the treatment process to trace underlying tensions which have produced mental illness in one member.
Morgan C 1986 Ensuring dignity and self-esteem for patients and clients. The Professional Nurse 2 (1) October: 12–14
How can they be preserved in relation to elimination, feeding, living style and dress for mentally handicapped people?
Murphy K 1986 Noises off. Nursing Times 82 (17) April 23: 16–17
Six out of 10 people aged over 70 suffer some form of hearing loss.
Peplau H 1987 Tomorrow's world. Nursing Times 83 (1) January 7: 29– 32
Discusses language skills, socialising activities, and health teaching.
Piff C 1986 Facing up to disfigurement. Nursing Times 82 (34) August 20: 16–17
What happens when your face is disfigured? The author explains what it means from personal experience.
Price B 1986 'Mirror, mirror on the wall'. Nursing Times 82 (39) September 24: 30–32
Discusses the relationship of body image to self-image.
Pyne R 1986 Tell me honestly. Nursing Times 82 (21) May 21: 25–26
Looks at the UKCC's Code of Professional Conduct as a means to help nurses safeguard their patients' interest.
Pyne R UKCC code of conduct. Nursing: The Add-On Journal of Clinical Nursing 3 (14) February: 510–511
Rankin-Box D 1986 Comfort. Nursing: The Add-On Journal of Clinical Nursing 3 (9) September: 340–342
Promoting comfort in daily nursing is revealed by actions, but it is insufficient to perform physical tasks well and be unresponsive to cues from patients indicating that they are anxious or uncomfortable.
RCN Association of Nursing Practice 1985 Guidelines for nurses working with the hearing impaired in hospital. Royal College of Nursing London
Rowden R 1987 The UKCC code of conduct: accountability and implications. Nursing: The Add-On Journal of Clinical Nursing 3 (14) February: 512–514
Rowden R 1987 The extended role of the nurse. Nursing: The Add-On Journal of Clinical Nursing 3 (14) February: 516–517
Scholes M 1986 Private and confidential. Nursing Times 82 (13) March 26: 59–60
What does the Data Protection Act mean for nurses? The implications are considered. One health authority formed its own code of practice.
Sharkey J 1985 Learning not to understand. Nursing Times 81 (16) August 17: 50
Suggests that some nursing programmes are

harmful to empathy and individuality. She believes that the ability to empathise makes the difference between an adequate nurse and an excellent one.

Shillitoe R 1985 I think, therefore I'm ill. Nursing Times 81 (8) February 20: 24–26
Be a good communicator. Make the treatment understandable. Help the patient feel competent. Involve the patient's family.

Sims S 1986 Slow stroke back massage for cancer patients. Nursing Times 82 (47) November 19: 47–50 (Occasional Paper 82 13)
A pilot study examines the effect of gentle back massage on the perceived well-being of six female patients having radiotherapy for breast cancer.

Swanwick M 1984 Early language development. Nursing: The Add-On Journal of Clinical Nursing 2 (22) February: 645–646
Pre-verbal communication skills. Infant modes of expression. Interpersonal skills. Development of speech.

Teasdale K 1986 Communicating with elderly people. The Professional Nurse 2 (1) October: 23–24
Gives four situations as subjects for discussion groups.

Tomlinson, A, Macleod Clark J, Faulkner A 1984 Role-play
1. Learning to relate. Nursing Times 80 (38) September 19: 48–51
2. Planning and preparing. Nursing Times 80 (39) September 26: 45–47

Tutton P 1986 Joining forces. Nursing Times 82 (47) November 19: 31– 32
Therapeutic touch: what is so amazing about it, is not that it works, but that we should be so doubtful about it.

Tutton L 1986 What is primary nursing? The Professional Nurse 2 (2) November: 39–40

United Kingdom Central Council for Nursing, Midwifery and Health Visiting 1984 2E Code of professional conduct. UKCC, 23 Portland Place, London W1N 3AF

Volpato D, Orton D, Blackburn D 1986 Making progress with Makaton. Nursing Times 82 (18) April 30: 33–35
Results of a project to introduce the Makaton method of sign language to a group of mentally handicapped women patients were disappointing. But project designers report that they did point the way to more effective methods of sign language teaching.

Vousden M 1986 Mind your language. Nursing Times 82 (34) August 20: 35
Our use of language often reveals more about our attitudes and prejudices than we realise.

Vousden M 1986 Computer breakthrough. Nursing Times 82 (16) April 16: 20
Computers are helping profoundly handicapped patients to communicate their needs to staff in a mental handicap hospital.

Walsh M 1986 On the frontline. Nursing Times 82 (37) September 10: 55–56
Describes the social and psychological factors behind violence and aggression in A. and E. departments and explains how to deal with them.

Walton L, Macleod Clark J 1986 Making contact. Nursing Times 82 (33) August 13: 28–30
A study of nurse interactions with two stroke patients found the nurses ill-equipped to communicate with them.

Waters V 1986 The sound of silence. Nursing Times 82 (23) June 4: 40-42
Everyone thought that Billy was mute; that is what he wanted them to believe. However, one nurse got through to him.

Watson P 1985 Towers of Babel? Nursing Times 82 (49) December 3: 22– 25

Wells R 1986 The great conspiracy. Nursing Times 82 (21) May 21: 22–25
Allegations of medical research involving the castration of old men without their informed consent have once more focused public attention on this dark side of health care.

Wilson-Barnett J 1978a Factors influencing patients' emotional reaction to hospitalisation. Journal of Advanced Nursing 3 May: 221– 229

Wilson-Barnett J 1978b In hospital: patients' feelings and opinions. Nursing Times Occasional Papers 74 (9): 33–36

Wright S 1985 Special assignment. Nursing Times 81 (35) August 28: 36–37
Several patients are allocated to a nurse for a spell of duty.

BACKGROUND INFORMATION

In the last decade the subject of communication between patients and nurses has gained high publicity because of several research reports which have been collected by Faulkner (1984). There are now several teaching packages about communication in nursing, one or more of which may be used in your school/college of nursing. In this text there will be a general introduction under the heading 'Communicating', followed by discussion under the sub-headings as they appear on page 13, before discussing 'Communicating and the process of nursing'.

Communicating

A nurse needs knowledge of the activity of communicating before she can help a patient to communicate. Until the last few decades, verbal language was considered to be the main component of communication; everyone was familiar with the 26 letters in the alphabet which form the basic units of the English verbal language. From various computations of the letters thousands of words have been constructed for general use, each having its own dictionary definition. The same alphabet is the base of several specialist 'languages' such as those used in medicine and nursing, and staff should refrain from practising their technical vocabulary on patients.

Words have to be interpreted in the context in which they are used. The word 'cup' when used as 'cup and saucer' suggests a mealtime; 'one cup' appearing in a recipe means a measure; 'the presentation of a cup' suggests a silver trophy for the winner.

The arrangement of words in a sentence affects meaning. For example, 'Put the cup on the saucer' has only one meaning, but if the six words are re-arranged to read, 'The cup on the saucer put' then the sentence has no meaning, yet if the re-arrangement reads 'Put the saucer on the cup' it has meaning which is different from the first arrangement of the six words.

When a baby discovers that he can produce voice he communicates his pleasure by 'billing and cooing' and his displeasure by crying reminding us that vocal sounds can transmit emotion. By a long process of associating the spoken word with an object or person, the infant eventually imitates the word successfully in response to the object or person. For this accomplishment there must of course be an intact brain capable of learning; an adequate hearing mechanism; an intact and properly functioning larynx, palate and tongue. There has to be environmental voice which can be imitated so that the child acquires an increasing vocabulary.

The quantity and quality of an adult's vocabulary can reflect his cognitive ability, although there are people who, whatever the level of innate intelligence, do not achieve their potential for a variety of reasons.

The adult's vocabulary may well be spoken in a particular dialect or accent, usually that of the place of residence during acquisition of speaking skills. It takes time for the ear to become accustomed to an unfamiliar dialect, and in these circumstances nurses can help patients by speaking slowly and clearly.

But words are never spoken in an emotional vacuum; they release and convey many emotions, and phrases such as 'You sound as if you're happy/unhappy' acknowledge this. Excited people (or any person in a situation which makes him feel nervous) often talk more than usual and words are spoken more rapidly; whereas sad and depressed people often speak slower than is their custom and the voice is flat and monotonic. On the other hand anger is often manifested by raising the voice, shouting and even screaming, indeed swear words may be used, and the episode is called one of verbal aggression. Sometimes *how* things are said is a more important clue as to the state of the speaker than what is actually said.

To achieve successful communication by use of spoken words one must ask what happens to them? They are heard (received) by the listening recipient who perceives (attaches meaning to) them. The words must therefore be known to the listener; everyone is aware of 'hearing' words in a foreign language, to which no meaning can be attached. Also all of the listener's previous experience, not only his familiarity with the words used, but also his attitudes, beliefs, values and prejudices make a contribution to the process of perceiving. This makes perception a selective process and people need to be aware of this so that they do not filter out any element of information which others are transmitting.

Listening is a skill in which the listener gives his whole attention to what is being said. In face to face situations additional information can be gained by observation, but there are people who are trained to listen in a face-less situation, the Samaritans being an excellent example. They are trained to interpret such phenomena as silences, sighs and sobs. For the distressed speaker, the very fact that there is an available listener who will not cut him off is therapeutic.

Verbal language is also used in reading and writing. It is easy to presume that all adults have developed adequate reading and writing skills but even in the developed countries there is current concern about the number of illiterate people.

Over the last few decades increasing attention has been paid to 'body language' — the information transmitted wittingly or unwittingly by facial expression, eye contact, body gesture, grooming, clothing, touching, activity, passivity, residence and mode of living. These factors are used in various combinations in expressing emotions, communicating interpersonal attitudes, indicating mutual attentiveness and providing feedback from listener to talker.

Argyle (1972) carried out an investigation to compare the effectiveness of verbal and non-verbal cues in the communication of interpersonal attitudes. A series of video-taped films of a female performer delivering different messages was prepared. The way in which the messages differed from each other in content was the first source of experimental variation. Judges who rated the messages independently before they were filmed agreed that one was 'superior', that is it talked down to people, one was 'inferior', that is it apologised, and the third was neutral in relation to the other two. Three different ways of delivering the messages provided a second source of variation. These were the non-verbal cues. The performer read each message, no matter what its content rating, in a 'superior' manner, with head raised, unsmiling and haughty; in a 'neutral' manner, with a slight smile; and in an 'inferior' manner, with a nervous, deferential smile and head lowered. The filmed performances were presented in random order to a group of subjects, who were asked to fill in a set of rating forms according to the impression made on them. It was discovered that nonverbal cues had over four times the effect of verbal cues on shifts in ratings. In other words, the **manner of delivery** had **greater impact** than the **content of the message**. The investigators suggest that it is possible that we have an innate pattern for communication and recognition of cues for interpersonal attitudes, just like the non-human primates.

Idioms in our language are indicative of the fact that we recognize these varying means of social interaction. We talk about a look enough to kill; we say that an audience looks interested or it looks bored. We talk about people making eyes at each other; about the come-hither look; about the cold stare that rebuffs an unwelcome approach by another person. There is the nod or wink in the sale room that is accepted by the auctioneer as evidence that one has made a bid. There is a special tic-tac language of the bookmakers on a race course. There is the conductor who is in constant communication with the members of the orchestra without speaking one single word. We talk about thumbing a lift, and so one could go on quoting instances of non-verbal communication. Such phrases as 'I might as well speak to myself, or to the wall' show that we can be conscious of failing to produce a reaction in the person with whom we are attempting to communicate.

A great deal of attention is now being paid to establishing communication between parents and their newly born infant; it is called 'bonding' and can be described as the flow of feeling between parent and child. It is achieved by the parents touching and getting to know their baby. In other words, by using the sensory-information-gathering systems, a warm and secure relationship is established.

After this brief consideration of communicating it is unfortunate that the process of nursing, which has a large communicating component, has come to be mainly associated with documentation. In an over-zealous acceptance of the fact that the main objective in using the process of nursing is to individualise nursing and document it, we may have overlooked the fact that many communicating activities which occur and recur in a ward or wherever a nurse works, do not need to be documented. Nevertheless they can contribute to individualised nursing. They are a part of the background knowledge and skills which students acquire gradually throughout a 3-year programme. An introduction to them follows.

Listening skills

Nurses should be able to create an atmosphere in which patients when talking to nurses will not be cut off. The patient stops talking if the nurse, while 'listening', shows that she finds the subject incredible, embarrassing, painful, repulsive and so on; this can be unwittingly conveyed to the patient by non-verbal communication. The patient stops talking if, by interjection, it is evident that the nurse considers her thoughts more important than those of the patient: for example, the patient states that his fingers are painful this morning and the nurse counters that it is rheumatism, it is a damp morning and her fingers are painful. The patient's look denotes that he is sorry he has spoken and he retires to bear his painful fingers as best he can.

The patient stops talking if the nurse, after listening cursorily, tries to give answers without taking the trouble to find out what the patient really wants to know. If these answers take the form of vague statements the patient may be so disheartened that he fails to make any further attempt at communicating with the staff; if the answers pass the responsibility, the nurse can help by asking the appropriate person to talk with the patient. This saves the patient having to make another first move to communicate about the subject. Whenever the patient asks a question, for example, 'Will I get better?' it is appropriate for the nurse to invite discussion of his fears by asking him what he thinks and feels about being ill and recovering. The nurse who listens carefully will be able to identify the patient's fears which may be due to ignorance or misinformation, both of which can be remedied.

Communicating non-verbally

Non-verbal communication is of tremendous importance to a patient, portrayed by the way in which he watches everything that goes on in the vicinity. It is important that he does not receive contradictory messages, for example polite words with a rough touch; polite words with banging of the requested article on to the locker; polite words with an angry look. He will experience some sort of emotional response to such untoward non-verbal messages. The 'difficult' patient may be responding to staff who deliver contradictory messages to him. By the development of the conveyance of accurate non-verbal communication it is possible to fulfil a patient's greatest need by being silently with him.

Communicating by name badges

Not all people possess an outgoing personality capable of communicating easily with a stranger. A new patient may have impaired sight, so that the wearing of identification badges does not relieve staff of the social obligation of introduction when attending to any patient for the first time. The badges relieve the patient of remembering so many names. For those with adequate vision a glance at the badge gives them the confidence to address each staff member by name thus helping to establish a **personal** relationship. However, if the patient wears bifocal spectacles, reading vision is only corrected for objects at a distance of 30 to 40cm, making the reading of a name badge very difficult.

Communicating with anxious patients

Even stalwart people experience some anxiety in the strange hospital environment. In one study, patient anxiety was measured and found to be highest in the first 24 hours (Wilson-Barnett 1978a). In another project Franklin (1974b) discovered that the majority of patients disagreed with the statement 'The nurses tell me what will happen to me'. And Wilson-Barnett (1978b) demonstrated that explaining to the patient exactly what was going to happen to him reduced his level of anxiety. Nurses have a responsibility to base their nursing practice on research findings; so helping newly admitted patients by giving information about what will happen to them during the ensuing 24 hours is an essential nursing activity.

The nurse must be alert to the fact that anxiety and previous misinformation can prevent understanding. It is therefore wise to make a summary of the main points at the end of an instruction. Not only does this refresh the patient's mind about all the facts mentioned, but the information is more likely to 'sink in' when repeated. It is sometimes wise to use more words than are strictly necessary, as only the repeat may bring the message home, for instance, 'Private, do not enter'. 'Private' should be sufficient; 'do not enter' is redundant — but it reinforces understanding. This method is used on some paper towel dispensers: 'Do not unfold: use double'. These are more successful methods of communication than the giving of scanty information once only. Whenever a patient is instructed, some feedback must occur so that the nurse can assess the patient's understanding.

Communicating and displaced concern

It is important for nurses to understand that a patient while communicating may displace concern about himself to some minor matter. For instance, the complaint may be about a bad mattress, poor food, poor service, too many blood tests and so on. Should such complaints be justified, they are not displacement, but when they are unjustified, the staff should take the time and use their behavioural and conversational skills to determine what is the patient's real concern. This gives him an opportunity to ventilate his fears, for example about how long he will be off work, and ensuing conversation may dispel some of his unrealistic anxiety.

Offering to communicate

Each patient needs opportunity to talk with staff. Many people think that opportunity is there when the nurse carries out individualised nursing activities such as bedmaking and bathing. However, the patient's thoughts are likely to be concentrated on the activity, and if this is the only opportunity he is offered, he is less likely to tell the staff what he wants them to know (for example that he has a pain at the back of his eye even though he was admitted with abdominal pain), and he is less likely to ask the staff what he wants to know.

In some wards each patient is offered the opportunity to talk to the nurse in charge on the 'morning round'. The offer should be left wide open, for instance 'How are things?' so that the patient is free to talk about the things he wants to talk about. The questions, 'How did you sleep?', 'What sort of a night have you had?' and 'How are you feeling this morning?' mean that the nurse has chosen the subject of conversation. The question, 'Did you sleep well?', 'Have you had a good night?' and 'Are you feeling better?' not only mean that the nurse has chosen the subject of conversation but imply that she expects the patient to have slept well, had a good night and to be feeling better, according to the question asked. The last question is likely to antagonise the patient who does not feel any better. No one can 'feel' to order. A patient who fails to feel better in spite of adequate treatment may be labouring under a misconception, like not being able to work again. The nurse who is skilled in patient-directed conversation may elicit the misconception, correct it and thereafter the patient will recover rapidly.

Patient's lack of information

There are several reports of research projects carried out over the years which reveal that many patients felt they had not received sufficient information. It is well known that anxiety impedes retention of new information. It may help nurses to realise this if they think of themselves discussing an emotive subject such as an impending divorce with a lawyer, and the likelihood that they would not remember all the details, especially those spoken in legal jargon. The ability to decrease anxiety in patients is a necessary skill for nurses so that patients can have the confidence which comes from being well informed about what is happening to them.

Some patients are more approachable than others and it is very easy for nurses to congregate around the bed of a lively extrovert; but it is the withdrawn, the prickly and the disgruntled patients who are in the greatest need of attention; they challenge the skill of nurses and they must not be neglected. It is only by generous attention to them as individuals, coupled with imagination, that their hostility and isolation can be reduced. Many patients require time to become accustomed to the nurses to whom they are allocated on the different shifts.

WARD ORGANISATION TO FACILITATE THE PROCESS OF NURSING

But how can nursing work be organised at ward level so that nurses can have the time and the opportunity to establish satisfactory nurse/patient relationships? Task allocation whereby each nurse is assigned a task which contributes a fragment of the patient's nursing plan mitigates against it. More favourable patterns of nursing are:

- *patient allocation*
  several patients are allocated to a nurse for a spell of duty (Wright 1985)
- *team nursing*
  a small group of two, three or more nurses are assigned to several patients for each day shift.
- *primary nursing*
  a primary nurse is allocated to a patient for however long the stay. She writes the nursing plan, implements it when she is on duty and delegates to 'an associate' when off duty. She is therefore responsible and accountable for the patient's nursing (Tutton 1986).

Patients are likely to communicate their feelings and anxieties more freely when they have to establish and maintain a relationship with only a few nurses. Nurse and patient can more easily establish rapport; the nurse can learn to understand the patient as well as his disease. Relatives are much happier when they understand that they can approach a particular nurse who will be capable of giving all relevant information. These patterns of nursing also help with improvement of written communications as each nurse is responsible for writing the nursing record on the patients allocated to her.

In the past several dimensions of the patient's physical dependency were used for collecting data about nurses' work, from which the nursing workload was calculated, and from it the necessary number of nurses was estimated. The data collectors seldom took account of the 'talking with patients' discussed in the previous paragraphs. But if nurses have bred the image that 'work' is all-important, that 'being busy' is all that matters, and that talking with patients implies idleness, then it is not surprising that people carrying out job analyses use *physical* dependency as the criterion when deciding how many nurses are necessary to care for a given number of patients. Nurses have obviously managed to convey that nursing is made up of *physical* skills; they have not managed to convey the *equally important* part of their work consisting of *social, behavioural* and *interpersonal skills* which are essential if patients are to be helped to communicate.

EMOTIONAL INVOLVEMENT AND THE PROCESS OF NURSING

In carrying out all four phases of the process of nursing, each of which will be discussed later, knowledge about emotional involvement is necessary. Emotion is feeling: involve means to envelop, to include, to embrace, to interlace. Feeling is a diverse and complicated mental function, that usually discharges itself in action. Feeling is a powerful function, and can transform a personality. For example, a feeling of rage or revenge can cause a person to use a force he did not know he possessed, when striking another. On the other hand, a feeling of depression can cause a normally active person to be listless and apathetic, and the action resulting when depression becomes unbearable is suicide. (p. 45). One cannot 'feel' to order, it is a spontaneous reaction — as one responds to someone or something. One can learn about feeling by allowing oneself to experience the whole range of feeling without cutting off that particular feeling-process by turning too quickly to other things, or denying its existence. Learning to cope with one's feeling-responses is acquired by experiencing the feeling along its whole range; coping is not acquired by denial of or cutting off one's feeling-responses. These are individual processes and they contribute to each person's uniqueness.

Whenever one sees a patient, one responds in some way:

- one may say 'Good morning' in such a way and with such an accompanying facial gesture that he gets the message that it has been a pleasure to acknowledge him. In other words a feeling of pleasure has been aroused in the nurse and patient. There has been fleeting emotional involvement, and the action resulting from the feeling of each has been discharged with mutual satisfaction.
- one may say a perfunctory 'Good morning', and the other, having been ready to respond in a pleasant manner, is nonplussed by the production of such behaviour. Even if the perfunctory greeting is due to preoccupation, the nurse has managed to convey that her business is more important than the patient's feelings. If the perfunctory greeting is accompanied by non-verbal cues such as a superior attitude, then the patient can experience any one or more of a number of feelings: hostility, revenge, deflation or anxiety. The feelings aroused in each have not been discharged with mutual satisfaction.
- the nurse may cross to the other side of the ward to avoid having to make vocal acknowledgement. Yet by the act, she is acknowledging a feeling of discomfort at the possibility of an encounter. Rarely can one take this 'avoiding action' without the other being aware of it, so that some sort of feeling has been engendered in the other — it may be a feeling of relief, anger, deflation and so on.

Nurse and patient are each bound to experience feeling even at the first encounter for collection of assessment data, and this feeling can be utilised to produce a comfortable milieu in which exchange of information can be accomplished. A nurse can convey sympathy and support while encouraging a patient to identify problems being experienced in relation to communicating: while setting mutually agreed patient outcomes and the interventions each may need to carry out to achieve them. Discordant emotions between nurse and patient may well contribute to non-compliance in carrying out agreed interventions, for instance in practising tongue and lip movements to increase clarity of speech sounds after dysphasia.

Emotional involvement can be silently communicated, as when one holds the hand of a very ill patient, or a confused, frail, elderly person. It is neither sentimental nor romantic, it is an appropriate act of 'caring'.

Some nursing textbooks say that a nurse should not become involved with patients but if the nurse does not deny involvement with patients, relatives and colleagues, the emotional energy from the involvement can be put to creative use, if recognised and channelled in constructive ways. To be aware of one's emotions, and sensitive to the emotions of others is the first step in this constructive activity. If 'constructive' is one end of a scale, then 'destructive' is the other end of the scale. Thus to be unaware of one's emotions and insensitive to those of others has dire implications.

Menzies (1961) suggests that a defence system operates in general nursing. The nurse wishes to become involved with a patient, but if she does, she exposes herself to an anxiety-provoking situation. In order to avoid this potential anxiety, systems of defence are erected, which guard against involvement. For example at the individual level, the emphasis is on 'patient', not person, while at the organisational level the social system operates built-in constraints to prevent involvement — such as moving the student nurses around every two or three months. Menzies' argument is based on the assumption that there is a potential interaction situation, that both nurse and patient are **capable** of responding to each other. It is this response that leads to anxiety — if nurses are unable to cope with the feelings engendered by the response.

All the foregoing information will be a useful resource when students of nursing fulfil their clinical allocations so that they can acquire skills in — assessing patients' ability to communicate; helping them to continue to communicate during their indisposition; and helping patients who are experiencing particular problems in communicating.

COMMUNICATING AND THE PROCESS OF NURSING

Considering the complexities of communicating in nursing as discussed in the previous section of this chapter, it is pertinent to focus it to the patient. Whichever model, or explicit interpretation of what constitutes nursing, is used in your 3-year programme, the process of nursing is a method of focusing the subject of communicating to the patient. It will be discussed in the accepted four phases — assessing, planning, implementing and evaluating.

Assessing

If a patient is conscious and not too ill, assessing ability to communicate will be part of the initial interview when data are collected for the assessment form with the objective of identifying what he perceives as a problem. The communicating will be a two-way process between nurse and patient. Each is using individual sensory systems for perceiving, seeing, hearing and smelling.

If the patient is wearing day clothes they will communicate some non-verbal information to the nurse — appropriateness of clothes, for example a person with an over-active thyroid gland may wear flimsy clothes in the middle of winter. Style and colour will communicate attitude to expressing sexuality, as will hair style and colour, the use of make-up, perfume or after shave lotion. Facial expression and body gesture will communicate current mood, anxiety and so on. Eye contact/avoidance has to be observed and recorded factually. Visible perspiration is evidence of an over-active autonomic nervous system, probably as a reaction to anxiety. Of course any such inferences will have to be explored with the patient.

Verbal communication is assessed by such things as words used (vocabulary), sentence construction (syntax), punctuation by 'redundancies' such as 'I mean', 'You know', 'er' or any combination of these, giving the speaker time to collect thoughts for the next sentence, or it may be merely from habit. Is the speech fluent or hesitant? Is the person reticent or forthcoming in the exchange of information?

It is easy to think that the wearing of spectacles means correction of vision to 100%, but this is not necessarily so. There can be tunnel vision which causes a person to move the head in unaccustomed ways. If people are given a simple line drawing of a house and asked to draw a replica, some of them will leave out a particular part. Perhaps a patient's 'clumsiness' could be understood if nurses were alerted to visual field deficiencies. Also some people have spatial appreciation difficulties; they may think the plate has safely reached the table and let go only to find that it clatters to the floor. Many people learn to cope by feeling the surface on which they intend to deposit an article. Very thick lens in spectacles — right, left or both — should alert the nurse to discover what this means to the patient. It may well mean that spectacles must be worn before the person gets out of bed — and this could have implications for the night nurse who should not put the spectacles in their case and pop them in the locker in the interests of safety and tidiness. Squints and cataracts are usually observable and can be explored further so that what is written on the assessment form is with the patient's consent and describes the visual problem. Some artificial eyes are not visually detectable, some are; and even nurses vary in their ability to detect contact lens in situ. However once the nurse has absorbed a scheme, that sight is part of communicating, she will become more experienced at eliciting accurate information.

At the initial assessment the nurse has to

remember that many people are hard of hearing. It has an extra disadvantage in that it is an invisible impairment. The deficit may be in one ear only, in which case the patient will turn his head so that the good ear is picking up the nurse's voice. This act of non-verbal communication should be explored with the patient, and adequate information written about whether or not professional advice has been sought; whether he would welcome arrangements for having his hearing investigated; how he copes with the deficit, maybe by watching the speaker's face, lip reading, avoiding participation in large groups and so on. A nurse should always tactfully discover if a hearing aid is being worn, remembering that some of them are attached to the spectacle frame. More will be said about deaf patients later.

The foregoing is a beginning level appreciation of assessing the majority of patients' ability to communicate, but a word must be said about assessing people who for some reason or other are unable, or have difficulty in communicating. The following list is not exhaustive but it will give readers an idea of the many conditions which can impede the process of communicating:

aphasia
blindness
changed level of consciousness
cleft palate
deafness
dumbness
dysphasia
dyspnoea
foreign language
hard of hearing
laryngectomy
mental impairment
spasticity (cerebral palsy)
tracheostomy.

Assessing the speech and language deficits, including reading and writing, of patients who have any one of the dysphasias is the work of speech therapists. However there are relatively few of them and nurses can learn some of the basics by reading Fawcus 1 and 2; they both contain information about assessing the particular patient's problems. As Fawcus points out, no two patients have exactly the same problems!

Most items in the foregoing list are medical diagnoses. Nurses need to gain greater skill at collecting information about patients' problems, writing them in patients' language so that they form a large data bank which can be analysed. Analysis may well reveal a cluster of patients' problems around a medical diagnosis; these can then be correctly called a nursing diagnosis.

Planning

The majority of patients will not have a problem which requires a specific nursing intervention. This is not to say that among the patient population, as among the general population, there will be a minority of poor communicators, a minority of excellent communicators and a majority of average communicators. Here we are talking about a planned nursing intervention for a person's individual problem with communicating. From the foregoing it will be realised that very skilled assessment is necessary to identify the communicating problems of some people, and a speech therapist, if available, is the person to carry it out. The intervention will then be at her suggestion with the patient's permission and co-operation; some call this a 'contract'. The nursing intervention is then carrying out the suggestion and/or supervising the patient's practice. Currently the setting of goals/patient outcomes are somewhat crude, 'Will name six out of six everyday objects correctly by (end of first week)', 'Will speak a six word sentence by ... (end of first week)'. A pooled data bank, collected over the years, and analysed may help nurses to be realistic and precise in time-related goal setting.

Individualised planning may be necessary for people with a mental illness to increase their ability to communicate satisfactorily with other people. Planning might also include teaching a person about diabetes or coronary heart disease and what can be done to minimise the effect of disease on daily living. Patients with gynaecological conditions will need information about resumption of sexual relationships.

Generalised planning is also necessary to help

patients to communicate. Provision of telephone booths throughout the hospital and mobile telephones for bed patients are a help. Arrangements for delivery and collection of outgoing mail are essential features of helping patients to communicate. Encouragement is also provided by the availability of daily papers and a library service, radio and television and other communicating media. Provision of privacy for communicating in the form of single rooms, adequate space between beds in multi-bed areas, and adequate curtaining off of each bed can only be accomplished by generalised planning.

Implementing

Communicating is such an individualised activity it is impossible in a textbook to take any other than a generalised approach as to what might happen when nursing patients who have specific conditions which interfere with communicating.

For those who have any impediment in speaking the nurse should continue to talk with them as befits their age, level of intelligence and previous experience. Useful information to guide nurses in individualising their conversation with each patient will be found on the assessment form. A nurse needs to use her ingenuity to help the person to communicate with her. For sighted people a 'speaking clock' which can be easily made and adapted to individual needs is illustrated in Figure 1.1. Another means of communication, a finger alphabet, is illustrated in Figure 1.2; it is useful for communicating with deaf people. Relief of frustration can be achieved for some people by use of a word bracelet; once the person has attracted the attention of a nurse by ringing the bell, he can turn the bracelet to the word required — pain, drink, food, bedpan, radio and so on. A fairly recent innovation is the use of 'Bliss' symbols which offer an alternative means of expression; it has proved successful with many 'non-communicators'. Speech therapists have devised their sign language called 'Makaton' to help people who cannot communicate because of

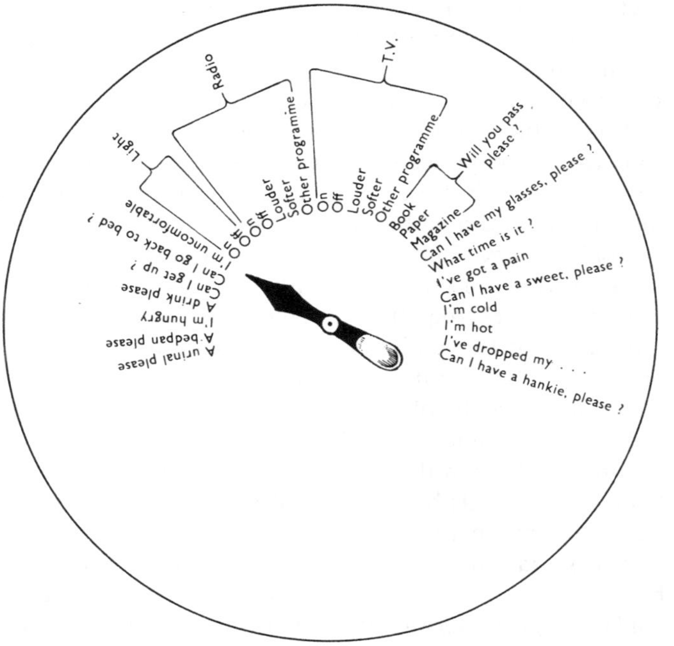

Fig. 1.1 A clock for communicating with a dysphasic person.

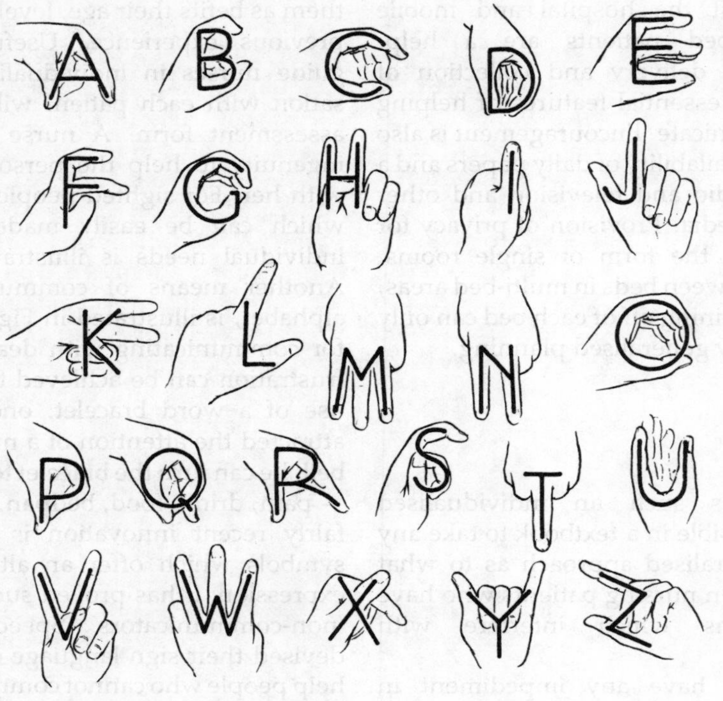

Fig. 1.2 A finger alphabet for communicating with a dysphasic person.

speech or hearing defects. The system can be modified so that spastic people, who often cannot control their movements, can also use it. Electronic devices to help patients with particular communicating problems are increasingly available, but are very expensive.

Aphasia literally means the absence or complete loss of language ability and dysphasia is impaired or partial loss of language ability. By custom the two words are used synonymously and dysphasia is currently used more frequently than aphasia. About one-third of the patients with a right hemiplegia are dysphasic but very few people with a left hemiplegia are dysphasic. In over 95% of right-handed people, the language function area of the brain is in the left hemisphere and in only one-third of left-handed people is most language function in the right hemisphere. Hence the association of right hemiplegia with dysphasia.

Some minor aspects of language are located in the right hemisphere, including swear words and language intimately related to music so that some severely dysphasic patients are able to sing appropriately and swear effectively.

Dysphasia has been divided into two types: sensory or receptive when there is impairment of language input or understanding; motor or expressive dysphasia when the impairment is of language output or expression. Nurses should be encouraged to distinguish fluent from nonfluent dysphasia. In fluent dysphasia the patient's conversation has many mistakes in it, of which he is largely unaware; he fails to recognise the incoherence and incongruity. He may be unable to name objects but can describe them. In non-fluent dyspyhasia the patient is very reticent in speech. Language comprehension is relatively less impaired so that he is aware of his language errors and this further inhibits his speech. Since information is received via all five senses it is important for the nurse to check the dysphasic patient's ability to see and hear and if necessary to arrange appointments at the ophthalmic and/ or audiology clinic. Poorly fitting dentures can also impede speaking, so they should be checked when appropriate.

A crucial element in helping the dysphasic patient is awareness of the degree of receptive impairment. When collecting assessment data the nurse should, without glancing at them, ask the person to point to different objects. The non-glancing is essential so that a correct response is to a verbal stimulus and not to a visual cue.

All those in contact with dysphasic patients, including the relatives, need to learn to exploit non-verbal communication; they can touch the part of the body which they want the patient to move; they can point at where they want him to move to, while at the same time asking him to move — so he receives tactile, visual and verbal cues.

Information about previous hobbies is helpful, particularly non-verbal games such as noughts and crosses, draughts and dominoes because many people continue to be able to play them. Such information will be found on the assessment form, and will help nurses on all shifts to individualise their interactions with the patient.

Conversation with the dysphasic patient is essential if he is to recover his language ability; the objective is to get the patient to participate. Everyday toilet articles, crockery and cutlery can be kept on a tray near the person and the nurse's time is best spent getting him to name each article in turn. It is important to give these people time to respond and lots of encouragement. The Chest, Heart and Stroke Association, Tavistock House North, Tavistock Square, London WC1 can be approached for details of aphasic (dysphasic) clubs for patients and their relatives. ADA (Action for Dysphasic Adults) publishes valuable booklets, a selection of which is in the Reading Assignment.

A nurse can help those people who are relearning speech by such simple means as positioning herself so that the person can see her facial gestures and speech movements. The person should be addressed by name frequently so that he can identify himself. A nurse should not be a nameless person to the patient, so she should use her name in conversation with him. He needs to be informed of the day, date and time, of where he is, what happened to him, when his visitors are coming, and so on. One needs to speak slowly and clearly and perhaps reinforce the information by writing it for him. Frequently his comprehension is unimpaired, so he is in the frustrating position of understanding all that is said, yet not being able to formulate the words for the reply (dysarthria). You might get some idea of how he feels if, in a small group, each of you in turn holds the lips, so that when you want to join in, you cannot. You will probably find yourself making frantic gestures to try to make yourself understood. You will feel anything but comfortable. Because of paralysis of the preferred hand many of these patients are deprived of the ability to keep in contact by the non-vocal method of writing. Again to try to experience the frustration of not being able to write with your preferred hand, try to write half a page with your non-preferred hand. Isted (1979) tells of his reactions to this affliction, and his account should be considered essential reading for every person who cares for patients who have suffered a stroke — and they may well be relatives in the home.

The blind or visually impaired patient needs special consideration. He has to learn to attach a name to a voice. He is deprived of using the identification badges of staff as an aid to memory. The staff should mention their name and their place in the ward team at the first personal contacts with the blind patient until he has confidence to address them by name from identification of voice. Footsteps will have warned the blind or visually impaired patient of the approach of a staff member. Deprived of sight the patient is less sure of when the conversation is finished and the staff member ready to leave. A patient appreciates being told that the nurse is leaving his bedside. Pressure on a patient's hand can be a token of farewell. Sighted patients can make their requests to appropriate staff. A blind patient, hearing a passing footstep, may be embarrassed to find that he has asked the doctor for a bedpan.

Deaf patients and hearing-impaired patients can be very anxious on admission to hospital. A hearing handicap is 'invisible'; it can have social and psychological sequelae leading to isolation and loneliness. Whenever a nurse admits a new patient she should be aware of the possibility and observe his facial expression for incomprehension. When speaking, the nurse must always face the patient with her face in a good light, so that the deaf person can have the advantage of seeing the expression on her face, and can observe the speech movements. Same-level eye contact is important so that both nurse and patient should be standing or sitting. The nurse should speak slowly and clearly and avoid a high pitch; if possible she should lower the pitch. Two excellent booklets are available to help both deaf patients and staff: *General guidance for hearing aid users*, Department of Health and Social Security, HMSO, and *Communication barriers in the elderly* published by Age Concern England, Bernard Swinley House, 60 Pitcairn Road, Mitcham, Surrey CR4 3LL. The Royal College of Nursing Association of Nursing Practice has also published a booklet 'Guidelines for nurses working with the hearing impaired in hospital' and it should be essential reading. It suggests that the logo of the 'Sympathetic Hearing Scheme' should be used to identify patients who have hearing difficulties.

For patients who do not speak the national language the British Red Cross Society has printed, in a question and answer format, cards in 35 languages; there is a separate set of ten for maternity work. Most hospitals have a list of people in the area who speak other languages and are willing to act as interpreters. However it has to be remembered that an interpreter can dilute a nurse/patient relationship. Body language, miming and drawing all help to convey the message to a patient.

The garbled and distorted speech of many spastic patients can be difficult for a nurse to understand; yet those who are in contact with them everyday have learned to interpret their vocal sounds. When such a spastic person needs to be admitted to a general hospital it is advantageous if someone who can interpret his speech can stay with him. Spasticity does not necessarily imply a low intelligence and it must be very frustrating when spastic patients fail to be understood by other people. A little patience and ingenuity on the part of nurses can go a long way towards defusing frustration in these patients by giving them a feeling of self-respect and helping them to be understood, an essential feature of communicating.

Tracheostomy renders a person incapable of speaking which must be a frightening experience. If he is capable of writing he can continue to communicate 'verbally' if given a pad and pencil, and nurses need to encourage his written contribution to the conversation of staff and relatives. For his psychological comfort he requires a non-vocal means of summoning a nurse.

When communicating with wheelchair or chairfast patients it is important that nurses, particularly those who are tall, remember that if they remain standing, the patient has diminished opportunity for observing their facial expression and eye contact. It is therefore common courtesy to offer same level face-to-face contact.

The foregoing background information, about people who are likely to have particular problems in relation to communicating, will in fact be used in all four phases of the process of nursing. The information is intentionally of an introductory nature and its purpose is to help nurses to consider nursing in a process context.

Evaluating

As said earlier, the majority of patients will not be experiencing a problem related to communicating which requires a specific nursing intervention that requires to be evaluated.

Experience and developing professional judgement will dictate whether or not 'deafness/hard of hearing' needs to have appropriate nursing interventions written on the nursing plan, since these conditions are not going to change. If the person's previous coping mechanisms are written on the assessment form, they will adequately guide nurses on the different shifts to communicate appropriately with the deaf/hard of hearing person.

Should there be temporary deafness from perhaps a middle ear infection, this problem will appear on the records (in some instances on the assessment form and in others on the nursing plan). On the nursing plan there will be a stated patient outcome and the nursing intervention to achieve it. Each time the intervention is carried out, it will be recorded in the patient's nursing notes, together with the gradual progress in regaining hearing. This will probably be finally checked at the audiology clinic, when solving of the problem will be recorded on the nursing plan together with cancellation of the intervention. The same scheme can be applied to blindness/ visual impairment.

For all the other groups of patients briefly mentioned on pages 25 to 28 nurses will need practice in writing problems as the patients experience them; this statement guides the patient outcomes and the agreed interventions to achieve them, and the consequent evaluation of whether or not the outcome is being or has been achieved.

Generalised evaluation as to whether patients were satisfied/dissatisfied with the level of communication during a stay in hospital has been carried out by several researchers. The reports are referred to in items included in the Reading Assignment and they are referenced so that those who need more information can find it. Unfortunately the results revealed inadequate information-giving and recommendations were made for teaching medical and nursing students' communication skills.

In this chapter, background information about communicating was discussed so that students of nursing could begin to develop a concept involving a principle of nursing, 'helping patients to communicate'. Communicating was then considered in a process context. The following application of the principle is a broad outline of the expected capabilities of a registered nurse, a list of topics for discussion and a writing assignment.

APPLYING THE PRINCIPLE

A registered nurse must be capable of:

- creating an atmosphere in which there can be free communication between staff, patients, visitors and all personnel visiting the ward
- offering special help to those who have communicating difficulties
- establishing, maintaining and terminating nurse/patient relationships
- applying the principle — helping patients to communicate — in a process of nursing context.

WORKING ASSIGNMENT

Topics for discussion

- empathy
- factors which can modify a patient's thinking and feeling when he is talking to the staff
- instruction
- learning from, and communicating with visitors
- how do you interpret the term 'becoming emotionally involved'?
- can one implement a patient's nursing plan without becoming emotionally involved?
- dispiritedness
- the Data Protection Act
- communicating with children
- confidentiality
- therapeutic touch
- informed consent
- UKCC's code of professional conduct.

Writing assignment

- write about the components of non-verbal communication
- define the following:

  aphasia
  body image
  cleft palate
  communication
  confidentiality
  counselling
  dignity
  dysarthria
  dysphasia
  dyspnoea
  dyspraxia

empathy
herpes simplex
laryngectomy
mentally handicapped
nurse/patient relationship
patient allocation
primary nursing
reality orientation
self-esteem
self-image
spastic
stress
team nursing
therapeutic.

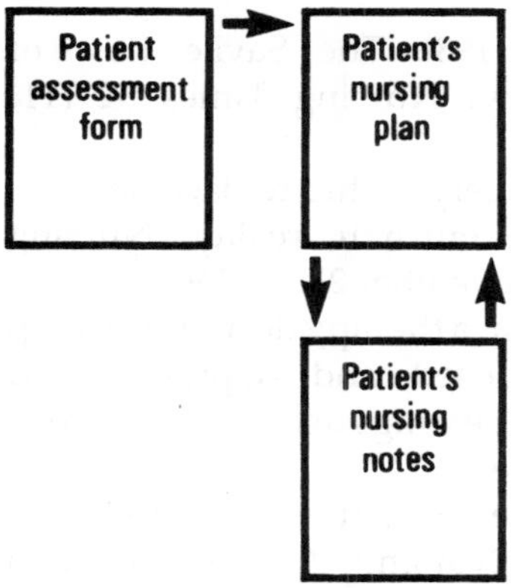

Reading assignment

Background information
Concept of health
Everyday living activities
Multidisciplinary habilitation/ rehabilitation team

Habilitation/rehabilitation and the process of nursing
Assessing
Planning
Institutionalisation
Antidote to institutionalisation — patient participation
Boredom
Antidote to boredom — visitors
Prevention of complications of bedrest
Implementing
Evaluating

Applying the principle
A registered nurse must be capable of:

Working assignment
Topics for discussion
Writing assignment

2

Helping to habilitate/ rehabilitate patients

READING ASSIGNMENT

Alexander M A 1977 Cerebrovascular accident. Nursing Mirror 145 (26) December 29: 25–26
The main problem was Mrs Brown's attitude which was one of depression and lack of motivation.

Brodie P 1985 Struck numb. Nursing Mirror 160 (5) January 30: 21–23
Describes how people with paraplegia and tetraplegia have to learn to do things with the help of others as they are rehabilitated to lead as normal a life as possible.

Burns D B 1979 Resettlement and employment of psychiatric patients. Nursing Times 75 (19) May 10: 799–801
Planned rehabilitation scheme has given many patients the prospect of leading a normal life in the community.

Cheadle A J 1978 Long-stay patient rehabilitation. Nursing Times 74 (33) August 17: 1382–1384
In many, the psychosis seems to recede in middle life and this makes the sufferer more responsive to efforts to rehabilitate him; nurses must help people to care for themselves.

Cronin W E 1978 Rehabilitation of a patient with myxoedema. Nursing Times 74 (33) August 17: 1364–1366
Illustrates how the quality of life at home can be improved by a short stay in hospital.

Curtis J 1979 Work: Living with disability. Nursing Times 75 (34) Supplement August 23:

19–20, 22–23
Describes the Disablement Resettlement Officer service and how nurses can co-operate with the service to get people settled back into work.

Daly J, Jones J, Rees J, Williams N 1979 Getting the elderly back on their feet after an accident. Nursing Mirror 148 (11) March 15: 28–30
Efficient instructions, good teamwork, consideration of the patient and his family as people, are essential ingredients in successful care of the elderly patient after accident.

Dainsborough A 1980 Miracles for the many. Nursing Mirror 151 (7) August 14: 28–29
Disablement is an international problem; report on congress on prevention and integration — priorities for the 1980s.

Fanshawe F 1978 Aids and equipment for the disabled. Nursing Times 74 (33) Supplement August 17: 3,4,6,8,11

Fanshawe E 1979 Access: Living with disability. Access. Nursing Times Supplement 75 (34) August 23: 3–4,7,8
The Chronically Sick and Disabled Persons Act of 1970 puts a duty on those involved with new buildings to provide access to and within new buildings.

Firth D, Chamberlain M A, Fligg H, Wright J, Wright V 1978 Health visitors in a rehabilitation unit. Nursing Times 74 (6) February 9: 249–250
Bridging the gap between hospital and home; patients had often forgotten what they had been told in hospital.

Frazer F W 1978 Community physio: a new colleague for the district nurse. Nursing Mirror 147 (16) October 19: 58–60
Assessment card used in studies; many district nurses have young paraplegics and patients with strokes or disseminated sclerosis on their lists, all of whom would benefit from physiotherapy.

Hawker M 1980 Return to mobility. The Chest, Heart and Stroke Association, London
Illustrations of bed exercises; getting out of bed; sitting in a chair; exercises when sitting, standing, walking, managing stairs, getting in and out of the bath/car, dressing and undressing — for the hemiplegic patient.

Heywood Jones I 1986 The Savile Row of prosthetic surgery. Nursing Times 82 (11) March 12: 55–58
Rehabilitative surgery — hip replacement.

Holden U P 1979 Return to reality. Nursing Mirror 149 (21) November 22: 26–29
Reality orientation, a therapy designed to help withdrawn, confused and depressed old people find their bearings again and improve their quality of life.

Keywood O 1978 Preparing the elderly to return home Part 1. Nursing Mirror 147 (10) September 7: 42–44
Defines rehabilitation; rehabilitative measures in hospital; basic requirements for life in the community after discharge.

Lambert J 1985 Adjusting to tetraplegia. Nursing Times 81 (6) February 6: 32–33
A personal account.

Lyttle P 1980 Winning her independence. Nursing Mirror 150 (18) June 12: 56–57
Describes Ena, and how she led a more complete life after attending a day hospital for rehabilitation of psychiatric patients.

MacInnes M S A 1977 Bilateral amputation of the legs — patient care and rehabilitation. Nursing Times 73 (27) July 7: 1033–1035
Illustrations of gadgets which helped a patient to regain his independence in daily living activities.

Maycock J 1985 Towards pain relief. Nursing Mirror 160 (3) January 16: 40–41
Pain can interfere with rehabilitation.

McLaren M 1977 Come on, Jiminy Cricket. Nursing Times 74 (37) September 25: 1433–1435
Illustration of a rehabilitation chart used to rehabilitate a patient in her home after a stroke causing a left hemiplegia.

Millard P H 1978 To rehabilitate or to vegetate. Nursing Mirror 146 (11) March 16: 14–16
All staff members work together to achieve the goal that the patient wants; always define the objective.

Newman D 1985 Essential physical therapy for stroke patients. Nursing Times 81 (6) February 6: 17–18
Contractures interfere with rehabilitation; they can be prevented.

Nursing Mirror 1981 Clinical Forum. The disabled. Nursing Mirror Supplement October 14

Partridge C, Wright B 1978 Helping patients to help themselves 1. Patients with stroke. Nursing Mirror 146 (23) June 8: 42–44
Achievement of a goal, however small, encourages an enthusiastic and optimistic approach to tackling the tasks ahead.

Partridge C, Wright B 1978 Helping patients to help themselves 2. Patients with bronchitis and rheumatoid arthritis. Nursing Mirror 146 (24) June 15: 40

Partridge C, Wright B 1978 Helping patients to help themselves 3. Patients with Parkinsonism and multiple sclerosis. Nursing Mirror 146 (25) June 22: 38
Inability to initiate movement; it's the taking off and the landing that's so difficult — in between it's not so bad.

Price B 1986 Giving the patient control. Nursing Times 82 (20) May 14: 28–30
Describes a patient rehabilitation model, indeed discusses it as a process. Uses the definition 'Any means of restoring the independence of a patient after disease or injury, including employment retraining.'

Robinson W 1977 Possum means 'I can!' Nursing Mirror 144 (50) February 3: 45–47
Describes a visit to the Possum factory where electronic aids for the disabled are produced.

Robinson W 1978 Aids for the disabled. Nursing Mirror Supplement 146 (7) February 16
Overview of services which local authorities are obliged to provide; describes aids for personal care, mobility, care of the home, leisure activities including holidays.

Sheahan J 1978 Caring for handicapped children at the Leon Gills Unit. Nursing Mirror 147 (12) September21: 32–34
Describes the fitting of prosthetic limbs to limb deficient children and the rehabilitation programme for those with spina bifida.

Stickland M R 1977 Problems of locomotion. Nursing Times 73 (47) November 24: 1841–1842
Although nurses may find it quicker to wash, dress and feed patients who are slow and clumsy, it makes a rod for their backs in the long run.

Sykes J 1985 A night out on crutches. Nursing Times 81 (48) November 27: 32–33
A student nurse wore a bandage and used crutches to visit an Italian restaurant to find out 'what it feels like'.

Tait A, Maguire P, Sellwood R 1980 Plan into practice: emotional aspects of mastectomy. Nursing Mirror 150 (4) January 24: 19–21
Appointment of a specialist nurse; discussion of the problems which she encountered.

Thursfield P J 1979 The hospital that doesn't say 'goodbye'. Nursing Mirror 148 (6) February 8: 50–52
Description of a comprehensive service to elderly patients discharged from hospital.

Turton P 1986 Relaxation techniques. Nursing: The Add-On Journal of Clinical Nursing 2 (39) September: 348–351
Relaxation as part of rehabilitation.

Waldron S 1983 Integration of handicapped pupils. Nursing Times 79 (15) April 13: 54–56
Rehabilitation of two handicapped children into a comprehensive school to the benefit of all the children.

Waters K 1986 Role recognition. Senior Nurse 5 (5/6) November/December: 15–16
Potential for nurses to develop a unique involvement in rehabilitation of the elderly.

Weaver S M, Armstrong N E, Brooke A K, Steward J 1978 Behavioural principles applied in a security ward. Nursing Times 74 (1) January 5: 22–24
Describes a programme of change: custodial principles breed their own problems; positive rehabilitation is more effective, humane and actually improves security.

Wells S 1983 Aiding rehabilitation. Nursing Times 79 (21) May 25: 56–58
An assessment flat was used by geriatric patients prior to being discharged home.

Wilson-Barnett J 1980 Rehabilitation for coronary patients: the nurse's role. Nursing Times 76 (15) April 10: 637–638
Restoration of physical health alone is not enough; psychological health is equally important.

Winship H 1977 Rehabilitation. Nursing Mirror 145 (17) October 27: 20–21

Describes Employment Rehabilitation Centres which are authorised by the government; work of Disablement Resettlement Officer (DRO).

Woodcock D 1978 Hospital resettlement officer in Wakefield. Nursing Times 74 (33) August 17: 1361
Working is to many patients a normal way of life and as such forms part of the 'total patient'. A future life at work is important.

BACKGROUND INFORMATION

Nurses' work has always had a habilitative and rehabilitative dimension, but in past years it has been implicit, for example preventing complications — of bedrest, and of the particular medical diagnosis from which the patient was suffering, which impeded the patient's habilitation or rehabilitation to optimal 'health'. In an attempt to make the dimension explicit, a concept of 'health' will be discussed, together with that of everyday living activities, and the multidisciplinary habilitation/rehabilitation team which contributes to habilitating and rehabilitating people to their optimal 'health'.

Concept of health

The concept of health is complex and multidimensional. Is a person 'healthy' whose body functioning is controlled within a normal range by drugs, for example a diabetic taking insulin, or a hypertensive person taking antihypertensive drugs? Such people may say that they 'feel well' yet their medical diagnosis will have been confirmed by various biological measurements. Consideration of these and other complexities led the World Health Organization in 1946 to define health as 'a state of complete physical, mental and social well-being, and not merely the absence of disease or infirmity'. Since 1946 the concept of health has broadened, after considering such questions as, Are babies 'healthy' who are born blind or deaf, or with a physical disability and/or mental handicap? Long lists can be made of the dimensions to be considered in developing a concept of health, but a manageable one might include 'a person who is functioning, within his capability, at the fullest:

- physical
- mental
- social
- vocational and
- economic aspects of living.'

For those born with a congenital defect, the composite plan carried out by several professionals, either in the home, school, health clinic or hospital, would be 'habilitation' to these goals. For those who had partly or fully achieved these goals, when their health status changed, perhaps because of acute or chronic disease, or injury, the goal would be 'rehabilitation' to their previous health status. It can be seen therefore that a habilitation or rehabilitation plan requires to be individualised. But what has to be individualised?

Everyday living activities

Along with the five broader aspects of living previously mentioned there are specific activities which have to be carried out in the process of living. The people in need of specific aspects of habilitation or rehabilitation are those who for any reason, for a short or long time, do not have the ability to:

- achieve a comfortable posture for sitting and sleeping
- breathe adequately
- brush teeth and gums
- comprehend the spoken and/or written word
- dress and undress
- feed independently
- groom hair
- hear adequately
- manicure nails
- move one or more limbs
- retain faeces in the rectum
- retain urine in the bladder
- see adequately
- smell adequately
- speak adequately
- stand and walk
- wash and bath.

After reading this list and consulting the Contents page, readers will realise that pertinent information is to be found in other chapters of this text. It is only for purposes of description that nursing knowledge can be divided into chapters; in reality each nursing activity is so complex that it requires a synthesis of knowledge from several chapters.

Multidisciplinary habilitation/rehabilitation team

With such a wide range of possible disabilities, helping the disabled is not the prerogative of members of any one discipline; it is in fact a multidisciplinary function and can involve any appropriate selection of the following:

- clinical psychologists
- disablement resettlement officer (DRO)
- doctors
- industrial therapists
- nurses
- occupational therapists
- physiotherapists
- social workers
- speech therapists
- vocational counsellors.

Whatever the composition of the professional team, long-term habilitation and rehabilitation is unlikely to achieve its goal without the patient and members of his family being given the opportunity to function as full members of the team and being constantly encouraged to do so. As a team member a nurse is encouraged to develop a positive attitude to rehabilitation and to realise that knowledge of rehabilitation is basic to all nursing interventions.

HABILITATION/REHABILITATION AND THE PROCESS OF NURSING

One objective of the process of nursing is to individualise the nursing contribution to the multidisciplinary approach to habilitation/ rehabilitation. Long term habilitation programmes will be necessary for those born with such conditions as spina bifida, Down's syndrome, mental handicap, physical handicap including absence of one or more limbs. Nursing personnel who are likely to have contact with these people and their families include midwives in the early days, then health visitors, school nurses, community nurses, practice nurses and later on occupational health nurses. And, of course, such people are just as likely as anyone else to develop a condition which requires hospital admission. For all of them, the long-term goal will be optimal independence for as many everyday living activities as possible, according to the particular circumstances. It could be that special equipment will be necessary for some activities when the concept of 'aided independence' is appropriate.

The rehabilitation requirements of people who have suffered amputation, paraplegia, tetraplegia, stroke and so on are well recognised. Whatever treatment is available for the physical disability, it may not achieve its goal if nurses fail to understand and provide psychological support to disabled patients and their families. Disablement whether of acute or chronic onset, and at whatever stage of the lifespan it occurs, means a change in body image and self-identity. Each person has a 'mental picture' of how he looks, behaves and relates to other people. Any interference with this self-concept is a shattering blow; a period of adaptation is essential to integrate into his self-concept the change and all that it means in the patient's life.

The initial reaction is usually one of shock which may manifest as withdrawal or excessive anxiety. There is inevitable *dependency* during which phase there can be alternating anger and depression as the patient begins to realise that life cannot be the same as before the disablement. During this phase the nursing intervention of listening and talking with him regarding his many fears about future living, permits him to realise that a different self-image can be developed.

Most patients in the early stages have to work through a phase of *denial* considered to be a healthy reaction because it gives time for the patient to begin to think positively about his changed self. The nursing intervention is to refrain from confronting him with too much too soon. The nurse needs to be responsive to the patient's emotional progress and proceed at his rate of acceptance of the change.

Many patients, particularly adolescents and young adults, pass through a phase of *turbulence* when they can feel depressed, are overtly hostile to staff and visitors, and try out various manipulative techniques. Firmness and consistency as part of all nursing interventions are important contributions to helping the patient achieve a more settled attitude to his condition.

The *working through* phase takes the longest and is a highly complex activity. In a society which values normality and attractive physique, disabled people can and usually do experience inferiority when they cannot do what society values as 'normal', and when they look 'different' from society's value of 'normal'. They have to re-examine society's values as well as their own. During nursing interventions they can be helped to become less comparison oriented, and more co-operative rather than competitive. Increasing independence, however slowly achieved, helps them to develop a new realistic and acceptable self-image incorporating the idea that disability and lack of worth are not synonymous.

A recently disabled person may be in hospital for several months while rehabilitating everyday living skills and it is unlikely that the nursing staff will remain unchanged from day to day. The written nursing records must therefore convey an accurate picture of 'where the patient is' in coming to terms with what has happened so that nurses on each succeeding shift will have a consistent approach.

Not all rehabilitation is carried out in hospitals, even including day hospitals. It is envisaged that in the future there will be three main groups of people needing progressive rehabilitation in the community:

- the increasing number of frail elderly people, many of whom live alone; they do not want to end their days in an institution, they want to continue living in their familiar environment and a planned rehabilitation programme could help to achieve this goal.
- patients whose lives have been or are being preserved by modern therapy, as for example, those who have survived severe injuries, and those who have chronic/disabling diseases. These patients cannot stay in hospital indefinitely: they block urgently needed hospital beds. But without a 24 hour community nursing service some of them are currently denied the possibility of being cared for in their homes, a privilege which many professionals think they should be offered.
- patients who are dependent on machines, for example home dialysis; at present these are few in number but they are likely to increase until such time as more donor kidneys become available.

Community nursing staff will therefore be involved in assessing, planning, implementing and evaluating the progress of these patients towards their long-term goals, and documenting the information so that relief staff can offer an equivalent nursing service.

The rehabilitation needs of patients after mastectomy or stoma surgery are recognised by the appointment of specialist nurses to attend to these needs. There is great emphasis on rehabilitation in the dialysis units. Several hospitals have a cardiac rehabilitation unit for patients who have had an acute episode of coronary heart disease and those who have had cardiovascular surgery. However a concept of rehabilitation should guide nurses as they carry out nursing activities for the majority of patients who are not in the previously mentioned categories in preparation for their dischage from the health service.

The foregoing paints a broad generalisation of the concept habilitation/rehabilitation. This has been necessary because the concept includes so many aspects of living which might require rehabilitation. It also incorporates the concept of quality of life, and a desirable quality has a very individual interpretation: it will, for example, be different for an ambitious as compared to a non-ambitious person. There has been an equally broad interpretation of the four phases of the process of nursing — assessing, planning, implementing and evaluating: examples of their use have only been given where relevant. However, use of the process has as its main objective individualised nursing. This is obviously impossible in a book, but the following text will be focused to each of the four phases in turn.

Assessing

The concept of habilitation/rehabilitation naturally guides the work of health visitors, paediatric nurses, school nurses, and those working with children. At the initial assessment it is pertinent to discover the exact stage which the child has reached in relation to what he can do regarding each everyday living activity and exactly what help he requires. This should be written factually, so that nurses on ensuing shifts can provide the much-talked about concept 'continuity of care'; and it will act as a baseline for ongoing assessment and evaluation. Of course for very young children, the secondary source of information, the parents or guardian will be used, but older children can be encouraged to give their version of what they can and cannot do and this can be verified by parents and so on. However, the older child may be admitted as an emergency and will not be capable of giving his version, so the secondary source will be used initially, and verified by the patient later.

For adolescents, young adults, adults and elderly people the initial assessment may realistically be guided by whether they are likely to be short-, medium- or long-stay patients. The notion of rehabilitation for people in each of these age groups is getting them ready for discharge from the health service, whether this is hospital or community. Assessment data about some or all of the following will be relevant — occupation, hobbies and other socialising patterns, type of residence; available support from family, friends, neighbours; and support services such as home helps, meals on wheels, physiotherapy, speech therapy and so on.

The usual interpretation of the purpose of collecting assessment data is to identify, with the patient wherever possible, the actual problems which he is experiencing in relation to the particular subject of assessment. But the patient may not be familiar with the concept of rehabilitation, and may be perturbed by conversation relating to his discharge so shortly after admission. However, if the nurse explores with him what he is expecting his admission to the health service — hospital or community — to achieve, it will help her to appreciate possible actual problems and any potential problems related to the general concept of rehabilitation with its notion of quality of life. Sometimes actual problems can impede both habilitation and rehabilitation, and of course much nursing time is spent in preventing the identified potential problems from becoming actual ones, so that the overall aim is achieved. Sometimes the identified problems will be associated with one or more of the everyday living activities and guidance about assessing them is contained in the appropriate chapters (see Contents page). Some actual and potential problems can be associated with a symptom which the patient is experiencing, for example suicidal behaviour (Ch. 3), pain (Ch. 4), dying (Ch. 6), pressure sores (Ch. 10) or incontinence (Ch. 11). Other actual and potential problems may be associated with particular treatments such as wounds (Ch. 21), plaster casts (Ch. 22), medications (Ch. 23) and operations (Ch. 24). Yet other actual and potential problems may be relevant because of admission to the health service, whether it is to hospital or in the patient's home (community). Such problems may be associated with the environment (Ch. 17), misidentification (Ch. 18), loss of personal possessions (Ch. 19) and community- or hospital-acquired infection (Ch. 20). In all chapters there is discussion of assessing as the first phase of the process of nursing.

This chapter illustrates well the relatedness of nursing knowledge and the fact that division into chapters can only be for the purpose of description. Each habilitative or rehabilitative nursing activity requires the appropriate synthesis of relevant knowledge from several chapters, and this synthesising ability can be best acquired in clinical practice, and becomes a part of professional clinical judgement.

Planning

Setting goals for patients' identified problems, and the plan of nursing interventions to achieve the goals, are discussed in each of the chapters, and though nurses have not always used the word rehabilitation, the nursing interventions are of a rehabilitative nature, and inclusion of the concept in a notion of nursing will probably increase awareness of the rehabilitative dimension of planned nursing interventions. In this section institutionalisation will be discussed, albeit briefly, because it is anathema to habilitation/rehabilitation, and planning is necessary to avoid it. This will be followed by patient participation as an antidote to institutionalisation. Because boredom is another experience which mitigates against rehabilitation, it too will be discussed and an antidote to boredom — visitors — and the planning necessary to make this a positive experience for the patients. This will be followed by the prevention of possible complications of bedrest which impede rehabilitation.

Institutionalisation

Change in previous life-style, including that of the physically disabled person, can decrease the opportunity for decision-making which encourages a passive role. The person becomes apathetic, withdrawn and dependent because of the unchallenging and unchanging circumstances. This is more likely to occur in hospital than at home and it is called 'institutionalisation.' One goal of individualised nursing is to prevent it.

Antidote to institutionalisation — patient participation

The concept of the process of nursing with its many subconcepts such as:

- assessing
- identifying with patients any problems they are experiencing with their everyday living activities which are amenable to nursing
- setting goals with patients for alleviating, solving or helping them to cope with insoluble ones
- agreeing with patients, nursing (and possibly patient) interventions to achieve the goals
- evaluating whether or not the goals are being or have been achieved

calls for patient participation and decision making throughout. This is a far cry from the 'nurse knows best what is good for the patient' attitude of yester year and calls for nurses' imagination and creativity in helping patients to structure their day so that they feel positive about it, thereby preventing institutionalisation and contributing to their rehabilitation.

Boredom

When a patient is removed from the pleasure-giving and self-fulfilling resources in his life, the enforced inactivity easily leads to boredom. Boredom tends to lower morale and Revans in his studies in the '60s and '70s found that patients in wards of low morale had a longer hospital stay. Lack of occupation leaves ample time for concentration on the illness and for introspection. Boredom is high on the list in the many 'patient satisfaction surveys' which have been carried out. Prevention of boredom is therefore an essential nursing intervention and a contribution to rehabilitation.

Antidote to boredom — visitors

Visitors can be an antidote to boredom and wise use of 'visiting' is an important nursing intervention to achieve rehabilitation of patients. 20 years ago there were rigid visiting rules in most hospitals. This varied from a monthly, to a weekly visiting period, to a half or 1 hour period twice weekly or daily. Several years ago the Government sent out circulars to hospitals advising implementation of more liberal visiting policies. There was, in many places, inadequate preparation of the staff and the public before introducing the policy. The public were never intended to visit even their near relatives continuously from first thing in the morning until last thing at night. Some relatives who interpreted 'free visiting' in this way felt guilty if they did not stay, and if they did stay, they and the patients found it a marathon task.

The objective of the change was that patients and their relatives could have *mutual choice* about the *time* and *duration* of *visits* subject to staff approval. It was hoped that this would spread the number of visitors in a ward at any one time, and the staff could continue their ministrations to those patients who were not being visited at that time. With visitors spread over a longer period, it could afford both visitors and staff a much better opportunity to *communicate with each other*. For each ill person there are anxious relatives or friends who need information, not only to keep their anxiety within reasonable limits, but also to teach them how they can help the ill patient to recover or to die peacefully.

Looked at in a wider context 'free visiting' could disperse 'traffic noise' and 'people noise' resulting from hoards of visitors arriving at the hospital at the beginning of, and departing from the hospital at the end of, a restricted visiting period. It could prevent visitors having long waits for buses and trains while too many visitors try to board too few vehicles. It could lessen traffic congestion near the hospital; this inevitably occurs at the beginning and end of a restricted visiting period. It could accommodate visitors travelling from a distance, whose train and bus times did not fit in with the restricted visiting time.

Those who visit a sick person in his home have to knock to gain access, and this can be refused. Maybe the visiting cards which used to be issued, two per patient, served a purpose. If they were re-introduced perhaps only one card would be issued to the next of kin for a very ill patient. Then by arrangement between the patient and charge nurse, more cards could be issued to fit the needs of that patient. Perhaps a son could visit for 10 to 15 minutes after lunch, a daughter could visit for a similar period in the early evening and a spouse could visit for 20 to 30 minutes later in the evening.

Except during that great influx of visitors at the beginning of a restricted visiting period, it is usual for a visitor to ask permission to see a patient. Should a reciprocal courtesy (it could be called a right) be extended to the patient? How are nurses to know whether the patient wants to see that visitor unless they ask the patient? Extended visiting would facilitate this; with restricted visiting it is impossible for the patient to retain control over who visits him. Is this an infringement of a patient's rights?

With regard to the *visiting of children in hospital*, it is Government policy that parents should have liberal access to their sick child. Hospital facilities for this purpose vary tremendously throughout the country. Some have excellent 'rooming-in' quarters so that at least one parent can be there throughout each 24 hours. Yet there are still hospitals which have restricted visiting of children. There are several organisations concerned with the welfare of children in hospitals and their policy is to campaign for the rights of children in every hospital in the country.

Children can be distressed by Mummy, Granny or any adult member of their 'family' being taken away to hospital. This has been recognised over the last few years and hospitals are advised to adopt a policy whereby children can visit the adult in hospital and thus relieve the nagging fear that Mummy or Granny has gone away and left them.

Whatever visiting policy is decided by an institution, its success, and that means the benefit and pleasure that the patients derive from it, depends solely on its execution by individuals at ward level. Conducting a successful visiting programme is an important contribution to the rehabilitation of patients.

Prevention of complications of bedrest

Patients who are confined to bed even for a few weeks are at risk of developing several physical and psychological complications (Fig. 2.1) which

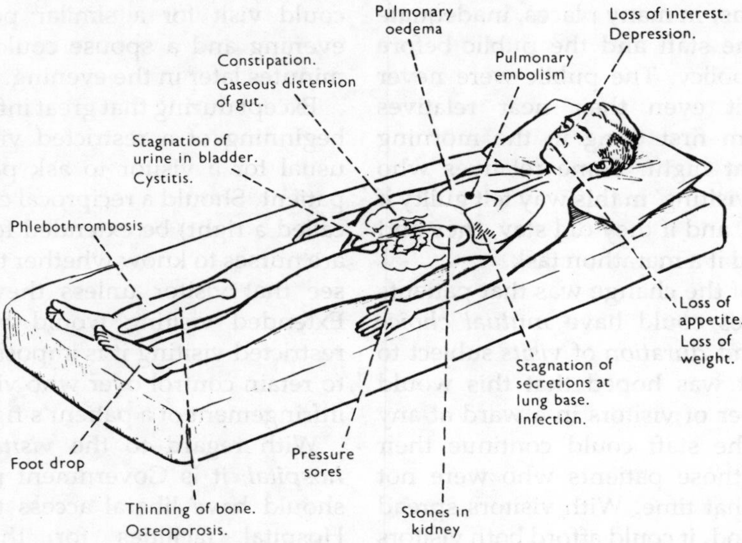

Fig. 2.1 Complications of bedrest

will undoubtedly hinder rehabilitation. Prevention is discussed at appropriate places throughout the text.

Implementing

Implementing, the third phase of the process, customarily means carrying out the planned nursing interventions. In the current interpretation of general nursing, the adjective 'rehabilitative' is unlikely to be used to describe nursing interventions, even though many of them do have an implicit 'rehabilitative' dimension in that their goal is optimising the patient's independence in a particular everyday living activity; they are discussed in the appropriate chapters (see Contents page). With the current emphasis on health (see Preface) it is possible that in the future the concept of habilitation/rehabilitation will be explicitly incorporated into the language of nursing. Meantime students of nursing will benefit from bearing in mind the concept while implementing the planned nursing interventions to achieve the goal of optimal independence in everyday living activities, to achieve discharge from the health service and to improve the quality of living.

The goals may be short-, medium- or long-term, for example rehabilitation programmes for patients recovering from a severe stroke, or spinal injury may last many months, or even a few years as the muscular co-ordination gradually increases. However, it is usual to break the final goal into tiny steps so that as each step is achieved, the patient is encouraged and reassured that progress is being made towards optimal independence. The programme involves the gradual withdrawal of nursing help, but this must be skilfully adjusted to the patient's increasing capabilities. Such phased activities not only call for the nurse's adaptability but they also require the use of clinical judgement. It is misjudgement to continue doing things for patients because it is quicker than letting them take the time to dress themselves, for example: it is also misjudgement to expect patients to carry out activities which they are not yet physically and psychologically capable of doing.

Evaluating

Evaluating, the fourth phase of the process, is accepted as observing, measuring whether or not the agreed goals have been achieved. Evaluating related to particular everyday living activities is discussed in the appropriate chapters (see Contents page). Evaluating independence for self-injection of insulin and pain-relieving drugs is mentioned on page 286; caring for a stoma on page 185, Refs.; complying with a medication programme on page 297 and these have an implicit interpretation of rehabilitation.

This chapter has considered the invaluable contribution which nurses can make to the multidisciplinary team by applying the principle — helping to habilitate/rehabilitate patients — in a process of nursing context. It has been shown that the principle informs all nursing activities. However, not all people have the motivation to want to go on living, so in the next chapter 'helping suicidal patients' will be considered.

APPLYING THE PRINCIPLE

A registered nurse must be capable of:

- helping immobile patients to prevent complications which interfere with rehabilitation
- helping patients to achieve their goal of optimal independence for living
- helping some patients to cope adequately with reduced independence in some areas of living
- helping patients to be satisfactorily discharged from hospital to home
- preventing institutionalisation
- applying the. principle — helping to habilitate/rehabilitate patients — in a process of nursing context.

WORKING ASSIGNMENT

Topics for discussion

- patients' boredom and its prevention
- hospital visiting policy
- rehabilitation
- institutionalisation
- aided independence
- habilitation
- health
- body-image
- self-esteem
- assertiveness
- aggressiveness
- quality of life
- patient participation.

Writing assignment

- state the physical complications of bedrest
- state the stages of adaptation to a changed body-image
- state three main groups of people needing progressive rehabilitation in the community
- define the following:

amputation
body-image
community nurse
dialysis
Disablement Resettlement Officer
Down's syndrome
habilitation
health visitor
mastectomy
mental handicap
midwife
occupational health nurse
paraplegia
physical handicap
practice nurse
rehabilitation
self-concept
spina bifida
stoma
tetraplegia.

3

Helping suicidal patients

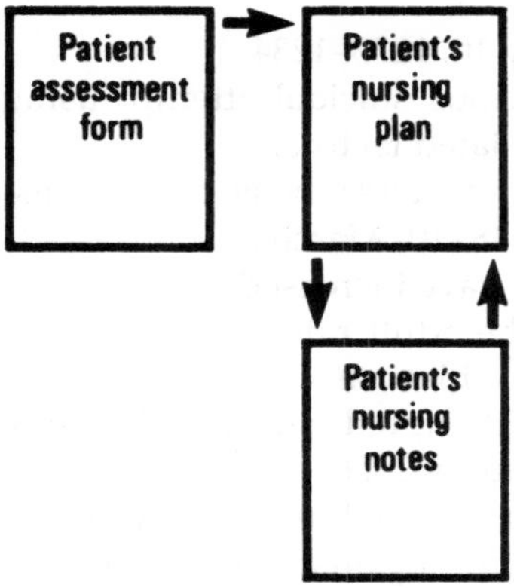

Reading assignment

Background information
Personal individuality
Suicide

Suicide and the process of nursing
Assessing
Planning
Implementing
Evaluating

Applying the principle
A registered nurse must be capable of:

Working assignment
Topics for discussion
Writing assignment

READING ASSIGNMENT

Andrews R, Jenkins J S, Sugden J 1985 Origins of sadness as a response. Nursing: The Add-On Journal of Clinical Nursing 2 (34) February: 995–998
Discusses depressive illness and its treatment, types of suicide. Table of high risk factors for suicide. Nursing is discussed using the headings Assessment and Planning Care.

Ashton J 1986 Preventing suicide in hospital. Nursing Times 82 (52) December 31: 36–37
Examines the unit incident files from 1981 to 1986 in an attempt to find some correlation, if any, between the suicide incidents. Identifies criteria which management and staff could apply in the prevention of suicide.

Bhagat M, Shillitoe R W 1978 Attempted suicide. Nursing Mirror 146 (6) February 9: 26–27
Helps nurses to understand suicidal attempts: without understanding it is difficult to help these patients and makes it easier to act with hostility and indifference.

Brooking J, Minghella E 1987. Parasuicide. Nursing Times 83 (21) May 27: 40–43
At least 100 000 people in Britain take an overdose or deliberately harm themselves each year. Studies at one hospital suggest that psychiatric community nurses might be more effective than psychiatrists at treating these patients.

Brown E A, Miller L 1978 Psychiatric problems in A and E departments. Nursing Times 74 (33)

August 17: 1369–1371
Self-poisoned and self-mutilated regarded as 'not a patient' so the very basis for a professional relationship is threatened; suicidal patients impair the satisfaction many nurses get from nursing.

Cowley S A 1978 We may need the bed. Nursing Times 74 (6) February 9: 248
Suicide patients are unpopular; description of the feelings with which nurses have to come to terms; overdose units.

Hamadah K 1977 Depression. Nursing Mirror 145 (19) November 10: 13–15
Depression is a disease which affects many systems; epidemiology; clinical picture; treatment.

Heywood Jones I 1985 Suicide — who's to blame? Nursing Times 81 (9) February 27: 44–45
Report of an investigation by the ombudsman of a complaint by a loving wife that her husband was not properly supervised despite her repeated warnings to the staff.

Ives G 1979 Nurse could you care more? Nursing Times 75 (35) August 30: 1475
Attitudes of hospital staff detract from the care given to suicidal patients.

Johnstone F 1987 Self-poisoning. Nursing: The Add-On Journal of Clinical Nursing 3 (16) April: 602–606
Comprehensive account of common drugs used in overdose: diagnosis and assessment: treatment: psychological aspects and recent advances in management.

McBean I 1979 Who should treat the parasuicide adolescent? Nursing Mirror 148 (115) April 12: 10
Responding letter to Reynolds (1979): Edinburgh findings show a diminishing number of patients who are mentally ill.

Moore I 1986 Ending it all. Nursing Times 82 (7) February 12: 48–49
Gives comparative figures for male and female suicides, aged 15 to 75+ for 1971, 1976 and 1980. Discusses aspects of the elderly and suicide and asks should nurses intervene in what some regard as a 'fundamental human right'?

Pyle P L 1980 An attempted suicide. Nursing Times 76 (28) July 10: 1233–1234
Analysis of a vicious suicidal attempt using Stengel's list of related factors.

Reynolds D 1979 Youngsters who go off the rails. Nursing Mirror 148 (10) March 8: 16–18
Teenage suicides have increased steadily over 10 years while the adult rate has decreased; counsellors or psychiatrists?

Roberts L 1977 Attempted suicide. Nursing Mirror 144 (3) January 20: 65–66
Suicide no longer a crime but regarded by the church as an offence against natural law and therefore a sin; find out what the cry for help means.

Rushforth D 1985 Deliberate self-harm. Nursing Times 81 38 September 18: 51–53
Discusses a recent DHSS recommendation which would expand the nursing role with this group of patients.

Stevens B C 1977 Preventing fatal overdoses. Nursing Mirror 145 (24) December 15: 47–48
An experienced nurse is invaluable in evaluating the depth and sincerity of a patient's depressive feelings and she has a crucial role in the prevention of suicidal behaviour.

Vousden M 1986 A friend in need. Nursing Times 82 (21) May 21: 16– 17
Describes the work of the Samaritans, of whom there are 21 000. It is estimated that there are around 200 000 suicide attempts or gestures a year.

Wright B 1986 Caring in crisis. A handbook of intervention skills for nurses, Churchill Livingstone. Edinburgh
Chapter 5: Table 5.1 Beck Suicidal Attempt Scale; Table 5.2 Incidence and aetiology in assessing risk.

Wright R I 1979 Self-poisoning trends and management. Nursing Times 75 (46) November 15: 1966–1968
Discussion of the size of the problem; drugs taken; possibility of crisis poisoning centres.

BACKGROUND INFORMATION

In order to help a suicidal patient a nurse needs to realise the background to the stigma which some people still attach to suicide. A circular issued to hospital authorities by the UK Government in 1961 stated that as attempted suicide was no longer a legal entity, it was to be treated as a medical and social problem. It was suggested that all cases of attempted suicide brought to hospital should receive psychiatric investigation before discharge but unfortunately many people still attach stigma to such an investigation. In the past some religions denied their ritual of burial to those who had committed suicide affirming that the act was sinful. It is therefore not surprising that people, including all entrants to nursing, develop their particular set of values and beliefs about the act of self-destruction.

Personal individuality

In the process of self-development, genes and environment both play their part so that some people are of quiet temperament, others are ebullient; some are gregarious while others prefer mainly their own company; some are confident, others lack self-confidence and so on. And no one 'feels' the same all the time. Throughout each 24 hours people experience a variety of emotions, possibly opposite ones. Long before children acquire verbal language they can communicate feelings such as:

	pleasure	displeasure	
	satisfaction	dissatisfaction	
positive	tolerance	intolerance	negative
	calmness	anger	
	contentment	discontent	
	achievement	frustration	

Gradually most children learn how to handle these emotions in a socially acceptable way producing a feeling of self-worth. Even so, some personalities are more adequate than others in the process of living. Some people are plagued with feelings of self-doubt, worthlessness and hopelessness and they seek help; others, unable to request help, appeal indirectly by attempting suicide to call attention to their plight.

Suicide

Stevens (1977), in her study of fatal overdoses, suggests that socially isolated, depressed persons who are deprived of secure emotional and financial support are especially prone to serious suicidal acts. 79% of the study population of 500 had a psychiatric history — mainly of depression. Stevens suggests that:

> Verbalisation of depressive hopelessness should be carefully assessed whenever possible in the light of the patient's usual personality structure and methods of communicating feelings to others. An experienced nurse is, in our opinion, invaluable in evaluating the depth and sincerity of a patient's feelings.

She goes on to say that nurses can play a vital role in the detection of patients who are especially at risk, and thereby in the prevention of many premature tragic deaths. She considers that her article is not only relevant to psychiatric nurses but to the many district nurses and hospital-based members of the profession who nurse elderly patients, many of whom possess the necessary tablets because they are dependent on sleeping pills to relieve insomnia.

From epidemiological research more females than males inflict deliberate self-harm, the highest proportion occurring in the 16 to 24 age group. Poisoning is the preferred method, accounting for 90% of all incidents. Non-fatal suicide attempts account for approximately 250 000 hospital admissions each year (Andrews et al 1985). Most people who attempt suicide are young and healthy, consequently it is difficult to understand their reasons for such a desperate act. When faced with situations which they cannot understand, nurses, just like other people, tend to react with hostility or indifference. Bhagat & Shillitoe (1978) describe the sort of people who attempt suicide in the hope that nurses will learn to understand them and offer appropriate help in an open and accepting way that recognises the distress of these people.

Ives (1979) says that nurses and medical staff in casualty departments and medical wards are often unsympathetic to the overdose patient; they feel that attending to self-inflicted injury is a waste of their valuable time. Ives emphasises that no person will attempt suicide, however seriously or otherwise, without there being great stress in his life which he is unable to handle himself.

Cowley (1978) points out that self-poisoned and self-mutilated patients are admitted to general hospitals where many members of staff have been inadequately prepared to cope with them. She thinks that group discussion of helping suicidal patients gives general nurses an opportunity to air their grievancies and worries, and explore their attitudes to these patients. She suggests that members of the Samaritans could discuss their work in helping to prevent suicide.

Brown & Miller (1978) who work in a psychiatric day hospital, offered to meet any of the Accident and Emergency staff in a local general hospital to discuss the problems encountered in their work. The patients who had attempted suicide, or had inflicted mutilations upon themselves were agreed by all nurses to constitute the biggest overall burden in terms of work and effort. They aroused the strongest feelings in the nurses and doctors, mostly negative feelings of resentment, anger and bewilderment. Brown & Miller discuss the idea that these people are not perceived as 'patients' by the professional staff and that this threatens the very basis for a professional approach. They quote instances of disintegration of such an approach when medical staff have urged self-destructive patients to 'do it properly next time'. They discuss at some length how nurses and doctors, called upon to treat these patients in general hospitals, might be helped and supported to develop adequate skills in helping suicidal patients.

Finally it is all too easy for the young and robust nurse to assume that all patients are motivated to recover from illness. An important motivating factor is having someone who cares whether or not one recovers. There are patients who do not have this motivating factor; many of them are old, they feel lonely and unwanted; they have lost their self-esteem. Their lack of motivation for living can be communicated non-verbally by such non-co-operative behaviour as not drinking, considered by some people to be a form of suicide. It is no use telling such patients that they ought to drink and that they have something to live for, because they do not see it like this. The only way that a nurse can help such patients is by conveying to them by her warmth and sincerity that she cares whether or not they live. When these patients have been supported through this period of lack of motivation and they have recovered their self-esteem, the nurse can offer the help of the social services to overcome the loneliness which they will experience after discharge from hospital.

SUICIDE AND THE PROCESS OF NURSING

From the articles in the Reading Assignment and the foregoing text, you will have gathered that the large majority of young people who have attempted suicide by poisoning are admitted as an 'emergency' to the Accident and Emergency department of a general hospital and after immediate treatment are transferred to a medical ward. In those cities which have a Poisoning Treatment Centre, it will be the route of admission. A minority of patients from both these sources are transferred to a bed in the psychiatric unit of a general hospital or in a psychiatric hospital. It is likely that in the emergency situation only relevant biographical details will be written on the patient assessment form, and the treatment prescribed by the doctor, whether or not it was carried out by a nurse, will be recorded in the medical notes. The nurse will collect together this information as appropriate on the nursing records before the initial assessment interview with the patient.

Assessing

It is impossible to 'individualise' collection of data for an assessment form in a text; it can only guide by offering background information. Obviously the time and place of an initial interview will need to be selected with sensitivity and awareness of when the patient will be ready to talk. Collection of factual information about the remainder of biographical detail, which cannot be gleaned from any other sources, and which was not collected in the Emergency department, should be non-threatening to the patient. However if this information reveals widowhood, separation or divorce the subject needs to be explored with great sensitivity, and indeed it may be preferable to return to the subject at a later interaction with the patient. Wright (1986) illustrates the Beck Suicidal Attempt Scale which provides a useful scheme for the nurse to bear in mind during the initial, and ongoing assessment.

The information requested on the assessment form about everyday living activities will probably provide a relaxed opportunity for nurse and patient to exchange information. When it seems appropriate, information about sleeping habits needs to be guided by knowledge of insomnia — time of going to sleep, time of wakening and so on. This can naturally lead to information about sleeping pills, anti-depressants, tranquillisers and so on. The words used by the patient for the drugs may signal awareness/unawareness of the clinical condition of depression, should this be relevant. Have the drugs been brought to hospital? This is obviously more relevant in instances of non-emergency admission, as is discerning whether or not the patient has any sharp instrument among his possessions. The patient's current mood and nonverbal communication will need to be assessed and reported factually.

From the Reading Assignment it is evident that suicide attempts in the young age group are not usually connected with the problem of mental illness but with problems of inadequacy in dealing with life events such as disagreement with parents about leaving home to live independently; disagreement, even severing of, an important relationship with a person of the same or opposite sex. Again it requires great sensitivity as to whether or not the patient is ready to talk about these aspects of living.

The above mentioned data are relevant only to the occasion on which they were collected, but nevertheless provide background information throughout the patient's stay in hospital, and should be used by staff on each succeeding shift to individualise conversation with the patient.

Planning

In this phase of the process of nursing it depends on what the patient perceives as a problem. It may be that realisation of the foolishness of the act means that nurses will assume a supportive role while the patient's goal may be reorganisation of his values and beliefs about the important people in his life. On the other hand, if the newly admitted patient continues to express suicidal intent, the nursing plan will contain the necessary precautions to be taken unobtrusively to prevent this happening.

If there are several of these patients, then generalised ward planning will place them together, so that they are more easily observed particularly during the night, and at staff change-overs as patients have been known to take advantage of these times.

The patient's nursing plan will probably contain nursing interventions related to the medical prescription of treatment such as electroconvulsive therapy (ECT), psycho-therapy, cognitive therapy and medication, all of which are described in the Reading Assignment. The documentation system used in this text provides for recording these separately from those arising because of problems with everyday living activities to help nurses to identify the nurse-initiated part of nursing. The prescription for medication will be written on the medication Kardex and need not be re-written on the nursing plan, but observing the patient for particular side-effects will be written on the nursing plan. The desired patient outcome from taking the medication will also appear, possibly with a date appended, to guide nurses as to when any change is likely to be evident.

Depressed (and therefore potentially suicidal) patients may appear to have problems with their everyday living activities such as communicating, observing socially acceptable standards of personal hygiene, including clothing, taking adequate nourishment and being constipated. However, the patient may not perceive all of these as problems and this highlights the possibility of 'nurse-perceived' problems which are not 'patient-perceived', and the problem of whether or not nurses have any right to document them.

The nursing plan, written in conjunction with the patient, informs nurses on all shifts of what will be carried out and when. It will, where relevant, contain outcomes which have been agreed with the patient and a date on which to evaluate whether or not the proposed outcomes are being or have been achieved.

Implementing

Implementing has been conceived as specific nursing interventions related to the patients' problems with everyday living activities, and as they are implemented it will be recorded on the patients' nursing notes. But what of the patients who do not have a particular problem? Nursing includes facilitating these patients carrying out their everyday living activities. In the 1970s nurses were relieved of most of the domestic work, preparing for and collecting in from meals, and clerical work so that they would have more time to spend with patients. Suicidal patients will benefit from nurses spending as much time as possible with them.

Evaluating

There will be some evaluations specifically requested by the nursing plan on a particular date. As evaluating, like assessing, is an ongoing activity there will probably be some relevant summative information in the patient's nursing notes which serves to show the relatedness of the different parts of the documentation system (in this book patient assessment form, patient's nursing plan and patient's nursing notes). Evaluating means having some base-line data against which current data can be measured or compared and so on, consequently only general comments have been made here.

It must be emphasized that reading the items in the Reading Assignment is necessary to acquire a basic level of knowledge required to fulfil the principle — helping suicidal patients. The chapter helps students to structure the knowledge gained into a process context.

APPLYING THE PRINCIPLE

A registered nurse must be capable of:

- consistently conveying warmth and sincerity to a patient manifesting lack of motivation to recover
- establishing and maintaining a professional relationship with patients who have attempted suicide
- tolerating suicidal patients' resentment, hopelessness and unreliability and still show a positive regard for them
- being available to listen to suicidal patients' account of their world as they perceive it
- applying the principle — helping suicidal patients — in a process of nursing context.

WORKING ASSIGNMENT

Topics for discussion

- the unco-operative patient
- the suicidal patient
- deliberate self-harm
- attempted suicide
- parasuicide
- the ombudsman
- ECT (electroconvulsive therapy)
- psychotherapy
- cognitive therapy
- nurse-perceived problems which are not patient-perceived
- should nurses intervene in what some regard as a fundamental right?
- Beck Suicidal Attempt Scale

Writing assignment

- write an essay on suicide
- define:
  epidemiological
  insomnia
  side-effects.

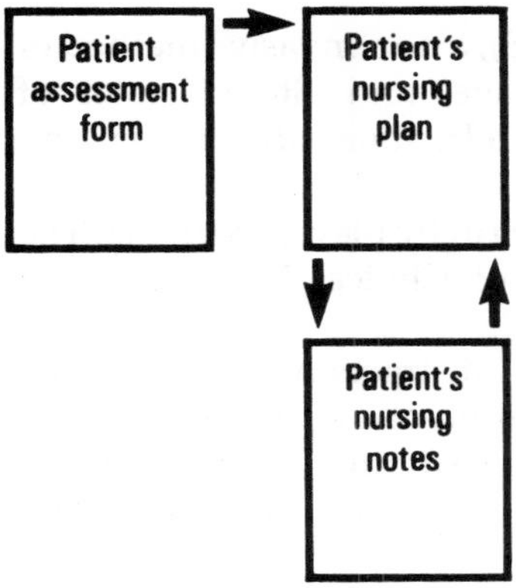

4

Helping patients to cope with pain

READING ASSIGNMENT

Akinsanya C 1985 The use of knowledge in the management of pain: the nurse's role. Nurse Education Today 5: 41–46
A list of words describing pain; physiological factors; psychological factors; measurement of pain; conclusion.

Alagaratnam W 1981 Pain and the nature of the placebo effect. Nursing Times 77 (43) October 28: 1883–1884
There is abundant evidence that placebos can be as potent as drugs, and in some cases even more effective.

Allan D 1981 The use of transcutaneous nerve stimulation in patients with severe pain. Nursing Times 77 (40) September 30: 1721–1722
This system of pain relief has the advantage of not requiring habit-forming analgesics.

Beales J 1986 Cognitive development and the experience of pain. Nursing: The Add-On Journal of Clinical Nursing 3 (11) November: 408–410
The function of cognitive involvement; Pain-modulating mechanisms; Selective attention; The affective component; Cognition and pain in children; Implications in chronic illness; Implications for patient care.

BNDU 1984 Nurses and pain. Nursing Times 80 (19) May 9: 58
Illustrates and describes a pain chart used at Burford Nursing Development Unit.

Bourbonnais F 1981 Pain assessment: development of a tool for the nurse and the patient. Journal of Advanced Nursing 6: 277–282

A tool was developed which incorporated many of the variables affecting the pain response in order to sensitize nurses to the need for careful pain assessment.

Carus-Wilson E, Griffen C, Banks A 1983 Controlling chronic pain. Nursing Times 79 (17) April 27: 51–53

Continuous injection intramuscularly of a pain-relieving drug using a syringe driver.

Castledine G 1985 Pain: a decade of nursing. Nursing Practice 1 16– 19

A survey of nurses' contribution to pain relief in the last decade.

Chung S, Dickenson A 1981 The last piece in the puzzle. Nursing Mirror 152 (6) February 5: 40–41

Endogenous pain killers and the acupuncture mystery.

Copp G 1984 Nursing interventions in postoperative pain. Nursing Mirror 159 (13) October 10: vii–xv

A concise account of the pain experience: a list of words used to describe it; a pain 'ruler' as a measurement tool.

Fordham M 1986 Psychophysiological pain theories. Nursing: The Add-On Journal of Clinical Nursing 3 (10) October: 362–364

Has two Tables giving the physiological, subjective and behavioural characteristics of acute pain and chronic pain.

Fordham M 1986 Neurophysiological pain theories. Nursing: The Add-On Journal of Clinical Nursing 3 (10) October: 365, 366, 368–370, 372

Discusses specific theory, pattern theories, gate control theory and endorphins.

Francis V 1984 Mind-body dualism. Nursing Mirror 159 (9) September 12: 30–31

Mind and body: do they function independently or in harmony with each other?

Gartside G 1986 Alternative methods of pain relief. Nursing: The Add-On Journal of Clinical Nursing 3 (11) November: 405–407

Discusses transcutaneous electrical nerve stimulation (TENS), a non-invasive method of pain relief; massage, and altered states of consciousness — relaxation, distraction and visualisation.

Gollop S 1986 Joe the rugby player. Nursing: The Add-On Journal of Clinical Nursing 3 (11) November: 424–425

Describes vividly distraction therapy used during the application of a leg plaster.

Gollop S 1986 Pain: a summary. Nursing: The Add-On Journal of Clinical Nursing 3 (10) October: 382–383

Pain and its relief become a partnership between the sufferer and the helper.

Goodinson S 1986 Pain relief: pharmacological interventions. Nursing: The Add-On Journal of Clinical Nursing 3 (11) November: 395–399, 401– 403

Three Tables — narcotic analgesics; non-steroidal anti-inflammatory drugs: co-analgesic drugs.

Gurrie H 1984 Psychological pain assessment. Nursing Times 80 (34) August 22: 38–39

Describes how a tool was developed to measure psychological pain — the assessment speedometer.

Hayward J 1975 Information — a prescription against pain. Royal College of Nursing London, p 106

Holmes P 1987 Breaking the pain barrier. Nursing Times 83 (6) February 11: 51–52

Describes work in progress at Liverpool's Walton Hospital Pain Clinic.

Nursing Mirror 1985 Research Supplement: Pain relief. Nursing Mirror 160 (5) January 30: i–viii

Investigates nurses' understanding of the use of narcotics; the effectiveness of transcutaneous electrical stimulation in relieving the pain syndrome.

Latham J 1986 Management of pain: good communication. The Professional Nurse 1 (9) June: 234–236

Three situations for discussion. A Table of problems which can result from bad communication and practice, and another showing the benefits of good communication and practice.

Latham J 1987 Syringe drivers in pain control. The Professional Nurse 2 (7) April: 207–209

Syringe drivers can play an invaluable role in pain control, but they must be used carefully and only in appropriate situations, with all mixtures of drugs checked for compatibility.

Mayer D K 1985 Non-pharmacologic management of pain in the person with cancer. Journal of Advanced Nursing 10 (4) July : 325–330

Morris R 1986 A personal account: life goes on with chronic pain. Nursing: The Add-On Journal of Clinical Nursing 3 (10) October: 375–376

Numbers L 1986 Pain: an introduction. Nursing: The Add-On Journal of Clinical Nursing 3 (10) October: 358–359

Nursing 1986 Use of the London Hospital pain observation chart. Nursing: The Add-On Journal of Clinical Nursing 3 (11) November: 415–419, 421–423
Several illustrations of the chart and how it is used.

O'Neill J 1985 Nursing assessment of the cancer patient who has protracted pain. Nursing Practice Spring 1 (1): 20–25

Ostrowski M J, Dodd V A 1977 Transcutaneous nerve stimulation for relief of pain in advanced malignant disease. Nursing Times 73 (32) August 11: 1233-1238
Three theories of the underlying mechanisms of pain: the specificity theory; the pattern theory; the gate control theory.

Prestt D 1986 Acute pain: a personal experience. Nursing: The Add-On Journal of Clinical Nursing 3 (10) October: 373–374

Sofaer B 1983 Pain relief: the core of nursing practice. Nursing Times 79 (45) November 23: 38–42

Sofaer B 1983 Pain relief — the importance of communication. Nursing Times 79 (48) December 7: 32–35

BACKGROUND INFORMATION

Pain prevents rest and sleep (p. 62), and like sleep, the phenomenon of pain is not yet fully understood. Ostrowski & Dodd (1977) discuss three theories of the underlying mechanisms of pain — the specificity theory, the pattern theory and the gate control theory. Pain is a protective mechanism; it is the most common symptom which brings a patient to a doctor or to a hospital. Pain is an *experience*; knowing in detail the sensory pathway from the inflamed boil to the brain has nothing whatever to do with 'understanding' about the experience of pain. It can occur at the site of trouble, when it is called local pain. It can be experienced at a distance, when it is called referred pain, for example pain from a gall-bladder can be felt at the tip of the scapula. It can be experienced in a limb which has been amputated when it is called phantom pain.

Pain can be experienced as an acute episode, which, when the cause has been dealt with will cease to be experienced. It can be chronic, and while this may be more 'bearable' than an acute attack; a constant nagging pain lessens the quality of living. It is difficult to feel cheerful, hopeful and optimistic while experiencing pain continuously.

After reading the relevant articles from the assignment, students will not be in doubt about pain's complexities and will realise that there are still many 'missing parts' which require to be identified before we can completely understand the phenomenon.

PAIN AND THE PROCESS OF NURSING

Even in the past 5 years nurses have developed more and different tools which can be used in the assessing and evaluating phases of the process of nursing. Of course pain is a subjective experience; it is what the patient says it is, and nurses need to practise empathy and to refrain from being judgemental in interacting with patients who are experiencing pain. There is ample evidence in the research reports in the reading assignment that nurses rate pain at a lower level than the patient who is experiencing it. When the same tool is used in the assessing and evaluating phases, information about the effectiveness of a pain relief programme for a particular patient will be available.

Assessing the experience of pain

When a patient states that he is experiencing pain the following proforma can be used to inspect the area:

- is it swollen? If so, is the swelling symmetrical?
- is the swelling smooth and diffuse? nodular? fluctuant?
- is it mobile, i.e. do the skin and underlying tissues move easily over it?
- is it immobile, i.e. appears to be adherent to the skin and underlying tissues?
- does it pit on pressure — evidence of oedema?
- is there tenderness? With tension headaches there is often tenderness of scalp, neck and shoulder muscles.
- is there any change in colour? Redness, pallor, cyanosis, bruising?
- is there any change in local temperature? Increased? Decreased?
- is pus visible?

A general inspection is then called for:

Position adopted? Knees drawn up is suggestive of abdominal pain. Severe and extensive pain makes the patient rigid and afraid to move. With pleurisy the patient lies on the affected side while complaining of a stabbing pain on breathing in. The patient with pain in the hip everts the leg and flexes the knee in an attempt to get relief. The photophobic patient turns away from the light.

General expression? Face pinched, anxious, drawn; often pale with fright, especially if pain has come on suddenly. Pupils dilated. Cold or hot sweat. Teeth and fists clenched. Grunting. Writhing in pain.

The nurse then needs to question the patient to elicit facts about the type and duration of pain, not forgetting — has the patient had it before? If so, what made it better? Does any position or movement make it better or worse? Questions should discover if there are any other accompanying symptoms, for example feeling hot and sweating, cold and shivering, headache, nausea, vomiting, diarrhoea, constipation, retention of urine, frequency of passing urine, or pain on passing urine.

The temperature, pulse and respiration are taken at the onset of an attack of pain. If the pain is due to acute inflammation, these recordings are usually above the patient's normal and this is reported to sister or doctor immediately.

Relevant information from using this proforma will be recorded on the assessment form if the pain is being experienced on admission. Pain in itself is a problem for the patient; it will undoubtedly interfere with sleep which is another problem; if pain is being experienced in the spine and/or hips it may interfere with the patient assuming a comfortable posture for sleeping, which is yet another problem. And, of course, pain may present the patient with problems in several other everyday living activities. The problems which are identified *with* the patient, will be written on the nursng plan, together with the agreed patient and nursing activities to alleviate/solve them.

Should pain occur during the patient's stay in the health service (hospital or home) the information from using the 'pain assessment proforma' (p. 51) will be recorded on the patient's nursing notes and any problems agreed by patient and nurse, together with any patient/ nursing interventions to alleviate/solve them, will be written on the nursing plan.

There is increasing interest in developing, testing and using proforma (tools) for assessing pain. Mayer (1985) mentions a modified McGill-Melzack Pain Questionnaire which includes an assessment tool and a flow sheet. There is also a daily diary which the patient could maintain for ongoing assessment and evaluation.

The article by Copp (1984) contains an illustration of a pain assessment tool with the following instructions:

> The following are factors and questions to consider in pain assessment. Parts one and two are visible observations of a patient experiencing pain. The remainder of the tool consists of questions to ask the patient, or for you to consider. If followed in the order presented, this tool can be used as a systematic approach to pain assessment.

There is also interest in trying to 'measure' pain. Hayward (1975) developed a pain thermometer (painometer) with a longitudinal scale, at one end of which was 0 for 'no pain', and at the other, 10 for 'the pain is as bad as it could possibly be'. The patient points to the number which equates with the current experience of pain and it can be recorded on a graph with the time. This gives a visual record of the patient's pain pattern and it can be compared with the times of pain interventions.

Copp (1984) gives an illustration of a 'pain ruler' on similar lines, with the measurement also ranging from 0 to 10. When used at the initial assessment the data provide a baseline against which further 'measurements' can be evaluated. Since pain is a subjective experience, the level applies only to that patient, but is useful to 'measure' the lows and highs relative to implementation of different interventions.

Planning to achieve pain relief

A very careful plan needs to be worked out for the patient who is in continuous pain and for whom science has not yet found a cure. Holmes (1987) discusses how people with intractable pain can live at home and visit a special Pain Clinic at intervals.

The broad objective in planning is to achieve analgesia without sleepiness during the day so that the patient can take what nourishment he desires, have necessary nursing attention to keep him fresh, and free from sores, and able to converse with staff and visitors. Planning will also take into account the resources available such as acupuncture, hypnosis and so on.

Interventions to achieve pain relief

This is the area which has expanded most in the last decade. No longer is it thought that the first line of defence is administration of a drug by whichever route, though this is still an important intervention for pain relief. After reading relevant articles from the assignment, reading the text of this chapter so far, and consulting one or maybe more dictionaries, the student should be acquainted with the following interventions arranged alphabetically:

- acupuncture
- biofeedback
- cold application
- counterirritants
- distraction
- heat application
- hypnosis
- ice packs
- imagery/imaging
- massage
- meditation
- progressive muscular relaxation
- relaxation
- transcutaneous nerve stimulation
- yoga
- zen.

There is no doubt that in the near future, either initial or further research will be carried out regarding these pain relieving interventions and they will be reported in the nursing journals.

Evaluating pain relief

From what has been written so far, and remembering that pain is a subjective experience, that is, no one person's pain experience can be compared with another's, the painometer would seem to offer the best evaluation of the pain relief experienced by an individual patient, but it has to be remembered that baseline assessment data must be available against which evaluation of pain relief interventions can take place. There is immediate evaluation as the current score is compared to the previous one.

Since pain can interfere with so many everyday living activities, evaluating how the patient is managing these activities against the information on the assessment form will be an indirect evaluation of pain relief. Examples are:

Type of pain	Everyday living activity
arthritic	mobilising expressing sexuality sleeping working carrying out hobbies
cystitic	eliminating urine
dysphagic	eating and drinking
haemorrhoidal	eliminating faeces
pleuritic pneumonic	breathing

This is not an exhaustive list; it is meant to alert nurses to the relatedness of the knowledge in the various chapters of this book and therefore ipso facto to the complexity of nursing.

In this chapter, pain as a subjective experience has been discussed. The student of nursing, by reading relevant articles from the Reading Assignment, will be aware of the various theories attempting to explain pain. The principle — helping patients to cope with pain — has been discussed in a process of nursing context.

Pain relief is an important factor in promoting rest and sleep, which subject will be considered in the next chapter.

APPLYING THE PRINCIPLE

A registered nurse must be capable of:

- identifying patients who are experiencing pain
- carrying out a pain relief plan to the patient's satisfaction
- acting as a role model to students who are learning to help patients to cope with pain
- assessing a student nurse's contribution to a pain relief plan
- teaching student nurses about pain and an individualised pain relief plan.
- applying the principle — helping patients to cope with pain — in a process of nursing context.

WORKING ASSIGNMENT

Topics for discussion

- pain
- quality of living
- painometers
- empathy
- pain relief process
- pain relief clinics.

Writing assignment

Define the following:

acupuncture
endogenous
local pain
referred pain
phantom pain
acute pain
chronic pain
relaxation
distraction
visualisation
syndrome
proforma for assessing pain
interventions to achieve pain relief

which everyday living activity is affected by:

arthritic
cystitic
dysphagic
haemorrhoidal
pleuritic
pneumonic
} pain?

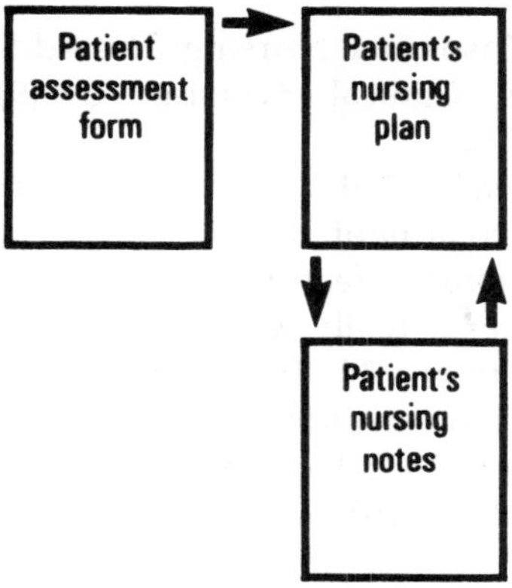

Reading assignment

Background information
- *Consciousness*
  - *Exercising*
  - *Relaxing*
- *Sleeping*

Sleeping and the process of nursing
- *Assessing*
  - *Sleep problems*
- *Planning*
  - *Generalised planning*
- *Implementing*
- *Evaluating*

Unconsciousness and the process of nursing
- *Coma*
- *Convulsions (fits)*
- *Induced unconsciousness*

Altered states of consciousness and the process of nursing
- *Confusion*
- *Dementia*
- *Induced altered states of consciousness*
  - *Alcohol abuse*
  - *Drugs abuse*

Applying the principle
- *A registered nurse must be capable of:*

Working assignment
- *Topics for discussion*
- *Writing assignment*

5

Helping patients to rest and sleep

READING ASSIGNMENT

Allan D 1986 Raised intracranial pressure. The Professional Nurse 2 (3) December: 78–80
Raised intracranial pressure in neurologically impaired patients is life threatening. Vigilant nursing can help to reduce brain damage and death.

Allan D 1986 Nursing the unconscious patient. The Professional Nurse 2 (1) October: 15–17
The quality of recovery and rehabilitation is almost entirely dependent on nursing skills.

Allan D 1984 Glasgow coma scale. Nursing Mirror 158 (23) June 13: 32, 34
A well-tested method of assessing levels of consciousness.

Allan D 1984 Glasgow coma scale. Nursing: The Add-On Journal of Clinical Nursing 2 (23) March: 668–669

Anon 1984 The day the strangers came. Nursing Times 80 (26) June 27: 51–54
Written by a senior nurse who had an alcoholic crisis.

Bahr R T, Gress L 1985 The 24-hour cycle: rhythms of healthy sleep. Journal of Gerontological Nursing 11 (4) April: 14–17
Developing nursing strategies.

Barker C 1984 Severe head injury. Nursing Mirror 158 (14) April 4: S8–S14 (NICG Journal 4)
Glasgow coma scale. Nursing care plan. Criteria of brain death.

Booth K 1985 Babies' sleeping patterns. Health

Visitor 58 (1) January: 17–18
A study of parental opinions and low sleeping infants.

Booth P, Dale B 1984 Managing a drink problem. Nursing Times 80 (25) June 20: 49–51
Few health authorities have policies for dealing with employees who have a drink or drugs problem.

Bouton J 1986 Falling asleep. Nursing Times 82 (50) December 10: 36– 37 Specific reference to how children's nurses should respond to the child who wakes in the night.

Brown R 1986 Disorders of sleep. Nursing: The Add-On Journal of Clinical Nursing 3 (9) September: 333–334
Respiratory disorders during sleep; sleep apnoea syndrome; the parasomnias; restless legs syndrome; sleep walking; nightmares and night terrors; bed wetting.

Browne K 1984 Confusion in the elderly. Nursing: The Add-On Journal of Clinical Nursing 2 (24) April: 698, 700–702, 704–705
Also describes the dementing person (organic brain syndrome).

Canavan T 1986 The functions of sleep. Nursing: The Add-On Journal of Clinical Nursing 2 (23) March: 682–683

Carter D 1985 In need of a good night's sleep. Nursing Times 81 (46) November 13: 24–26
Reviews the small literature on sleep in hospitals and concludes that nurses should implement appropriate nursing measures to assist sleepless patients.

Edgil A E and others 1985 Sleep problems of older infants and pre-school children. Paediatric Nursing 11 (2) March/April: 87–89

Findley L 1984 Altered consciousness. Nursing: The Add-On Journal of Clinical Nursing 2 (23) March: 663-664, 666
Delirium; stupor, coma; concussion; hypnosis.

Hayter J 1983 Sleep behaviour of older persons. Nursing Research 32 (4) July/August: 242–246

Hayward J 1975 Information — a prescription against pain. Royal College of Nursing London

Hearne K 1986 Dream sense. Nursing Times 82 (1) January 1: 28–31
Describes dream theories over the ages and what recent research reveals.

Jahanshahi M 1986 Insomnia. Nursing: The Add-On Journal of Clinical Nursing 3 (9) September: 328-332
What is insomnia? What causes insomnia? Assessment and treatment.

Johnson J 1985 Drug treatment for sleep disturbances: Does it really work? Journal of Gerontological Nursing 11 (8) August: 8-12
Report of research on an elderly population.

Kennedy J, Rogers C 1985 How much do you drink? Nursing Mirror 161 (18) October 30: 35–37
The nursing profession needs to look to its own education as well as that of the general public.

Lareau S C, Bonnet M H 1985 Sleep disorders: insomnias. Nurse Practitioner 10 (8) August: 16–17, 20–24

Macmillan P 1980 A noisy noise annoys. Nursing Times 76 (27) July 3: 1163
Trundling trolleys, clatter, voices, shoes.

McNeil B J and others 1986 'I didn't sleep a wink'. American Journal of Nursing 86 (1) January: 226–227
A study of patients' sleep patterns.

Muncy J H 1986 Measures to rid sleeplessness. Journal of Gerontological Nursing 12 (8) August: 6–11

Murphy F, Bentley S,Dudley H A F 1977 Sleep deprivation in patients undergoing operation: a factor in the stress of surgery. British Medical Journal 2: 1521–1522

Ogilvie A J 1980 Sources and levels of noise on the ward at night. Nursing Times 76 (31) July 31: 1363–1366
A list of noise sources in two wards; noise induces sleep deprivation which could lead to unnecessary anxiety and stress, prolonged wound healing and extended hospital stay; noise is made by staff — loud talking, heavy footsteps and noisy procedures.

Oswald I 1974 Sleep. Penguin, Harmondsworth

Oswald I, Adam K 1983 Get a better night's sleep. Martin Dunitz, London

Parker V 1984 Amnesia — towards a cure. Nursing: The Add-On Journal of Clinical Nursing 2 (24) April: 695–696
Short- and long-term memory. Memory drugs. Memory jogging

Roberts M 1986 A book at bedtime. Community Outlook June: 23–24
A sleep clinic to help families establish a bedtime routine and firm rules for night-time behaviour.

Roper N, Logan W, Tierney A 1985 The elements of nursing, 2nd edn. Churchill Livingstone, Edinburgh, p 177 (alcohol), p 185 (illicit drug-taking)

Shuldham C 1984 Communication — a conscious effort. Nursing: The Add-On Journal of Clinical Nursing 2 (23) March: 673–675
Communication with the unconscious patient.

Smith S 1985 Drugs and sleep. Nursing Times 81 (6) February 6: 36–37
Describes the action of benzodiazepines and barbiturates; should be used as last resort.

Stead W 1985 One awake, all awake! Nursing Mirror 160 (16) April 17: 20–21
A research project suggests ways in which night nursing can procure less disturbed sleep for patients.

Sugden J, Saxby P 1985 The confused elderly patient. Nursing: The Add-On Journal of Clinical Nursing 2 (35) March: 1022–1025
The assessment of confusion. The management of nursing care. Protocol for assessment.

Thornton P, Walsh J, Webster J, Harries C 1984 The sleep clinic. Nursing Times 80 (11) March 14: 40–43
A behavioural approach was used to solve children's sleeping problems.

Turpin G 1986 Psychophysiology of sleep. Nursing: The Add-On Journal of Clinical Nursing 3 (9) September: 313, 315–317, 319–320

Tyerman A 1984 The problem of personal identity in neurological rehabilitation. Nursing: The Add-On Journal of Clinical Nursing 2 (23) March: 679–681
Personality change; self-concept change; reconstructing personal identity.

Wardle J 1986 The chronology of sleep. Nursing: The Add-On Journal of Clinical Nursing 3 (9) September: 325–326
Sleep in infancy; sleep in childhood; sleep patterns in adult life.

Watts C A M 1977 Sleep and sleeplessness. Nursing Mirror 145 (12) September 22: 16–17
Description of sleep; jet lag, effect of sleeping tablets.

Webster R, Thompson D 1986 Sleep in hospital. Journal of Advanced Nursing 11: 447–457
Reviews sleep and its relationship to nursing practice.

Wilcock A, Chun Wan O 1984 Total patient care. Nursing: The Add-On Journal of Clinical Nursing 2 (23) March: 675–678
A perceptive study of a patient who had had a stroke, and was unconscious.

BACKGROUND INFORMATION

Everyone would wish to sleep soundly and to awaken feeling refreshed. Many lay people have a vague sort of notion, if not a belief, that when people are feeling poorly, sleep will help to make them better, so that those who are sick are not wakened but allowed to waken naturally. However registered nurses have to be capable of distinguishing sleep from unconsciousness, each a very complex concept. Many conditions can interfere with sleep, and unconsciousness can have many causes. 'Altered states of consciousness', a term fairly recently introduced into the nursing vocabulary, can result from particular pathology, or from abuse of substances such as alcohol and hard drugs. These then are the concepts which will be discussed in this chapter.

Some of the articles in the Reading Assignment will only be needed as you encounter patients with the different conditions. The annotations should help you to locate the information you need when you currently require it. Before discussing sleeping it is pertinent to consider, albeit briefly, the concept of 'consciousness', not least because we are all aware that we are 'conscious' for two-thirds of each day.

Consciousness

The concept of consciousness has been a subject of the mystics and philospophers throughout the ages. People in the world of the arts strive to help others to increase their conscious awareness of the chosen subject, be it a painting, a piece of music, or a piece of sculpture. But increasingly in the last few decades it has become a subject for investigation by scientists in various disciplines. The concept is very complex; it implies that a person is consciously perceiving the environment via the five senses and responding to the perceptions. There are varying levels of perceptual awareness and people who have developed a high level are said to be 'sensitive' to their environment and respond to it in a mature and appropriate way. In the two thirds 'conscious' period of each day, healthy people are carrying out activities which are either exercising mainly the mind or the body, or they are relaxing.

Exercising

With today's emphasis on healthy living, people are being encouraged to exercise in whatever form appeals to them — jogging, swimming and walking are easily available to most. As well as promoting a sense of well-being, exercise tones up the muscles and stimulates all the other body systems, relaxes the mind, and the ensuing 'healthy tiredness' is conducive to sleep.

Relaxing

Over the last few decades interest in relaxation has grown apace. Increasing public awareness of the possible ill-effects of such things as tranquillisers and sleeping pills has caused those people who are aware of tenseness as a reaction to the rapid pace of, and problems in, their everyday living activities, to turn to one or more of the relaxations available. These range from the various well-tried yoga 'philosophies' which, as well as teaching sequential postures, include methods of achieving a relaxed way of living. Other relaxation regimes achieve their objective by teaching people to tense voluntarily a group of muscles and at the height of tension to relax immediately or 'let go' so that they will recognise the different feeling associated with tenseness and relaxation. Some people achieve relaxation by becoming involved with appreciating a picture, a piece of music, a play, a film, a poetry reading or whatever.

Current interest in relaxation is not only related to rest and sleep but also to the relief of pain (p. 53) and to the lowering of stress levels: the level can be visually displayed on a biofeedback machine and the person, under guidance, can learn to relax and lower the reaction to stress. This has been of benefit in treating not only insomnia, but also hypertension and irritable bowel syndrome.

Interest is also growing in such complementary activities as aromatherapy, massage, reflexology, and the application of a cloth wrung out of hot, then cold water, as a means of relieving tenseness in a particular part of the body to relax it. Some nurses are using such remedies and the teaching of patients about relaxation as 'nurse-initiated activities'. It is evident that readers will learn more about this developing area of knowledge by reading the nursing journals.

Sleeping

Even when all family members are living under the same roof, the relaxing, resting and sleeping habits of each individual may well vary. Familiarity with the environment is an important factor especially when considering sleeping habits. This is evidenced by the fact that few people sleep well the first night in a strange environment, even though the change may have been anticipated with pleasure, for example holidays, or visiting friends.

One experiences a feeling of strangeness about the room itself, the position of the bed in the room especially in relation to the door and window, the bed itself — its height, resilience of mattress, number and type of pillows and weight of bedclothes. Some people like the lightest possible covering compatible with the desired warmth and use a continental quilt to achieve this. Others like to feel the weight of bedclothes even in warm weather. Some people like the upper bedclothes tucked under the mattress, others abhor the 'straight jacket' that this produces and prefer 'untucked' upper bedclothes so that they can tuck them around their own person.

Unfamiliar noise disturbs more than familiar noise, for example a city dweller may sleep through the gear-changing of heavy traffic and yet be awakened by the birds' dawn chorus when visiting the country. Some people find familiar sounds soothing, for example the ticking of a clock.

Some people like a warm bedroom, others prefer a cool one and would not dream of having it included in a central heating plan.

Some people sleep with the blinds down or the curtains drawn, others raise the blind and/or withdraw the curtains before getting into bed. Some close the bedroom window to sleep and only open it a fraction on the warmest night; others keep their window open even on the coldest night.

Many claim to be bad sleepers and haunt their doctors who resort to prescribing sleeping tablets.

Many husbands and wives sleep in double beds; others prefer twin beds. It is apparent from census statistics that many young people must be sharing a bedroom with a sibling since two- and three-bedroomed houses outnumber any others in Britain.

Many people have a bedtime snack, including an alcoholic nightcap as there is a belief that this helps to promote sleep.

Most people visit the lavatory and perform some sort of toilet just before going to bed. Many people turn on their electric blanket before going to bed, or take a hot water bottle to bed with them.

Given the complexity surrounding the approximately one-third period of each day spent sleeping, it is important for nurses to realise that each person is socialised into a pre-sleep routine which is necessary for comfort and relaxation, both prerequisites for sleep.

The last three decades have increased our knowledge about it; this has been achieved from research work carried out in various sleep laboratories. Human beings 'learn' a 24-hour pattern of sleep/wakefulness and this is referred to as a 'circadian rhythm'. The mechanism responsible for the repetition of this 24-hour rhythm is termed the 'biological clock'.

Sleep is a recurrent state of inertia and unresponsiveness during which the sleeper does not appear to react to external stimuli. Although consciousness is lost temporarily, a sufficient new stimulus such as the telephone ringing will arouse the sleeper (Oswald 1974). In this respect sleep differs from the altered consciousness of anaesthesia and coma, to be discussed later in the chapter.

Two dimensions of sleep are recognised, each having different functions. Orthodox sleep is the phase during which the growth hormones are secreted. It is readily apparent that this is an essential phenomenon to permit growth from infant to adult; but it continues to be essential since adults shed many thousands of cells from the skin and mucous membranes daily and they have to be replaced; worn out elements in all the other body cells have to be constantly replaced. It therefore becomes obvious that orthodox sleep is essential for any person who is recovering from an operation or any form of trauma or illness. Some people prefer to call orthodox sleep 'obligatory' sleep. Rapid eye movement, REM sleep, on the other hand, is thought to be connected with the brain's function as a 'computer' — sorting out the day's events. The items that need to be retained in the memory are kept available in a 'current account'; less vital matters are assigned to the 'deposit account' and the mental garbage is discarded completely (Watts 1977). REM sleep is often referred to as dream sleep.

These two dimensions, obligatory (nonREM) and REM sleep occur consecutively and make up a sleep cycle, of which there are four to six in any one sleep period, usually the night. In one cycle, once the threshold of sleep has given way to true obligatory sleep, this lasts about 90 minutes and is followed by approximately 20 minutes of REM sleep. Laboratory work shows that if volunteers are awakened each time they are in REM sleep, the end result is far more upsetting than loss of obligatory sleep; the victim feels mentally exhausted, tense, irritable and unable to concentrate. Beginning nurses may not appreciate that this knowledge about sleep can be used in clinical practice: it will be discussed later.

SLEEPING AND THE PROCESS OF NURSING

As more and more research is being carried out about patients' sleeping in hospital, it is becoming clear that nurses do need to consider using the four phases of the process of nursing to amass an adequate data bank which could be used retrospectively with a variety of objectives.

Assessing

From the previously mentioned varied backgrounds patients come to hospital. It is therefore imperative that nurses bear these factors in mind while collecting information from a newly admitted patient about individual sleeping habits and routines.

Several items in the Reading Assignment discuss nurses' inadequate information about the patient's sleeping habits. Webster & Thompson (1986) after giving a comprehensive review of the nursing literature on the subject of sleep in hospital, discuss the measurement of sleep and state:

> However polygraphic recordings are much more expensive, time-consuming and, in large scale studies, impractical to perform. Alternatively, subjective reports are constrained by bias and rely heavily on the subject's memory. However, it has been shown by various sleep researchers that subjective reports do correlate significantly with objective assessments. (References given)

They end their article:

> Unfortunately, many nurses are not skilled at assessing patients' sleeping habits and there is possibly a need for the development and utilisation of instruments designed to evaluate sleep on a day-to-day basis in the ward.

Nurses need to be aware of the potential problem of sleep disturbance in hospital and use their knowledge and experience to keep it as just that — a potential problem which manifests itself as a real problem as infrequently as possible.

Consequently to help beginning nurses to realise what factual information is required on which to individualise the nursing plan some suggestions will be given. When written, they look formidable and nurses may ignore them on this score. But the first time is the worst! Most nurses' experience is that as they become more proficient it takes less time. Not all questions need to be asked of every patient; most people like talking about themselves and much of the information may be given in answer to just one question! Careful prompting will then fill in any gaps which the nurse carrying out the initial assessment considers will be useful, according to such things as expected length of stay, in order to individualise the nursing plan. The initial assessment data will not need to be written again and it should be available to nurses on the different shifts. Any further information from ongoing assessment will be written on the patient's nursing notes which will be available to all nurses. Now to those suggestions about possible topics for factual information:

- pre-sleep routine including any medication
- usual time of going to bed
- usual time of going to sleep
- single or double bed
- type of bedclothes
- number of pillows
- type of pillows (allergy)
- any wakening during the night
- reason for wakening
- number of wakenings
- length of awake period
- if anxiety-producing, what helps to get off to sleep again
- usual time of morning wakening
- refreshed/tired on waking
- patient's classification of himself as:
  good } sleeper
  moderate } sleeper
  poor } sleeper
- daytime naps
  — number
  — usual time of
  — usual length of
  — where — chair, bed.

The purpose of collecting assessment data is firstly to help those patients who do not have a sleeping problem to continue their individualised sleeping habits; and secondly to help in identification of any sleeping problems which the patient is experiencing. These will now be discussed.

Sleep problems

Knowledge about sleep problems is growing all the time clinical psychologists investigate them. The classification system which they use includes 'Insomnia' which then proceeds to use the words 'primary', 'secondary' and 'subtypes' (Jahanshahi 1986). In this text, however, the subject will be discussed at an introductory level using the broad headings — sleeplessness, restlessness, drug dependence and sleep deficit. Included in the Reading Assignment are items which give more detail about sleep problems and as readers encounter patients suffering from them, they can refer to the particular articles.

Sleeplessness Some people experience a lag between the time of going to bed and falling asleep. The sleep researchers report a range of 30 to 90 minutes, with a preponderance of 30 minutes (Jahanshahi 1986). The suggested assessing proforma (p. 60) would give base information against which any change can be evaluated. If the patient usually takes a long time to fall asleep, as long as he remains unconcerned about it, and the nurse does not suspect very high levels of anxiety and/or discomfort, nursing intervention is not required, but it would be reasonable to let him wake naturally and not conform to the wakening at 06.00 hours which is still common in many wards.

Some people have one or more wakeful periods in a night's sleep. This is likely to continue while in hospital; should it become worse, the nurse can offer to help and she will be guided by what the patient thinks would be helpful in getting off to sleep again. If the increased wakefulness is due to worry, a hot drink and a chance to talk about the worry will probably be an acceptable nursing intervention, which will be reported on the patient's nursing notes.

Early morning wakening can be a problem and if reported on admission it will be recorded on the assessment form, to alert the night nurse to observe for it. It is characteristic of the elderly and it may not be anxiety-producing. Any nursing contribution will depend on the ward's geography. A patient in a single room can continue to cope by doing what he does at home, perhaps reading until the ward's wakening time. Continued early wakening should alert the nurse to observe any withdrawn behaviour, pre-occupation or depressed mood, then she should explore these with the patient. The clinical condition of depression is eminently treatable and the nurse could encourage the patient to report the symptoms to the doctor, or gain permission to be an intermediary.

It must be obvious to the reader that assessing a patient's sleeping is not confined to the night period because behaviour resulting from sleep disturbance can be manifested during the next day. The need for concise factual documentation is self-evident.

Restlessness Restlessness is a complex but as yet little understood concept. Most of us can identify it and have experienced periods of restlessness. However, when it occurs related to the sleep period, it is usually perceived as a problem. When it occurs in bed, the person is aware of all the muscles being in a tense, tingling state and letting go to achieve a lessening of tension is almost impossible. If it occurs in the pre-sleep period, sleep is impossible. Another form is an inability to stay still and is characteristic of hyperactivity (hyperkinesis). When it occurs in bed we talk about 'tossing and turning'. The term 'restless legs syndrome' has been coined and used in the last few decades. It is described as a sensation of discomfort in the legs and an irresistible urge to move them. It causes such concentration on the phenomenon that sleep onset may be severely affected. This suggests that distraction therapy like concentrating on favourite music could be successful.

Drug dependence If a nurse, at the initial assessment of sleeping (p. 60), discovers that the patient is in the habit of taking a tranquilliser or a sedative type of medication, further information should be elicited about the time of day at which it is taken, how regularly it is taken, for how long it has been taken, the kind of sleep produced, the state on wakening, and any side-effects experienced. The groups of drugs in question are those most frequently prescribed by GPs. Nurses should be aware that extensive research in this area led Oswald (1974) to write:

> To stop requires a willingness to put up with broken sleep and nightmares for a couple of weeks and then further weeks before sleep is fully normal.

More recent research (Oswald & Adam 1983) discovered that after taking sleeping pills for several nights, when they were discontinued the person slept badly, and return to a natural sleeping pattern took 6 to 8 weeks. This is important information for nurses counselling patients about discharge which occurs in the majority of instances before 6 weeks.

Sleep deficit There is evidence that many patients who enter hospital for surgery accumulate a considerable sleep deficit (Murphy et al 1977). Equipment and voices of staff were the main causes of noise disturbing sleep, and the researchers wrote:

> We recommend that from time to time sound engineers should use the simple methods that we have used ... to show the staff how much they pollute the environment. Furthermore, the staff should be educated against noise pollution as part of good hospital procedure.

Nurses can help patients to sleep by minimising noise when on duty. They can wear shoes which do not cause excessive noise when walking; they can close doors quietly and prevent them from banging; they can handle equipment quietly and most of all they can modulate their voices and refrain from talking in the vicinity of patients. Should the noise be of external origin as from traffic, Swedish wax earplugs may be useful to those patients who can wear them.

Carter (1985) examines the comprehensive evidence on the sleep of hospital patients and states that

> research findings indicate that many hospital patients do experience difficulty in obtaining what they themselves consider to be adequate sleep, and a number of factors thought to contribute towards patients' sleep problems have been identified. Some might argue that asking patients about their sleep is too subjective, but as Johns[24] points out, an individual's report of his sleep is a fundamental reflection of his personal experience.

Helping patients to cope with pain was described in the previous chapter but here it is relevant to consider criteria for evaluating particular pain-relieving interventions related to sleep; they include such observations as:

- time of onset of sleep
- character of sleep
- duration of sleep
- mood on wakening
- refreshed/unrefreshed on wakening
- general appearance } next day
- general behaviour } next day
- mood } next day
- appetite } next day
- fatigue } next day

Again, baseline data must be available against which these criteria can be evaluated. It cannot be stressed too strongly that evaluation can only be as good as the sleep assessment prior to the pain-relieving intervention.

Planning

Where no actual or potential problem exists, sleeping does not appear on the patient's nursing plan; if adequate information has been recorded on the initial assessment form, the nurses can plan to 'individualise' the nursing by using it. Relevant details such as whether the patient had a nap or naps during the day — when, in chair or bed, how long; and a factual account of the night's sleep will, if relevant, be recorded in the patient's nursing notes. Should a problem arise then it will be written on the nursing plan together with the planned nursing intervention to deal with it. The carrying out of this intervention will be recorded on the patient's nursing notes. When the problem is solved this will be recorded on the nursing plan and the nursing intervention cancelled.

If drugs have to be resorted to, they are prescribed by the doctor and written on the medication Kardex which requires the date, name of the drug, dose, route and intended time of giving which would probably be 'when necessary' (PRN). There is usually space for recording the time of giving and signature of the giver. This information need not necessarily be duplicated on the nursing plan, as long as the medication Kardex is considered to be a nursing document as well as a medical one. However the ongoing assessment of the hours which the patient sleeps and the report he gives about the sleep, and his behaviour throughout the next day must be written on the patient's nursing notes. This is a medically prescribed nursing activity, but the nurse should know how long it takes the medication to act, and arrange for the patient to be settled for the night in time to give him maximum sleep and to prevent him having a 'hangover' in the morning. Should such a patient want to pass urine during the night, using a bedside commode or bedpan/urinal is safer than struggling to the lavatory in a dazed state.

There is no point in withholding sleeping tablets to see if sleep comes naturally, *unless this is the patient's wish*. It can result in the patient forcing himself to stay awake, afraid that he will not get his tablet. Should a patient who is 'written up' for a sleeping pill fall asleep naturally, the doctor does not expect the nurse to disturb the patient. Hospital policy varies as to who checks these drugs and each student must know and adhere to the policy in the hospital in which she is working.

The drugs used for the induction of restfulness and sleep are classed as sedatives, hypnotics and narcotics. The nurse must be familiar with any side-effects which they may produce so that she can recognise and report them. (It also has to be remembered that some drugs produce daytime sleepiness as a side-effect; antihistamines and tranquillisers come into this category.)

Generalised planning

Most patients are used to a divan type of bed. Except in the few hospitals that have adjustable height beds, we ask them to 'climb' into a bed to get out of which many patients may find equal difficulty. This can be anxiety producing if the patient is in the habit of visiting the lavatory during the night. For the frail elderly person, easily disorientated by strange surroundings, planning should make available an adjustable Hi-Lo bed; when set at 'Lo' for the night, frail patients are more likely to be able to get out without accident.

The 'strangeness' of the bed is increased by mattress protection in the form of a polythene cover or long 'mackintosh' and in some instances by a draw 'mackintosh' and sheet. These tend to make the patient hot and sweaty thus contributing to restlessness. Nurses should feel sufficiently confident in their assessing ability only to use 'mackintosh' protection and drawsheets when they are absolutely necessary.

There are bound to be unfamiliar sounds in a hospital ward. Only a few people are used to lifts banging and telephones ringing during the night. Some of the old central heating systems are anything but noiseless especially during the night, and a word of warning may prevent patients lying awake wondering what is causing the strange sound. Forward planning should ensure that management is aware of these sources of noise pollution in the wards so that they can be considered in any future upgrading programme. There are always a few patients who require medicines, injections, turning and other treatments during the night and nurses should plan to carry out these activities as quietly as possible.

Unconscious and very ill patients sometimes make peculiar noises which are frightening to the other patients. If the nurses plan so that one of them is always present in the ward it lessens such fear. Occasionally a patient becomes delirious or obstreperous during the night; a patient may become confused as a result of drugs. The presence of a nurse is essential to prevent accident, for example a patient falling out of bed. If staff and circumstances permit, it may be best to move the patient into a single room. Here daytime conditions can be simulated by turning on the light; this avoids shadows which increase confusion; the staff can speak clearly — whispering increases confusion. On the other hand, moving the patient may increase confusion; in this case it is better to re-orientate him in the ward, a short period of disturbance there being preferable to a longer period of disturbance in a side ward.

Sometimes a ward has to admit a patient during the night. An empty bed is usually left near the door for this purpose to cause the least disturbance to the rest of the patients. A patient can collapse during the night necessitating resuscitative measures, presence of medical and extra nursing staff. Sometimes a patient dies during the night and if this has been anticipated, the bed will have been placed where it will cause the least disturbance.

When these things happen during the day the increased sound and activity are absorbed into the general pattern of daytime sounds and activities. In the comparative silence of the night they become more sinister to patient and nurse alike. The nurse's initiative, ingenuity and resourcefulness convert what could have been a major upheaval in the ward into a minor one.

The daily rhythm is bound to be changed for each patient on admission to hospital. Early wakening of patients and lack of opportunity to rest during the day are complaints made from time to time in the professional and daily press. It is evident that many hospitals do not yet meet their patients' requirements in this respect. As nurses, not only should we be aware of our patients' requirements but we must be capable of playing our part in fulfilling them. Many people need to be consulted, for instance medical, domestic and catering staff, before a satisfactory hospital policy of later wakening of patients can be formulated. We must be willing to experiment with shedding the workload throughout the day so that we achieve a more rational waking and sleeping hour for patients.

The Department of Health and Social Security issued, in 1976, a report on *Organisation of the inpatient's day*, in which the following statements still have implications for nursing:

- the time at which patients are wakened should be reviewed periodically (para 38)
- an early morning drink should be readily available as part of the regular meal and drink service. There should be no compulsion for patients to be wakened for it if they prefer otherwise, unless there is a medical need (paras 39–41)
- the patient's condition should determine whether or not a protective mattress covering is necessary. Old-style rubber mackintoshes should not be used (para 45)
- every effort should be made to provide a quiet rest period for patients during the day (para 48).

Stead (1985) conducted a similar survey of 78 patients, ranging in age from 14 to 96 years, 43 were male, 34 female and one did not reply. The patients were nursed in all areas of the acute unit. 55 patients said that ward lights switched on at 06.00 h was 'about right'. They complained mainly about general noise, and noise caused by other patients who were ill and required frequent attention during the night.

Implementing

Most people have a favourite position in which they fall asleep. When circumstance fails to permit the assumption of this position there is usually interference with sleep at first. The dyspnoeic patient may like an adjustable height bed-table with a pillow, on which he can rest his arms. The patient in a plaster cast may find that he can sleep better with the foot or the head of his bed raised. The patient in a high bed with a leg on traction may feel more secure with pillows on which to rest his arms. The nurse must be prepared to experiment with these patients until together they find a solution to the patient sleeping in an unaccustomed posture and it should be recorded on the nursing plan.

Students of nursing in a 3-year programme may see little relevance of knowledge from sleep research to everyday practice, but nurses can help patients who require treatment during the night by avoiding the time at which they are likely to be in REM sleep. Contrary to expectation, Hayter (1983) advises that for those patients who require to nap during the day, the morning period is more beneficial than the afternoon. Students will undoubtedly meet patients who describe themselves as having a sleep problem. Her research also found that daytime napping does not lessen the night sleep period.

Ideas about nursing interventions for the different sleep problems are contained in the appropriate paragraphs describing them. Specific information about the carrying out of planned nursing activities to help the patient sleep will be recorded in his nursing notes and this may provide summative information when evaluating whether or not the nursing interventions have achieved what the patient perceives to be 'a good night's sleep'.

Evaluating

Evaluating, the fourth phase of the process can only be as good as the assessment data, so the patient assessment form will have to be consulted, together with the patient's nursing plan and nursing notes. The majority of patients will have a potential problem of not being able to sleep. It is a nursing responsibility to prevent it from becoming an actual one. When a patient has an actual sleep problem, a sleep diary or a sleep questionnaire may be used as an ongoing assessment and evaluative tool, and of course it will be used each 24 hours. The sleep of every patient should be estimated at the nurse's first morning encounter each day. 'Did you sleep well?' infers that the nurse expects that the patient has slept well. 'How did you sleep?' is preferable and leaves the patient some choice in formulating an answer. 'How was your night?' is even more open ended and enables the patient to paint the picture of what had enabled him to sleep well, perhaps 'nurse made me a drink of hot chocolate after which I slept soundly': or the picture may be of what had prevented sleep — perhaps 'my pyjamas were wet with sweat; nurse helped me change them, brought me an iced drink and I went off to sleep again.'

UNCONSCIOUSNESS AND THE PROCESS OF NURSING

Until fairly recently it was presumed that the unconscious person's sensory systems were not functioning. However, it is now realised that this is a simplistic notion of unconsciousness; it is a very complex concept. There is evidence that some unconscious people hear and are aware of what is going on around them but are unable to signal their awareness, though they can recount their experience on regaining consciousness. This has tremendous implications for nursing practice. Three forms of unconsciousness will be discussed — coma, convulsions and induced unconsciousness (general anaesthesia).

Coma

The terms 'unconscious patient' and 'comatose patient' can be used interchangeably. The commonest causes of coma are head injuries and strokes (cerebrovascular accident CVA). The difficulty of understanding what unconsciousness is contributes to inhibiting the nurse in implementing planned nursing interventions with their social dimensions, for the unconscious patient, in the same way that she would implement them for the conscious helpless patient. It is recommended that all nursing interventions should be carried out within the perceptual framework of assisting the patient in his state of unconsciousness to re-orientate himself to his surroundings. To make the 'surroundings' as familiar as possible the nurse needs to acquire from the relatives detailed information about the habits and routines of the patient's everyday living, his life-style and background, his social activities, his work and so on. These factors can then be built into conversation with the patient, one-sided though it will be in the early stages, helping him to re-orientate himself to his surroundings.

The level of functioning of the senses can be assessed and evaluated by using the Glasgow coma/responsiveness scale (Fig. 5.1). It has been tested for reliability and validity and can therefore be confidently recommended as a competent observation/management record (tool) when nursing comatose patients; the lower the score, the greater the 'unconsciousness'. As the score increases, so the patient will respond to the constantly repeated re-orientation implementation of addressing him by name, telling him the time, the day, the month; where he is and what has happened to him.

Readers can identify three articles in the Reading Assignment which give further information about using the Glasgow coma scale. Raised intracranial pressure can occur in patients with head injuries and when a student encounters such a patient in the ward, the relevant article can be consulted. Allan (1984), Shuldham (1984), Wilcock & Chun Wan (1984) all give useful and sensitive information about nursing the unconcious patient.

Convulsions (fits)

Convulsions are characterised by involuntary contraction of muscles resulting from abnormal

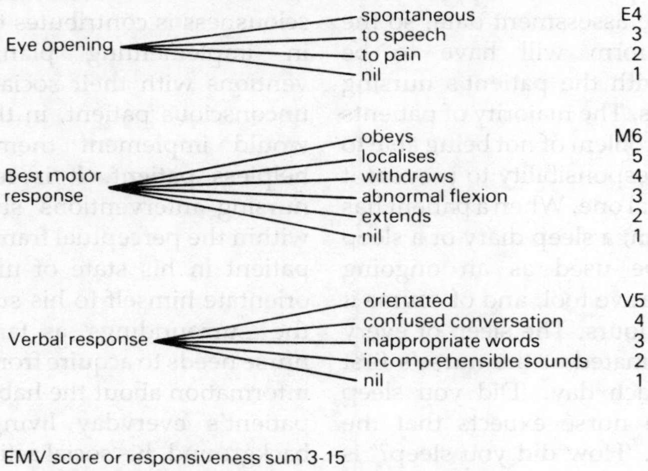

Fig. 5.1 The Glasgow coma/responsiveness scale

cerebral stimulation. There can be transient unconsciousness, and the safest position is to have the patient lying on one side with the face turned down so that there is no danger of the tongue obstructing the airway and any secretions will gravitate into the mouth thereby avoiding their inhalation (p. 211) A record must be made on the patient's nursing notes, of the time and duration of a convulsion, which muscles were affected and whether or not there was unconsciousness and incontinence, usually of urine, seldom of faeces. When convulsions occur in children they may herald an infection so the temperature, pulse and respiration should be taken and recorded on the appropriate chart.

Induced unconsciousness

Anaesthetics induce unconsciousness, a state referred to as anaesthesia. The anaesthetised person is rendered incapable of responding to his environment; since his eyes are closed it would seem impossible for there to be visual input, and there is very little available information about sensory input from touch, smell and taste. But some people have reported that during anaesthesia they were 'aware' of what was going on around them but were unable to signal their awareness. The implication for nursing is that in the vicinity of an anaesthetised patient all activities should focus on him *as a person*; the state of anaesthesia (induced unconsciousness) should not be the focus of nursing activities. On his return to consciousness it is important for the nurse to reorientate him by using his name and telling him the time, where he is and what has happened to him.

ALTERED STATES OF CONSCIOUSNESS AND THE PROCESS OF NURSING

Just as it is difficult to conceptualise consciousness because of its complexity, so it is equally difficult to conceptualise 'altered consciousness', a term fairly recently included in medical vocabulary. Two issues of the journal *Nursing* were devoted to the subject — Part 1, December 1979 and Part 2, January 1980.

There is not as yet an agreed classification of the conditions and diseases allocated to the term. Rationally, a patient in coma, having a convulsion, or an anaesthetised person is in an 'altered state of consciousness'. In this text, only confusion, dementia and induced altered states by alcohol and drugs will be considered. Either the title or the annotation in the Reading Assignment will guide readers to other conditions and diseases.

Confusion

A state of confusion may be episodic throughout daytime and the person may be completely rational in between the episodes. Biographical information on the Assessment Form will give each nurse background information about the patient's family, his social contacts and type of home; there should be a vignette about his everyday living activities including work, hobbies and personal interests which will help the nurse to 'individualise' conversation with him so that his memory is stimulated which usually reduces confusion. It is important to maintain this level of communication during the confused episodes, since one never knows when lucidity will again be evident.

Dementia

The adjective 'senile' is often used but it can occur in younger than expected people due to 'Alzheimer's disease'. There is gradual decline in mental ability, including loss of memory, progressing to inability to recognise time, place and even loved ones. The ability to carry out everyday living activities declines to the point where such people are totally dependent on others for implementing these activities in a humane and dignified manner.

Both confusion and dementia relate to resting and sleeping in that the patient may not remember, or be aware of pre-sleep routines; may not be able to identify 'his' bed; may not remember the habit of changing from day clothes to night attire and so on. Any night wakening may well be distressing to the patient; every attempt should be made in a gentle way to re-orient, so helping him to sleep again. Nurses should resist any temptation to treat these patients as an object of fun, or treat them as less than a human being. At all times they are entitled to be treated by people who have a compassionate and humane attitude to them.

Induced altered states of consciousness

Throughout the ages there has been interest in changing one's state of consciousness. Attempting to cope with inevitable 'low' periods is part of everyone's experience of living. Some people 'cope' by opting out, so they abuse such things as alcohol and drugs. Only a brief introduction to this vast subject will be given here and in the context of their relationship to resting and sleeping.

Alcohol abuse

Roper, Logan & Tierney (1985) outline the size of the increasing problem of alcoholism as studied by the World Health Organization. The WHO document indicated that in industrialised countries 30 to 50% of fatal road traffic accidents involve drivers with a high level of alcohol or other drug in the blood.

A student may well find survivors of road traffic accidents admitted to a ward after surgery. The patient will not be in a condition to discuss drinking habits at an initial assessment, indeed it may only be when a satisfactory nurse/patient relationship has been established that the nurse may pick up clues as to these. However, meantime, an abuser of alcohol is likely to develop symptoms of 'withdrawal' which will be apparent during ongoing assessment, and they are usually worse during the night. They include restlessness, agitation, hallucinations, delirium, disorientation, shaking and tremors, giving the full blown syndrome the name 'delirium tremens'. In such an instance the doctor will prescribe treatment (which will probably result in one or more delegated nursing interventions), and advise on follow up. The nurse should give full support to the patient in following the programme. In the absence of the full blown syndrome, the nurse may detect that the patient is interested in seeking help for his drinking problem. The nurse will learn about the local resources available so that she has positive information to offer such patients.

On the other hand, a student may only become acquainted with the notion of alcohol abusers by a visit to a special centre for treating people with this problem as part of the 3-year programme. Or she may do so during an allocation, for example to a medical ward or to the Accident and Emergency department. It is impossible to predict when and where this experience will be available to a student, so that during clinical allocations reference to appropriate literature is essential.

Drugs abuse

There is now a large literature on this condition which can run such a tragic course. It affects mainly the young age group to which the majority of students of nursing belong. Only a brief introduction is given here to alert readers to the fact that drug abusers can be admitted to hospital for reasons other than drug abusing. The physical evidence of solvent abusers is a lingering smell of the particular solvent on the clothes and hair, and redness, spots or even blisters around the nose and mouth. Should these be present at the initial assessment, the term 'solvent abuser' is not recorded on the form, but the facts which the nurse has observed. They should alert the night nurse to observe specially the patient's resting and sleeping patterns which might well be different from the information given by the patient at assessment. The night observations will be recorded on the patient's nursing notes. Information on the assessment form and the night nurse's recording will alert the day nurses to specially observe daytime behaviour which can be changed by solvent abuse, and record it on the patient's nursing notes. Should the data reveal a problem with resting and sleeping or daytime behaviour it will be confirmed with the patient and it, together with the nursing and possibly patient intervention to solve/alleviate the problem, will be written on the nursing plan. Carrying out the interventions will be recorded on the patient's nursing notes and when evaluation reveals that the goal has been achieved, this will be added, and the nursing intervention cancelled on the plan. The supposition was that this patient was admitted for a reason other than solvent abusing, so this example of using 'process' thinking and recording will end here.

Roper, Logan & Tierney (1985) give an introduction to the various drugs, some of which can be taken by other routes, but here an overall view will be given of the injected drug abusers. A long-sleeved pyjama jacket may conceal the injection sites and any surrounding redness or sepsis, so the arms may need to be observed for example when taking the blood pressure, but the facts will be recorded on the assessment form which will be available to the night nurses. 'Process' thinking and recording as instanced in the previous paragraph, will be put in motion.

This chapter has discussed, albeit at a primary level, a wide range of subjects which focus on the principle of nursing — helping patients to rest and sleep — and it was considered in a process of nursing context.

APPLYING THE PRINCIPLE

A registered nurse must be capable of:

- finding out about each patient's previous sleeping habits and explaining about things which have to go on in a ward during the night
- deciding which patients need waterproof mattress protection and removing it when no longer needed
- regulating the physical environment, including temperature of ward, ventilation, lighting and noise
- arranging the work so that the patients are wakened as late as possible and there is no evening crescendo which is not conducive to sleep
- observing quality and quantity of sleep and reporting these in factual terms. It is particularly important to report those patients who go to sleep, but awaken after 1, 2 or 3 hours. Early waking is characteristic of depression
- recognising the first signs of depression and boredom and taking steps to alleviate them

- creating a climate in which a patient feels free to tell the nurse about any factors which are interfering with sleep. The nurse must be capable of acting according to this information
- assisting patient into a suitable posture for rest and sleep
- teaching relaxation for the relief of tension
- talking with patients and encouraging staff to talk with patients without arousing the feeling that it is 'wasting time'
- assessing what effect lack of sleep is having on the patient, for example is he upset by it? Does he look tired and heavy-eyed? Does he nap during the day? Is it interfering with his appetite? Is he losing weight? Older patients often need less sleep. Little harm comes from lying restfully.
- deciding which drugs, treatment, and so on are essential during the night and giving precise instruction about these
- using foresight and leaving an empty bed and those patients needing most attention in an area which will create least disturbance to the other patients
- recognising when a patient is suffering pain. Being able to give physical relief. Offering heat or cold to the part as is appropriate. Following hospital procedure re household analgesics. Getting the doctor to prescribe other analgesics, administering and recording same, and noting effect on the patient's nursing notes. Knowing side-effects of drugs used
- administering sedatives, hypnotics and narcotics at the optimum time, recording same, noting effect and any side-effects on the patient's nursing notes
- making useful suggestions to a planning committee, so that disturbing environmental factors will be minimal in renovated or new buildings.
- applying the principle — helping patients to rest and sleep — in a process of nursing context.

WORKING ASSIGNMENT

Topics for discussion

- as a qualified nurse you visit a relative in a radiotherapy ward. In his locker you find a dozen tablets which you identify as Seconal. You ask where they came from and receive the reply, 'Oh! Nurse leaves one for me each night in case I can't sleep. I pop it in the locker in the morning.'
- you are on night duty. You see one patient standing by her neighbour's bed and hear her say, 'Take two of these, dearie, and you'll sleep a treat. My doctor gives me them.'
- a patient has had a hysterectomy and is written up for morphia to be given postoperatively and repeated when necessary. At 21.00 hours on the second postoperative day you find her wide awake and distressed by soreness and discomfort. Night sister's first round will be at 23.00 hours. What will you do?
- discuss the ethics related to obtaining information about a patient's drinking habits
- discuss the ethics related to obtaining information from patients about drug abusing
- patient in a single room: 'The biggest noise is voices in the corridor. Their tongues can wag. They're just like a lot of magpies.'
- consciousness
- unconsciousness
- altered states of consciousness
- preventing the potential problem — of patients not being able to sleep — from becoming an actual one.

Writing assignment

- Define the following:

  alcohol abuse
  analgesic
  antihistamine
  assessing pain relief
  assessment proforma for sleep pattern

biofeedback
biological clock
bruise
cerebrovascular accident
circadian rhythm
coma
confusion
convulsions
criteria for evaluating particular pain relieving interventions to produce sleep
cyanosis
delirium
delirium tremens
dementia
disorientation
drug dependence
drugs abuse
dyspnoea
evaluating pain relief
fluctuant
hallucinations
head injuries
hypnotic
Glasgow coma scale
induced unconsciousness
interventions for pain relief
meningitis
migraine
myalgia
narcotic
nausea
neuralgia
oedema
osteomyelitis
pain
painometer
pathology
planning for pain relief
photophobia
pleurisy
pre-sleep routine
pus
relaxation
reliability
restless legs syndrome
restlessness
sciatica
Seconal
sedative
side-effects
sleep deficit
sleeplessness
suffix — algia
suffix — itis
tonsillitis
tranquillisers
validity
vasoconstriction
vasodilatation

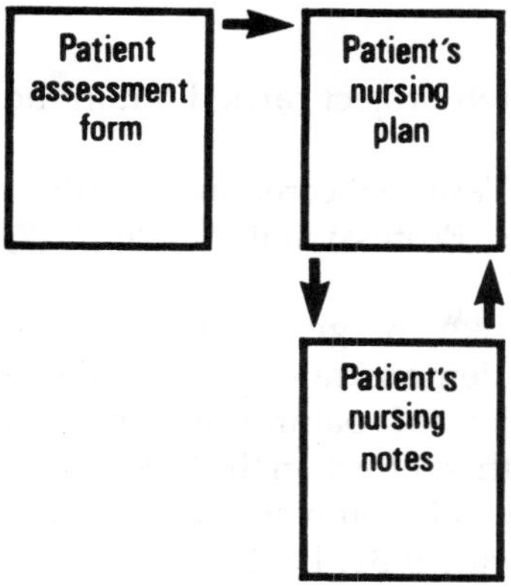

6

Helping dying patients

READING ASSIGNMENT

Adams J 1986 Time to bury the past. Nursing Times 82 (2) June 25: 46–47
Informs about current arrangements so that the poor are not denied the rite of a funeral.

Airrd R 1985 Comfort and pain relief. Nursing Mirror 161 (19) November 6: 36-37
A visit to a hospice to find out how best to help terminally ill patients make the most of their final days.

Allan D 1984 Brain death. Nursing: The Add-On Journal of Clinical Nursing 2 (23) March: 671–672
Discusses brain death and illustrates a form used to record brain death criteria.

Allsworth J 1985 Carer not caretaker. Nursing Mirror 161 (11) September 11: 19–21
Night nurse should be involved in devising and implementing 'care' plans; particularly important when nursing the terminally ill in general wards.

Ashdown M 1985 Sudden death. Nursing Mirror 161 (18) October 18: 22– 24
Sudden death has a traumatic effect on the victim's relatives. A nurse interviewed some bereaved people and found that their experiences in the A & E department are indelibly printed in their minds.

Barnard A 1985 Bereavement: A care study. Nursing: The Add-On Journal of Clinical Nursing 2 (43) November: 1286–1287

A sensitive account of helping a family when one of its members is terminally ill.

Bell I 1984 Bereavement in continuing care wards. Nursing Times 80 (37) September 12: 51–52
How do nurses help patients cope with the death of a fellow patient? Describes how the author tried to find out, and gives the reactions of both patients and staff.

Bennett P 1984 A care team for terminally ill children. Nursing Times 80 (10) March 7: 26–27
A nurse decided to care for her dying son at home but she experienced lack of communication between the carers. Figure 1 illustrates existing communication patterns and possible breakdown points, while Figure 2 suggests how communication should be achieved.

Blake A 1985 The loss of a baby. Nursing: The Add-On Journal of Clinical Nursing 2 (43) November: 1270–1274
Gives very practical advice that is required in such a tragic circumstance.

Blanchflower S 1984 Living with death. Nursing Times 80 (47) November 21: 34–37
Describes frustration in trying to nurse a patient who had not come to terms with imminent death, and regrets how poorly nurses are prepared for this role.

Bryan E 1984 When a twin dies. Nursing Times 80 (10) March 7: 24–27
Parents of a dead twin are mourning that child while celebrating the life of the other. Discusses some of the special problems parents face when a twin dies.

Calvert R 1984 Home from home. Nursing Times 80 (50) December 12: 44
Establishment of a hospice in Belfast and describes how domiciliary care is one of the most important parts of what the hospice service can offer the dying and bereaved.

Charnock A 1985 Sharing the sadness. Nursing Times 81 (40) October 2: 40–41
A dying child in an intensive care unit; how do nurses learn to become constructively involved?

Conboy-Hill S 1986 Psychosocial aspects of terminal care: a preliminary study of nurses' attitudes and behaviour in a general hospital. International Nursing Review 33 (1) January/February: 19–21
Report of a research project carried out in the UK.

Conboy-Hill S 1986 Terminal care: their death in your hands. The Professional Nurse 2 (2) November: 51–53
If nurses are to take charge of terminal care they will need to demonstrate special skills in the communication of painful information and in dealing with its effect on the individual.

Corr D 1984 The hospice movement. Nursing Mirror 159 (16) October 31: 19–22
Dying people need a caring environment and expert care from those who can help them maintain as near normal a life as possible.

Darbyshire P 1986 Licensed to kill? Nursing Times 82 (7) February 12: 22–25
In the case of patient killing, intentional or unintentional, the author argues for a more open system of communication.

Darbyshire P 1986 Angels of mercy? Nursing Times 82 (8) February 19: 49, 51–52
Withholding or withdrawing treatment from patients has serious legal, ethical and professional implications for the nurse; there is no legal defence for mercy killing and nurses need stronger guidelines.

Dicks B 1985 Care of the dying cancer patient. Nursing: The Add-On Journal of Clinical Nursing 2 (43) November: 1278–1279
The care we give should enable the patient to retain as much control over his death as he had over his life.

Field D, Kitson C 1986 The practical reality. Nursing Times 82 (12) March 19: 33-34
Report of an investigation into teaching hours spent on, and methods used in preparing nurses to deal with dying patients, death and bereaved relatives. It gives several references to work which found disparity between this and what happens in the real world of hospital practice.

Garland M 1986 Death of a dear friend. Nursing Times 82 (22) May 28: 58–59
A death in a psychogeriatric ward is the loss of a friend for the other patients and staff. Discusses two useful concepts, the head reaction in which we consider the dead person — it is good that he has escaped; and

the heart reaction in which we consider ourselves — how we will miss what the person has meant to us in their life.

Gray A 1984 When the bough breaks. Nursing Mirror 159 (19) November 21: 19–20
Cot death is the term used to describe the sudden inexplicable death of an apparently healthy infant. This article looks at current international research, which aims to find a common causative factor, and bring under control a modern tragedy.

Hannah G 1987 Lessons from the hospice. Nursing Times 83 (17) April 29: 37
Gives some practical proposals for more considerate nursing of the dying which could be implemented without disrupting the routine of busy wards.

Hickon H 1984 Caring for a terminally ill patient at home. Nursing Times 80 (44) October 31: 29–32
Describes the care given to a patient with carcinoma of the stomach and the total dedication of the family at this difficult time.

Iveson-Iveson J 1985 Part of the spiral of life. Nursing Mirror 160 6 February 6: 38
Nurses have to come to terms with the reality of the natural cycle of life and not suffer guilt when a patient dies.

Iveson-Iveson J 1985 A part of life. Nursing Mirror 161 (8) August 21: 43
Grief is the natural reaction to death, but it should be tempered with the knowledge that without endings, there can be no beginnings.

Janes G 1986 Planning for terminal care. Nursing Times 82 (17) April 23: 24–27
Cerebral secondaries from a primary bronchial carcinoma were diagnosed and the patient's prognosis was poor. Outlines the plan of care devised to nurse Will as his condition deteriorated. Thoughtful study.

Kent J 1986 A better way to die. Community Outlook May: 11, 13
Home care teams help patients and their families to adjust emotionally and spiritually to approaching death.

Lansdown R 1985 Coping with child death: a child's view. Nursing: The Add-On Journal of Clinical Nursing 2 (43) November: 1264–1266
Discusses ages and stages in the development of a concept of death, using actual situations to explain that children commonly know far more than we imagine.

Larder E 1985 Coming to grief. Nursing Times 81 (7) February 13: 55– 57
An acute psychiatric breakdown in a 46-year-old woman was precipitated by the sudden death of her husband. The author feels that use of the process of nursing would have helped this patient, but it was not being used in the hospital.

Limerick S 1984 Sudden infant death. 1. Epidemiology. Nursing Times 80 (10) March 7: 28–29
Examines the extent of the problem and known risk factors.
2. Research. Nursing Times 80 (11) March 14: 50–52
3. Prevention. Nursing Times 80 (12) March 21: 37–38

Lombardi T 1987 Helping clients to come to terms with loss. The Professional Nurse 2 (6) March: 178–180
Clients who are terminally ill or experiencing other kinds of loss need support. If we are to be effective in helping them, we need to develop our interpersonal skills.

Lovell H, Bokoula C, Misra S, Speight N 1986 Mothers' reactions to a peri-natal death. Nursing Times 82 (46) November 12: 40-42
Emptiness, disappointment, guilt and failure were some of the feelings reported by mothers in a small study which aimed to find out how they felt about the care they had received after the death of their babies.

Macmillan M 1986 Last offices in Scotland. Nursing Times 82 (22) May 28: 28–29
Letter to the Editor responding to Olivant's (1986) article 'Last offices' (March 19)

Manning H 1985 Sudden death. Nursing Mirror 160 (18) May 1: 19–21
Unless nurses explore what they personally think and believe about death, they cannot gain insight into what it means when someone dies suddenly.

McGarr P 1986 Final knowledge. Nursing Times 82 (14) April 2: 52, 54
Discusses the problem when nursing patients who are unaware that they are dying.

McGuinness S 1986 Death rites. Nursing Times 82 (12) March 19: 28–31
Reports a study on the way nurses in an Accident and Emergency department handled sudden death, and the radical changes which followed her initiatives.

McMeeking A 1985 Is death before birth a non-event? Nursing: The Add-On Journal of Clinical Nursing 2 (43) November: 1267–1269
Discusses this harrowing event in detail together with practical advice including when the event occurs in different cultures.

Nash A 1985 Bereavement: staff support. Nursing: The Add-On Journal of Clinical Nursing 2 (43) November: 1288
Discusses various ways in which this can be accomplished.

Neuberger J 1986 A crying shame. Nursing Times 82 (12) March 19: 22
Nurses should feel able to share the grief of those who have lost loved ones in hospital, yet those who show their emotions are still frowned upon.

Neuberger J 1987 Death is part of the process. Nursing Times 83 (10) March 11: 22
The point at which a patient is considered dead is now the subject of intense debate among the medical profession, especially in relation to organ donation. This article analyses the issues.

Neuberger J 1987 Caring for dying people of different faiths. The Lisa Sainsbury Foundation Series

Nursing Times 1986 UK baby deaths come high up WHO list. Nursing Times 82 (3) January 15: 10
The UK's infant mortality rate of around 11 deaths per 1000 live births is shown in a bad light when compared with WHO statistics showing mortality rates of 6 per 1000 live births in Sweden and Iceland and 10 in Singapore.

Nursing Times 1986 Stillbirth case causes concern to midwives. Nursing Times 82 (25) June 18: 8
Helping women who have had stillbirths to grieve may be affected by one woman in such circumstances who killed herself.

Olivant P 1986 Last offices. Nursing Times 82 (12) March 19: 32–33
Reviews some of the practical issues which relatives have to attend to. Organ donor cards are mentioned.

Parkes C M 1985 Terminal care: home, hospital or hospice? Lancet 1 January 19: 155–157
Report of a study, with special reference to pain.

Pilsbury C 1985 Am I dying, nurse? Senior Nurse 3 (1) June: 15–17
The author talks to health care staff about their reactions to such a question and asks whether the terminally ill receive enough honest communication.

Price B 1986 Peacefully at home. Nursing Times 82 (1) January 1: 22–24
Illustrates a social map of a patient, and a list of stressors for him and his family.

Ray G 1985 Look back in anger. Nursing Times 81 (16) April 17: 52
Deplores the casual attitude of some nurses towards expressions of anger and rage in the bereaved.

Roch S 1987 Sharing the grief. Nursing Times 83 (14) April 8: 52, 53
When a baby dies or is born damaged, both parents and professionals need help. Describes how a staff support group is providing help to both parents and carers.

Saunders C 1986 Care of the dying: The last refuge. Nursing Times 82 (43) October 22: 28–30
Provides a map of hospices in the UK and Eire at April 1984. Traces a history of their development.

Swaffield L 1985 Protecting the parents? Nursing Times 81 (31) July 31: 51–52
Does a child have the right to know he is dying? It is evident that many children do know something of their condition without having been told. Would a more open and honest attitude help all concerned in his care?

Teesdale J 1985 Stress and coping mechanisms in families of children with cancer. Nursing: The Add-On Journal of Clinical Nursing 2 (43) November 1280–1282
Gives practical advice for those caring for dying children and their families in each of the stages of grief and dying.

Teesdale J 1985 Acute lymphoblastic leukaemia — a nursing-care study. Nursing: The Add-On Journal of Clinical Nursing 2 (43) November: 1283–1285
But when death finally occurred there was an almost universal feeling of unshackling, of freedom to live without fear and pain again, both for themselves and their dead children.

Turton P 1986 Wall of silence. Nursing Times 82 (15) April 9: 23
The stress of caring for a patient uninformed about his illness falls particularly hard on nurses. She advocates a nursing voice in the decision to tell the full facts.

Turton P 1987 Last rights. Nursing Times 83 (17) April 29: 18–19
Should nurses obey a doctor's instruction to end a patient's life — or are there instances where a nurse should take the decision? The issues surrounding nurses' involvement in euthanasia have been raised in a recent case in Holland.

Waters A 1985 Support for staff in a paediatric oncology unit. Nursing: The Add-On Journal of Clinical Nursing 2 (43) November: 1275–1276

Waters V 1987 First impressions of grief. Nursing Times 83 (5) February 4: 46–47
The nurses' attitude has a profound effect on newly bereaved relatives. Suggests that the quality of empathy can help the nurse to provide comfort.

Webster M 1986 Easing emotional distress. Nursing Times 82 (44) October 29: 43–44
Discusses how nurses can help the terminally ill cope with their impending death.

Webster M 1986 Patients' coping strategies. Nursing Times 82 (43) October 22: 34–35
When caring for a terminally ill patient it is important to find out about his customary coping style when faced with a crisis or problem. Useful information to be gathered as part of a nursing history.

White C 1985 Jack: A study in anguish. Nursing Times 81 (41) October 9: 24–26
When and how to tell a terminally ill patient that he is dying raises many problems. Describes how one family tried to come to terms with this stressful event.

Wilkinson S 1987 Hidden loss. Nursing Times 83 (12) March 25: 30–31
When a woman has a miscarriage, few people, including nurses, feel equipped to offer consolation. 'You can always have another baby' is wounding. Positive help can be given by explaining the possible reasons for the miscarriage.

Woodhall C 1986 A family concern. Nursing Times 82 (43) October 22: 31–35
A study into whether the terminally ill would prefer to die at home or in hospital, reveals that in both settings, the family plays an important role.

Woolf J 1985 Equal to the task. Nursing Mirror 161 (1) July 3: 39– 41
Reports analysis of a questionnaire on student nurses' feelings towards the dying and bereaved.

BACKGROUND INFORMATION

So much has been written about death, dying and bereavement that all entries in the Reading Assignment have been changed. The new ones have been selected to cover a wide range of perspectives and the references in the articles will lead students to further reading. Before nurses can develop skills for helping dying patients, they need to examine their attitudes, values and beliefs about death, dying and bereavement.

Death, dying and bereavement

In the life of each individual there is only one certainty which is that he will die; it is the time of this event which is unknown. In schools, teaching about conception and birth has increased but death is still treated as a hush-hush subject although it is a 'fact of life'. And an individual cannot come to terms with a situation about which he is not allowed or not even encouraged to think.

Yet death impinges on the life of each human being; one reads or hears about the death of people one does not know, often in hostile or tragic circumstances; one learns of the death of known people. Sooner or later one experiences the death of a member of one's family and finally as the last link with life on this earth, one faces one's own death. And what of those one leaves behind — the bereaved?

In many ways the subject of bereavement has been released from taboo to a greater extent than that of death and dying. The media have helped to bring the subject to the attention of the public and there are several associations which help particular categories of bereaved people. The grieving process or syndrome is now well documented and the articles describe it and give helpful advice on dealing with it. They are recognisable by the title and/or annotation.

Death can be immediate and unexpected as when a child is killed in an accident; it can be sudden and unexpected, for example a person collapses and within 24 hours is dead; death can be expected because of the medical diagnosis but in the end it can occur suddenly, or a patient can be terminally ill for a period varying from a few days to several months. The articles in the Reading Assignment illustrate the different sorts of death which can be encountered. Several of the articles discuss the ethical dilemma of resuscitation in terminally ill patients.

In times past, and still in many instances today, death can be assumed when a person's pulse and respiration have ceased. However, the advances of medical technology are such that when one or more body systems fail it is possible to keep the patient 'alive' by use of a machine; this may be done with a view to removal of organs for transplant surgery and it has led to the acceptance in law of three definitions:

- biological death: death of the tissues
- brain death: irreversible brain damage
- clinical death: death of the person.

Most people would prefer to die in their own home in the presence of familiar people. The majority of people achieved this at the beginning of the century when the extended family was the rule rather than the exception it is today. A minority of patients currently die at home. Allsworth (1985) gives the figure of 33%. When management at home is impossible a few fortunate patients (7%, Allsworth 1985) are admitted to a hospice — a place which specialises in multidisciplinary care of the terminally ill. The atmosphere is similar to that of 'home' as opposed to hospital. Pain control is priority number one, followed by control of distressing symptoms such as constipation and faecal impaction, thrush in the mouth, nausea and vomiting. Each patient, together with family and friends, is encouraged to live one day at a time and to achieve as high a quality of living as possible during that day.

60% of deaths occur in general hospitals (Allsworth 1985). The satisfactory management of these patients and their families demands great patience, sensitivity and professionalism from all members of staff. The main purpose of 'acute' wards is to facilitate the patients' recovery and an active policy is formulated and carried out to achieve this. The needs of a dying patient and his relatives is an anachronism in this actively oriented atmosphere. Where a single room is available the patient can be removed from the bustle and hurry but it can increase the isolation and loneliness which many such patients experience.

A critically ill person may die in the ambulance before arrival at hospital; it is usual for the doctor to certify death in the ambulance, after which the body is conveyed to the city mortuary. These deaths are thereby not accounted to the hospital for statistical purposes. A critically ill person may die in the Accident and Emergency department before admission to a ward. He has usually been lifted from the stretcher on to the couch in the admission room, but is still fully clothed. The relatives may wish to see him like this for many of them will have great difficulty in believing that he is dead; or they may want to wait until last offices have been performed in a separate room; or they may wish to view the body in the hospital mortuary.

The extensive literature on death, dying and bereavement makes it clear that frank and open discussion of these subjects is therapeutic. Various television documentaries are enabling people to discuss the subject comfortably and without embarrassment, but as yet, this does not apply to the majority of people. Debate continues about who should be told that a patient has a terminal illness as witnessed by the titles in the Reading Assignment.

DYING AND THE PROCESS OF NURSING

Considering that — a baby can be stillborn; death can occur shortly after birth; there are sudden infant deaths; death can occur at any other stage in life, either suddenly from accident or disease, or as a result of a chronic disease which enters its terminal phase of a few days, weeks or months, it is impossible to discuss each of these unique experiences of death, dying and bereavement in a text. Only broad guide lines can be suggested, which with the carefully selected items in the Reading Assignment, together with the Topics for discussion (p. 79) should be sufficient to prepare student nurses for experience in their clinical allocations.

It must be difficult for beginning nurses to realise that in emergency situations the well-defined phases of the process of nursing may be going on 'in the experienced nurse's mind' simultaneously. This is likely to be so in Accident and Emergency departments. There are other instances when a patient in any other clinical area 'collapses' and immediate nursing cannot be divided into the accepted four phases of the process. However, the phases do have retrospective relevance and in many other instances are essential in day to day nursing.

Assessing

From your reading you will have gleaned that being terminally ill does not necessarily mean being bedfast, nevertheless the patient may be frail and easily fatigued. It may not be possible to collect all the necessary information for the Patient Assessment Form at one go. Furthermore the patient will be anxious and may be distressed that he no longer feels in control of his life.

The biographical data requested by the form will be of particular significance, for example next of kin, and here nurses have to bear in mind that patients can be estranged from next of kin, and may give the name and address of the person who looks after such everyday living activities as collecting the pension, washing, shopping, keeping the pet or the car and so on. Information about estranged relatives may only be mentioned in the ensuing days and patients' wishes regarding whether or not they need to be informed should be respected. Non-verbal signals may give nurses some clues as to what is going on in patients' lives.

Collecting the required health data needs great skill, sensitivity and an ability to recognise when it is inappropriate to carry on. The sort of questions to be borne in mind, not necessarily asked, are:

- does the patient know the medical diagnosis?
- does the patient know that it is a terminal illness?
- do the relatives know the medical diagnosis?
- do the relatives know that it is a terminal illness?
- what do they understand about terminal illness?
- what are they expecting from the hospital admission?
- what do they want the nurses to do when death seems imminent?
- what do they want the nurses to do in the event of death?
- does the patient have an organ donor card?
- if so, do the relatives know this?

These questions will not be asked directly; they are a guide to help nurses to pick up cues from the patient or relatives. When information about these 'questions' does become available in ensuing interactions with the patient and family, a factual note will be made in the patient's nursing notes so that nurses on succeeding shifts will be able to interact appropriately with all concerned.

Information about how the patient manages everyday living activities is very important so that for as long as possible he can make as many decisions as possible to maintain self-esteem and dignity. However this information, unlike the biographical and health data, is only relevant for the day on which it was collected. If there are any actual or potential problems they should be identified with the patient. A scoring system to identify those at risk of developing pressure sores should be used early in the patient's stay to act as base data against which evaluation can take place (p. 117). It is important to remember that all patients fear pain and in the case of the terminally ill, it may be appropriate to use one of the tools (painometer p. 52) for assessing its severity early on, as its succeeding use will guide any pain relief programme. Since some of the patients' problems which can occur in those dying of carcinomatosis are:

- constipation and faecal impaction
- thrush in the mouth
- vomiting

special attention should be given to formulating questions to elicit information at the initial assessment.

Planning

Ward planning will include selection of a bed sufficiently near toilet facilities to encourage independence for as long as possible. Ideally the quietest part of the ward should be used and if a covering rug is provided, the patient can have a nap on top of the bed as he feels inclined.

Individualised planning will aim to maintain quality for each of the days of life which are left for the patient. On the nursing plan, each of the identified problems with everyday living activities will have a goal agreed with the patient whenever possible and a nursing intervention to achieve the goal with date for evaluation. The carrying out of the nursing intervention will be written on the patient's nursing notes, as will any summative evaluation towards achieving goals.

There will also be nursing interventions arising from the medical prescription of drugs to control pain. The administration will probably be recorded on the medication Kardex, but if nurses need to be alerted to observe for any side-effects, this nursing intervention will appear on the nursing plan, and should a side-effect appear, it will be recorded on the patient's nursing notes. Should it be a 'problem' it will be transferred to the nursing plan with an appropriate goal and a nursing intervention to achieve it.

The British Medical Association is of the opinion that in all cases, death should be certified by a doctor before last offices (laying out of the dead) is started. There are sometimes difficulties about this, particularly in psychiatric hospitals, when death occurs during the night and the doctor does not certify it until the next day. In general hospitals in many cases, by personal arrangement between doctor and sister, the sister takes the responsibility, and arranges for last offices to be done and the body removed to the mortuary. When this was reported to the British Medical Association and Royal College of Nursing Liaison Committee, the British Medical Association reiterated its views that death should be certified by a doctor and any difficulties should be reported to the Association.

Implementing

All planned nursing interventions will be carried out and recorded on the patient's nursing notes. The records will probably include use of a painometer and a scoring scale for risk of developing pressure sores as well as periods of fatigue, rests on top of the bed, appetite, nausea and/or vomiting, state of mouth, bowel movement and any other appropriate observations (ongoing assessment). The state of partial dependence in an increasing number of everyday living activities is likely to occur, possibly changing to that of total dependence for some of them.

If family members show any inclination that they would like to help the patient in any of these activities it should be welcomed and guided by the nurse as to the patient's changing capability. Diversional therapy can take many forms — the patient may enjoy arranging the flowers brought by visitors and knowledge of the patient's occupation and hobbies will help nurses to individualise their conversation thus helping to make the day as meaningful as possible.

Evaluating

Suggestions have already been made about use

of objective measures. Subjective measures are likely to include gauging the patient's stage of acceptance of the inevitability of death; his attitude to the period of living before the event of death; ability to engage in activities to make each day meaningful; ability to maintain relationship with family/friends and so on. And the final evaluation will be, Was it a good death?

In this chapter, death, dying and bereavement were discussed as background information. As practice for readers, the principle — helping dying patients — was considered in a process of nursing context.

APPLYING THE PRINCIPLE

A registered nurse must be capable of:

- rendering help to the dying patient and relatives
- supporting staff and patients in the event of a patient's death
- applying the principle — helping dying patients — in a process of nursing context.

WORKING ASSIGNMENT

Topics for discussion

- death at home v. hospital
- dying
- bereavement
- the conspiracy of silence
- resuscitation of the terminally ill
- euthanasia
- last offices performed by nurses v. mortuary technicians
- the pros and cons of moving a dying patient from the ward to a single room
- empathy
- painometer
- scoring for risk of developing pressure sores
- three definitions of death accepted in law.

Writing assignment

- name some associations which help particular categories of bereaved people
- give a brief account of the grieving process
- give the three definitions of death accepted in law
- give some complications which can occur in patients dying from carcinomatosis
- define the following:

carcinomatosis
constipation
extended family
faecal impaction
infant mortality rate
nausea
stressors
sudden infant death
terminal illness
therapeutic
thrush
uraemia
vomiting.

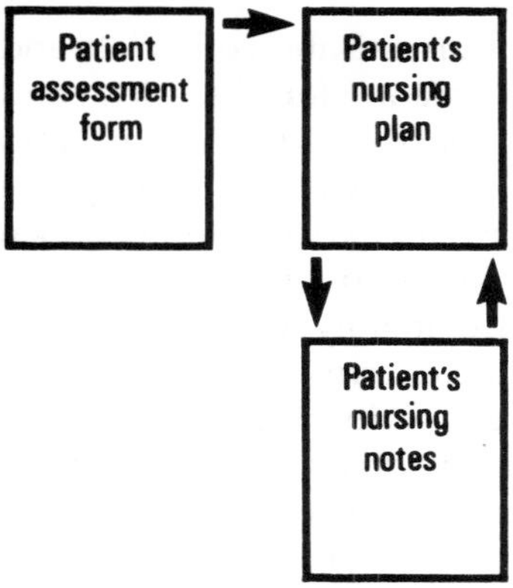

7

Helping patients to practise their religious/spiritual concepts

READING ASSIGNMENT

Barnes E 1961 People in hospital. Macmillan, London

Bentham I A 1976 My friend Kashmir Kaur. Nursing Times 72 (17) April 29: 665–666

Burkhardt M A, Nagai-Jacobson 1985 Dealing with spiritual concerns of clients in the community. Journal of Community Health Nursing 24 (4): 191–198

Burnard P 1986 Picking up the pieces. Nursing Times 82 (17) April 23: 37–38.
How does the nurse respond to the patient who is not clinically depressed but feels an increasing sense of futility? Dispiritedness is described and methods of treatment given.

Frye B, Long L 1985 Spiritual counselling approaches following brain injury. Rehabilitation Nursing 10 (6) November/December: 14–15

International Council of Nurses 1973 Code for nurses: ethical concepts applied to nursing. ICN, Geneva

Israel M 1977 The spirit of man. Nursing Mirror. 145 (26) December 29: 20–21

Kettle B 1976 At the bamboo roots — 1. Nursing Times 72 (32) August 12: 1228–1230

Kettle B 1976 At the bamboo roots — 2. Nursing Times 72 (33) August 19: 1274–1275

Lothian Community Relations Council 1978 Religions and culture. Lothian Community Relations Council, Edinburgh EH1 3LH

Lyall D 1978 Chaplaincy involvement in nurse

education. Nursing Times 74 (24) June 15: 1022–1023

McGilloway F A, Donnelly L 1977 Religion and patient care: the functionalist approach. Journal of Advanced Nursing 2:3–13

McGilloway O, Myco F 1985 (eds.) Nursing and spiritual care. Harper and Row (Lippincott nursing series).

Neuberger J 1987 Caring for dying people of different faiths. The Lisa Sainsbury Foundation Series

Peterson E A 1985 The physical ... the spiritual ... can you meet all of your patient's needs? Journal of Gerontological Nursing 11 (10) October: 23–27
Spiritual care of the elderly.

Richards F 1977 What they believe and why. Part 1 Roman Catholics, Jehovah's Witnesses and Christian Scientists. Nursing Mirror 144 (15) April 14: 65–66

Richards F 1977 What they believe and why. Part 2 The Jewish faith. Nursing Mirror 144 (16) April 21: 64

Richards F 1977 What they believe and why. Part 3 Muslims, Hindus and Buddhists. Nursing Mirror 144 (17) April 28: 67

Simsen B 1986 The spiritual dimension. Nursing Times 82 (48) November 26: 41–42
Report of a project which set out to discover: Do patients bring spiritual resources to the experience of illness and hospitalisation? Do patients experience spiritual need during illness and hospitalisation?

Speck P 1976 East comes west. Nursing Times 72 (17) April 29: 662– 664

Vogelsang J 1983 A psychological and faith approach to grief counselling. Journal of Pastoral Care XXXVII (1): 22–27
Discusses orientation towards an ultimate reality.

BACKGROUND TO RELIGION AND CULTURE

Whether or not a person subscribes to a formal religion he cannot escape the effects of religion on his culture. The major religions have played an important part in the development of national life by influencing the organisation of society and by the provisions made for its sick and disadvantaged members. Religion has also influenced the national laws which designate various activities as right or wrong and the legal system applies sanctions to offenders.

Some religions are mainly concerned with transmitting a specific doctrine of beliefs about spirituality, and the carrying out of particular rituals such as infant baptism, church service, confirmation, marriage service and burial service. The religious beliefs of adherents inform the concepts of right and wrong, and desirable behaviour such as being kind, considerate of others and charitable in both word and deed. In this way they influence everyday living but there are no special rules affecting, for instance eating and drinking.

Other religions, as well as transmitting religious beliefs, transmit relevant practices which directly affect a follower's activities of everyday living; for example the way in which food is prepared; the type of food eaten; periods of fasting; attending public worship; praying; handwashing; perineal toilet; and even the type of clothes worn.

But there are also people who have strong non-religious convictions which guide their concepts of right and wrong and some of them affect their everyday living activities; humanists, atheists, agnostics, vegans and conservationists are examples.

Spiritual concepts

In an increasingly secular western society, words such as 'spirit', 'spiritual' and 'spirituality' are used in a non-religious context. There are idioms in our language which acknowledge this, for example when speaking of a person who is undergoing a stressful experience, the summing up might be — but 'he's in good spirit.' In this context it seems to be concerned with hopefulness, optimism and positiveness. At the other end of the scale we speak of a person being 'dispirited' when he seems to have lost hope, is pessimistic and negative. The notion of the 'spirit' of man is usually taken to be his search for 'meaning'. Vogelsang (1983) maintains that 'everyone has an orientation towards an ultimate reality whether they are firm believers:

- in an established religious tradition
- in their own power to succeed
- in scientific truth or
- in life itself.'

Whether or not a person uses the word 'spiritual', it seems clear that personal beliefs, values and attitudes are probably the most sensitive part of one's 'being'. Not only do they inform one's concept of right and wrong but they guide the 'grey' areas of decision-making, for example, 'Should granny be admitted to a long-stay ward, or should she be looked after in her daughter's home, in which she, her husband and three young children live?' Simsen (1986) describes a study which she carried out and says 'The notion of the *spirit* of man (his concern with infinite realities and ultimate meanings) was seen as distinct from any *religious* framework within which these concerns might be expressed.'

RELIGIOUS/SPIRITUAL CONCEPTS AND THE PROCESS OF NURSING

Simsen (1986) posed two questions as a starting point for a descriptive pilot study. They were:

- do patients bring spiritual resources to the experience of illness and hospitalisation?
- do patients experience spiritual need during illness and hospitalisation?

The encompassing theme in analysis of the data emerged as 'the patient's search for meaning.' The tasks identified in this search were to:

- make sense of this experience
- get through it and
- move on
- find meaning
- experience meaning and
- anticipate meaning.

The skills identified for accomplishing the tasks were 'knowing, hoping and trusting.' Simsen goes on to say that 'Assessing these skills, enabling others to develop and exercise them, and encouraging the search for meaning, may well be more important to the patient than we realise.'

A nurse who practises a formal religion may find that she is shocked by a patient who subscribes to the values and beliefs of a non-religious cult. Similarly a nurse who subscribes to one of these non-religious cults may feel an intellectual antagonism to those of religious faith. All nurses have to remember that the patient is entitled to his values and beliefs and only if they have a negative effect on his health status do they need to be questioned. A nurse's services are given without regard to creed, race or colour and this is achieved by establishing empathy and by being aware of and sensitive to a patient's individuality and dignity. A nurse's function is to provide an environment in which each patient can continue to live by the principles which guide his behaviour.

In recognition of an increasingly cosmopolitan population, the Lothian Community Relations Council (1978) prepared for health service staff a booklet as a guide to patients' beliefs and customs. The members of religions and cultures which were included are:

- Buddhists
- Chinese
- Hindus
- Jews
- Muslims
- Sikhs.

The information is organised under the following headings (where appropriate):

- ablutions and toilet
- attitudes to medical staff and illness
- birth
- blood transfusions and transplants
- death
- diet
- family planning
- fasting
- ideas of modesty
- language
- names.

Assessing

Many patient assessment forms request the patient's religion. The question, 'What is your religion?' does not guarantee an accurate answer. In a desire to conform it may bring the first formal religion that springs to mind or it may bring the sect of the church attended as a child. This can cause embarrassment to a patient a few days later when the visiting chaplain asks him which church he normally attends. In some hospitals, to help the staff, including the chaplain, the inpatients' religion is designated as Anglican, Free Church or Roman Catholic by a different coloured cross attached to the name plate at the bedside.

While collecting initial assessment data the nurse, instead of asking the patient's religion, might say, 'Have you any beliefs and relevant practices that you fear may be interfered with while you are in hospital?' For example, if a patient always listens to the radio morning religious service, then the nurse can check that there is an available functioning radio and arrange treatment time to prevent interference with the practice. Another example could be the beliefs and practices pertaining to food, personal hygiene, covering for the head or legs and this serves to show the relatedness of the knowledge contained in the different chapters of this book.

If the patient makes statements like 'I don't know why this has happened to me' or 'I don't know what I've done to deserve this,' the nurse could reflect the statement trying to find out how the patient is currently perceiving the situation and whether talking about it brings any relief. If not, the nurse might ask if the patient would like to talk with anyone else, for example a social worker or a member of a non-religious or a religious foundation and the referral would be recorded on the assessment form. In the current state of the art, it is unlikely that nurses, together with patients, will identify any 'problems'. If the patient wants to participate in any available religious services or sacraments, or non-secular activities, a note will be made of this so that nurses on the appropriate shift will have this information and make the necessary arrangements.

Planning

Currently for the majority of patients there are unlikely to be any individualised interventions on the patient's nursing plan. As already mentioned, personal beliefs are such a sensitive and private part of 'being' that individualised planning cannot be captured in a book. However, in the case of dying patients, it is important that nurses know what the patient and family want to happen in the case of imminent death and in the event of death (Neuberger 1987).

Ward planning is necessary to arrange services on the ward, or to transfer patients to the hospital chapel or even to a local church in the case of long-stay patients, or to a secular meeting.

Generalised planning of course is behind the availability of preferably a non-denominational chapel, the upkeep of the building, provision of hospital chaplains, an organist, domestic staff and so on.

Implementing

Part of the implementing phase of the process of nursing has already been referred to, and this shows how knowledge cannot be put into little 'boxes' and that the phases of the process are not demarcated.

Evaluating

In the context of the process of nursing, the evaluating phase means observing or measuring the data collected on the appointed date, and comparing it with that collected at the initial assessment. From the literature, it would appear that this is not done in relation to helping patients to practise their religious/spiritual concepts. This may be because nurses are not yet sufficiently skilled, and have not yet collected an adequate data bank from which relevant knowledge can increase. The proforma which have been used to measure patients' satisfaction with their stay in hospital have not included this item.

In this chapter complex spiritual concepts

related to secularity, religion and culture have been briefly introduced. A principle of nursing — helping patients to practice their religious/spiritual concepts — was discussed in a process of nursing context.

APPLYING THE PRINCIPLE

A registered nurse must be capable of:

- eliciting information from patients about those beliefs and relevant practices which can be catered for in hospital
- helping patients to express their perception of meaning in illness
- applying the principle — helping patients to practice religious/spiritual concepts in a process of nursing context

WORKING ASSIGNMENT

Topics for discussion

- the concepts of right and wrong
- the spirit of man
- the effect of Christian beliefs on everyday living activities
- the effect of non-Christian religious beliefs on everyday living activities
- the effect of secular beliefs on everyday living activities
- beliefs and customs surrounding birth in different religions and cultures
- beliefs and customs surrounding death in different religions and cultures
- ethics

Writing assignment

- the patients' beliefs, are they of relevance to nursing?

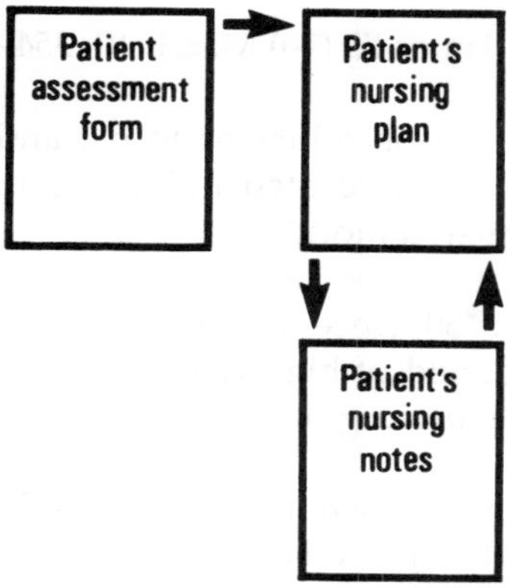

8

Helping patients to keep the body clean and well groomed

READING ASSIGNMENT

Allbright A 1984 Oral care for the cancer chemotherapy patient. Nursing Times 80 (21) May 23: 40–42
Suggests some of the ways nurses can help to prevent patients suffering during therapy.

Bergstrom E, Cooper D, Simonsson J 1985 Bathrooms designed for the disabled. Nursing Mirror 160 (25) June 19: 21–24
Describes and illustrates well-designed bathrooms and lavatories which can be built into a patient's home.

Cheater F 1985 Xerostomia in malignant disease. Nursing Mirror 161 (3) July 17: 25–27
Cancer patients commonly suffer from a dry mouth, which can lead to infection and tooth decay; explains why and suggests ways to maintain oral hygiene in such patients.

Creamer E 1985 Scabies. Irish Nursing Forum 3 (4) Winter: 10–12
A serious and not so serious look at the subject of scabies infestation.

Davis W M 1970 Self aids. Thistle Foundation, 22 Charlotte Square, Edinburgh EH2 4DF

Dealey C, Berker M 1986 Action speaks louder than words. Nursing Times 82 (29) July 16: 37–39
Reveals negative attitudes in some members of staff to introducing research based policy regarding patients' wash bowls.

deMont A 1985 Don't let your hair down. Community Outlook September: 16–17

Looks at what is available over the counter for headlice and dandruff.

England P M, Oxley D E, Staveley L P, Taylor M G 1979 An experiment in health education. Nursing Times 75 (35) August 30: 1491–1492
Mentally handicapped patients learn to care about their own personal hygiene; evaluate abilities rather than IQ.

Geissler P, McCord F 1986 Dental care for the elderly. Nursing Times 82 (20) May 14: 53–54
Gives practical measures carers of the elderly should take to ensure that their clients' oral health is maintained.

Finlay I G 1986 Oral symptoms and candida in the terminally ill. British Medical Journal 292: 592–593
Candida is easily isolated from the mouths of 29 to 50% of healthy adults and is a normal commensal.

Gooch J 1987 Skin hygiene. The Professional Nurse 2 (5) February: 153–154
A literature search suggests review of practice. Discussed under the headings — skin changes, bacterial hazards, equipment used and suggested practice.

Greaves A 1985 We'll just freshen you up, dear... Nursing Times (Journal of Infection Control) 81 (36) 27: 3–4, 7–8
A research report shows that washbowls can cause a patient to be microbiologically dirtier after the bath than before.

Hadley A, Sheiham A 1984 Nursing Times 80 (27) July 11: 28–31
Smile please! If the measures described were adopted, subsequent generations would only know about dental disease from history books.

Hallett N 1984 Mouthcare. Nursing Mirror 159 (21) December 5: 31–33
A sore mouth adds considerably to the distress of the terminally ill patient. Examines the management of oral hygiene and the value of specific cleansing agents.

Hilton D 1980 Oral hygiene and infection. Nursing Times 76 (29) July 17: 1270–1272
Patients suffering from terminal illness develop distressingly unhealthy mouths; they suffer emotionally as well as physically.

Howarth H 1977 Mouth care procedures for the very ill. Nursing Times 73 (10) March 10: 354–355
It is the person who is reluctant to eat and drink who becomes dehydrated and therefore develops a dry crusted mouth.

Johnson A 1985 Dental care during pregnancy. Nursing Times 81 (50) December 11: 28, 31
Pregnancy is a period of high risk for dental disease. Offers a basic guide to prevention and treatment.

King J 1984 A multidisciplinary approach. Nursing Times 80 (27) July 11: 32–33
Primary health care workers have an important role in advising people about dental health.

Lewis I A 1984 Developing a research-based curriculum: an exercise in relation to oral care. Nurse Education Today 3 (6): 143–144
A working party concluded that the project has demonstrated to the participants the need for both nursing practice and nurse education to be research-based.

Maunder J W 1983 The louse and the law. British Pest Control Association, Cambridge, UK
An essential discussion paper if nurses are to understand their legal position in relation to lousiness.

Munday P, Gelbier S 1984 Provision of dental health education in nurse training. Nurse Education Today 3 (6): 124–125

Nursing Mirror 1985 Get ahead of the lice. Nursing Mirror 160 (9) February 27:4
Headlice affect 250 000 children in the UK every year. They are a chronic problem, since they thrive on the cleanest heads and do not discriminate between sections of society. Gives details of where to get leaflets in many languages for those attending minority groups.

Roberts G Keeping caries at bay. Nursing Times 82 (5) January 29: 48–50
Preventing dental caries in children.

Roberts S 1987 Getting to know you... Nursing Times 83 (14) April 8: 36
Describes two different experiences of bedbathing — a frail elderly person, and an obese 70-year-old who had been labelled a 'difficult' patient.

Roberts A, Besterman A 1986 The oral mucosa.

Nursing Times (Senior Systems 5) 82 (33) August 13: 51–54
An excellent account, well illustrated, of abnormal mouth conditions.

Roberts A, Besterman A 1986 The digestive system. Nursing Times (Senior Systems 4) 82 (28) July 9: 55–58
Decline in sense of taste; anorexia; the mouth; dentures; dental treatment for patients in poor health; gum diseases in the elderly; common changes in elderly jaws.

Thurston R, Beattie C 1984 Nursing Times 80 (34) August 22: 44–46
Gives new thinking on why diabetic people are particularly prone to develop problems with their feet.

Wagnild G, Manning RW 1985 Convey respect during bathing procedures. Journal of Gerontological Nursing 11 (12) December: 6–10
Describes how patient well-being depends on it.

Wallace J, Freeman P A 1978 Mouth care in patients with blood dyscrasias. Nursing Times 74 (22) June 1: 921–922
Battery operated automatic (oscillating not rotational) toothbrush; small head reaches all parts of mouth; pressure on gums even; less bleeding from gums and less thrush; patients independent.

Wells R, Trostle K 1984 Creative hairwashing techniques for immobilised patients. Nursing 14 (1) January: 47–51

Wickenden J 1985 The little head louse. Guidelines for parents on the prevention, detection and treatment of head lice. Department of Applied Biology, University of Cambridge, UK

Wilson M 1986 Personal cleanliness Nursing: The Add-On Journal of Clinical Nursing 3 (2) February: 80–82
Bedbathing discussed under the headings — aims; environment; control of infection; guidelines for procedure; observation; teaching; communication; social interaction; evaluation.

BACKGROUND INFORMATION

For the majority of people, to feel clean, sweet-smelling and well groomed are essential dimensions of well-being. The many activities involved in achieving this objective are carried out independently and in privacy with pleasurable satisfaction; they are built into the daily routine to give a sense of stability and safety, and they are usually congruent with family and societal expectations. They include skin cleansing; care of the nails, hair, feet, mouth and teeth. They are necessarily dependent on available facilities and it is important for nurses to remember that there are still thousands of houses in Britain which do not have a fixed bath. But even with equivalent facilities members of the same family can develop an individual routine related to personal cleansing and grooming.

Congenital mental and/or physical handicap has in the past prevented people so afflicted from achieving independence in these activities. However, there is growing evidence that with individualised programmes, a considerable number of congenitally handicapped people can become independent or at least achieve their 'optimum independence' requiring a minimum of help from others (England et al 1979). Other people, having achieved independence, may for a variety of reasons lose some or all of it and may well require nursing help with their particular problems, identified from their assessment data. Davis (1970) contains descriptions and illustrations of many self aids to help handicapped people achieve maximum (aided) independence.

Bacterial colonisation of the skin begins shortly after birth; the microorganisms, though present in large numbers (Roper 1976), are not usually pathogenic, but since they can reproduce in 20 minutes, they can be a threat should there be a break in the skin's continuity. Furthermore the organisms can become attached to the skin scales which are constantly being shed on to clothing and into the atmosphere. It is for these reasons that, for most people, a daily bath, shower or all-over wash is recommended.

WASHING/BATHING AND THE PROCESS OF NURSING

Putting skin cleansing in the context of the

process of nursing usually means discussing it in the phases of that process, commonly accepted as assessing, planning, implementing and evaluating. Yet the sum of these, is greater than the phases, as evidenced in the foregoing background information. Each of the phases is ongoing and may be overlapping which compounds the complexity of 'nursing' to be discussed later. A relevant environment must be provided in which skin cleansing can be accomplished safely for the patient, and remembering the possibility of nosocomial infection (Ch. 20). The process of nursing has to be applied to neonatal infants, other infants, toddlers, children, adolescents and adults of any age, whether they are able or disabled, in their homes or in hospital.

Patients are also admitted in emergency; they may have collapsed or had an accident at work, at play, in the home or on the road. Consequently nurses will encounter some patients in their work clothes and with the grime of work, or blood from trauma on their skin, and this has implications for understanding the process of nursing.

Assessing

The usual interpretation of this first phase of the process is of an initial interview with the patient, the objective being to discover his usual pattern of skin cleansing and whether or not he perceives any problems with it. But this cannot be the case for all patients.

When patients are admitted in a state of unconsciousness, information will usually be collected from the next of kin. A nurse has to remember that skin cleansing is a private activity and should the patient live alone, detailed information may not be available, even from near relatives. But it should be as detailed as possible because creating the previous 'familiar' environment helps unconscious patients to return to consciousness. In these instances the patient cannot verify his problem but it is that of total dependence for skin cleansing. The goal will be to cleanse the patient's skin in a style as near to his usual style as possible; to prevent body odour, especially if there is increased perspiration; and to maintain intactness of the skin. The nursing intervention to achieve this will probably be a daily bed-bath; morning and/or evening washing of the face and hands, followed by application of the usual toiletries for each individual patient — a familiar smell may help to lighten the level of unconsciousness.

Of course it is only for the purpose of description that assessing an unconscious patient's skin cleansing activities can be considered on its own. In reality it will be used in conjunction with assessing risk of developing pressure sores (p. 117), level of unconsciousness (p. 66) and hazards of bedrest (Fig. 2.1, p. 40), yet another example of the relatedness of nursing knowledge.

Some patients who are admitted with the grime of work and/or blood from trauma on their skin, have to be prepared for the operating theatre. It is unrealistic to expect that these very ill patients who will probably be experiencing acute pain are fit to give information for the assessment form, from which the nursing plan is prepared with its nursing interventions. However, the nursing 'activity' of bedbathing is essential preoperatively with the objective of minimising the number of microorganisms on the skin prior to its incision with a scalpel, so lessening the risk of nosocomial infection (Ch. 20).

It is still customary in some hospitals for nurses to carry out an 'admission bath' in the bathroom or in bed as appropriate: this need not imply that the patient is dirty but it affords the nurse an opportunity to assess the patient's skin for such things as:

- athlete's foot
- birthmarks
- bruises
- bunions
- callouses
- chilblains
- corns
- deformities including nails
- infestation
  - — head lice
  - — body lice
  - — scabies

- pressure sores
- rashes
- scars
- ulcers.

It is especially important that any observed abnormality is described objectively on the patient's assessment form, preferably signed by the nurse. Particularly for bruises and pressure sores it is an additional precaution to have a witness.

At the initial assessment the nurse may discover that the patient is in the habit of using an aid to maintain independence even if it is just a non-slip mat in the bath. He will obviously have a problem of increased anxiety if one is not provided, or cannot be procured in hospital, and the problem may have to be solved by relatives bringing in his own, and the patient accepting responsibility for its safe keeping.

Any other problems being experienced in relation to washing/bathing will be identified and verified with the patient and written as the patient describes them, either on the assessment form or the nursing plan, whichever is the custom, but writing it twice should be avoided.

Planning

For each identified problem, a patient outcome/goal/objective — whichever word is used where you are working — will be decided with the patient whenever possible. In the case of children in long-stay areas the plan will be to habilitate them to the maximum degree of independence in the circumstances (p. 35). For those who had achieved independence before the accident or illness then the goal will be to rehabilitate them to the maximum independence of which they are capable (p. 36). There are thousands of possible variations and these can only be coped with by each patient having an individualised nursing plan.

The generalised planning in the area where you work will be responsible for the environment in which washing/bathing takes place. The planners may be faced with older hospitals which were built when patients were confined to bed for most of the time, consequently they are short of bathrooms and sinks and the means of providing privacy, warmth and freedom from draughts. These can be constraints on the quality of washing/bathing procedures, but they challenge nurses to keep the planners informed of deficiencies, so that when money is available it will be spent to patients' advantage in upgrading programmes.

Generalised planning is behind the equipment available for washing/bathing particular patients; non-slip mats have been mentioned. Figure 8.1 shows one of many available attachments to help disabled patients get into and out of a bath. Figure 8.2 shows a chair which permits showering of patients who cannot cope without the support of a chair.

There are now several mechanical hoists which can be used to bring bedfast and chairfast patients to the bathroom for an immersion bath (Fig. 8.3).

There are several models of 'open-ended' baths into which patients can be wheeled and the end of the bath replaced; the seals are watertight. Careful control of the temperature of the water is important — as it runs into the bath while the patient is in the bath. Likewise the bath is emptied of water, before the end is taken off and the patient removed. Advertisements in the nursing journals carry details of all lifting and

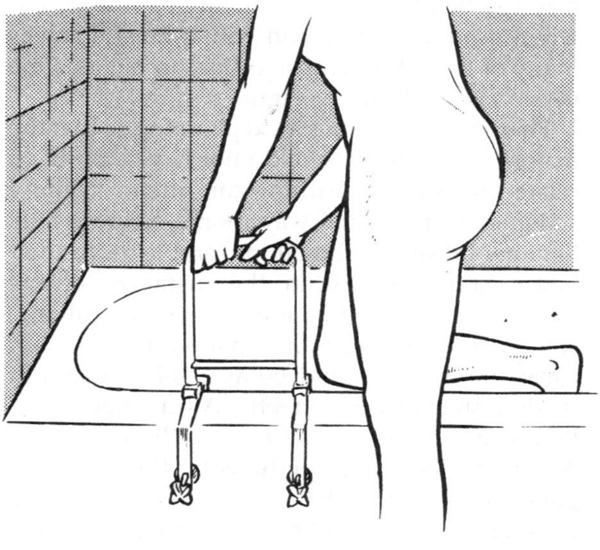

Fig. 8.1 An attachment to help patient into and out of bath

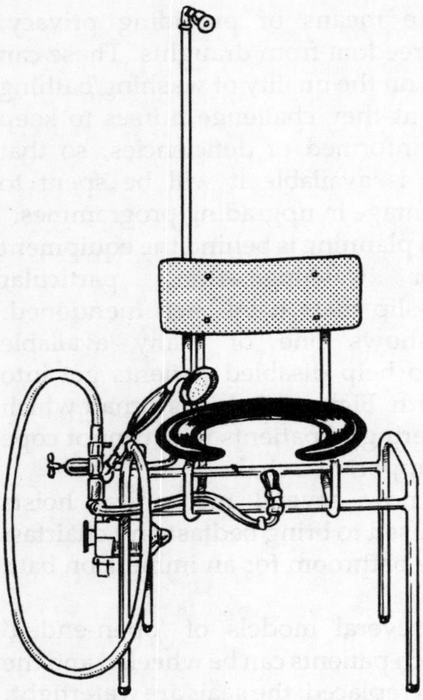

Fig. 8.2 Chair for showering

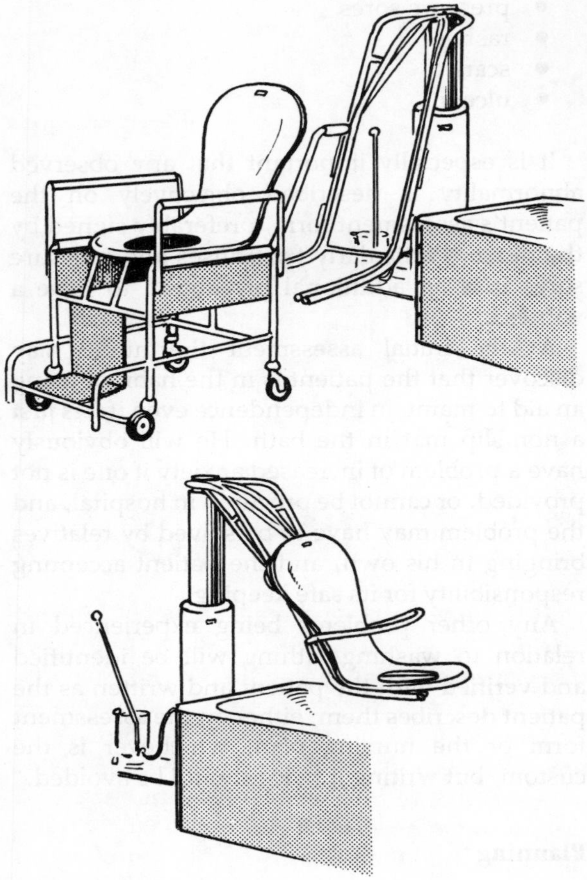

Fig. 8.3 A chair-type bath lift

bathing equipment. It is worth scanning these each week to keep up to date with what is available.

Lifting patients and stooping over a low bath are hazardous to the nurse's back. A new Hi-Lo bath can be fitted into almost any bathroom and when used in conjunction with a hoist it solves many of the lifting and stooping problems. One version is illustrated in Figure 8.4.

There has to be some ward planning so that the majority of patients who do not have a problem related to washing/bathing can attend to these activities in the usual way. Some of these may have mobilising or breathing problems so their beds should be within the distance (of the sanitary facilities) they are capable of walking; some may need to sit on a chair while washing. Clean tumblers should be available for mouth rinsing after brushing teeth. All members of a family cannot use the bathroom at the same time. A rota can be made, perhaps by the ambulant patients, so that the facilities can be used throughout the day at times which are congruent with other ward activities.

There will be ward policy agreed with the control of infection committee about cleaning baths and sinks, use of bath mats and so on, so that patients do not acquire a nosocomial infection (Ch. 20). The policy must extend to wash bowls used by bed patients. Greaves (1985) is a report of an investigation into the misuse of wash bowls and Dealey & Berker (1986) describe the difficulties which they experienced in trying to use Greaves' research-based recommendations in the wards.

Implementing

The implementing phase of the process of nursing is putting 'the plan' into effect. Customarily the nursing plan is predicated on the patient having a 'problem', in this instance

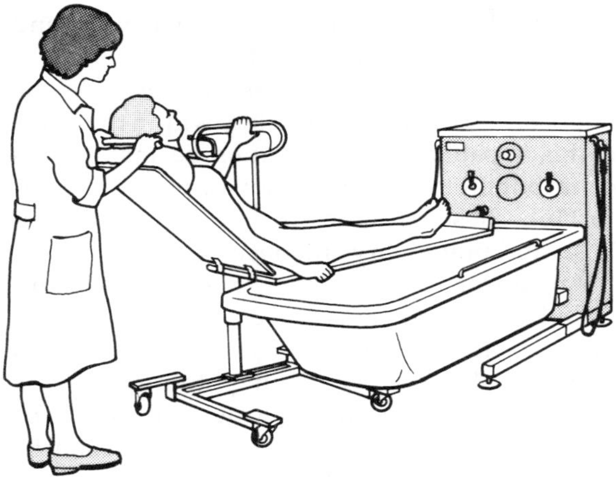

Fig. 8.4 A Hi-Lo bath

with washing/bathing. But not all patients have a problem — we have already referred to the fact that ambulant patients who do not have a problem can continue to carry out washing/bathing activities if the necessary toilet facilities are provided, and they are acquainted with where and when these activities can be carried out. Information about the individuality of these activities will be on the assessment form and it does not need to be duplicated on the nursing plan.

Helping a patient with an immersion bath engages the nurse in touching those parts of another body which are taboo except to those in a close relationship. The nurse's sensitivity to this and to the possible disparate age of her and the patient will help her to be 'professional' and thereby lessen any embarrassment which the patient might experience; this permits him to retain his dignity in an abnormal situation.

The patient's problem may be that he cannot manage to get to the bathroom, and have an immersion bath without help. The help required will be stated on the nursing plan, and the goal may be that the patient feels refreshed, and is free from the smell of stale perspiration. The intervention may achieve the goal but the patient may be fatigued and this should be written in the nursing notes. It may not change the nursing intervention, particularly if walking to the bathroom with assistance is part of the rehabilitation programme (Ch. 2). The appropriate nursing activity is to help the patient into a comfortable position for resting either in a chair or bed, and later to enquire how the patient feels — not, 'Do you feel rested?' or 'Do you still feel tired?' However, the information may change the nursing intervention to a wheelchair as the means of transport if the patient, who may be terminally ill, agrees, so that his energy is conserved for the bathing process.

The patient's problem may be that he is bedfast because of the medical diagnosis, but nevertheless he may be capable of attending to his washing/bathing activities in bed, if a bowl of hot water is provided and he has the necessary accessories (soap, flannels, deodorant etc.) so that the appropriate nursing activity is discovering whether or not this is the case — the patient may have been admitted as 'an emergency' and may not have had the opportunity to have these accessories brought to him. Some patients can attend to their nails, feet, perineum, hair and teeth but this should not be taken for granted.

The nurse may need to give some assistance, for example washing and drying the back, or the toes of a leg that is in plaster. In other instances washing the back can be a form of physiotherapy. Such patients need praise and encouragement from the nurse. At the end of the procedure the nurse returns to make up the bed and leave the patient warm and comfortable. The towel and face cloth need to be dried (Fig. 8.5). A soap dish should be provided to avoid soggy soap being smeared over the toothbrush and tube of toothpaste in the toilet bag. A hot drink may well be acceptable to the patient after a bath.

When the patient cannot manage and the nurse has to do the washing (Fig. 8.6) and drying, there is enforced regression to the stage when the patient was a naked baby and toddler and his clothed mother did the bathing. It is acknowledged that in this situation the child voices his most intimate thoughts. Repetition of this behaviour can result in a smutty story or intimate details of life. An adult's conception of himself bathing is usually of being alone and

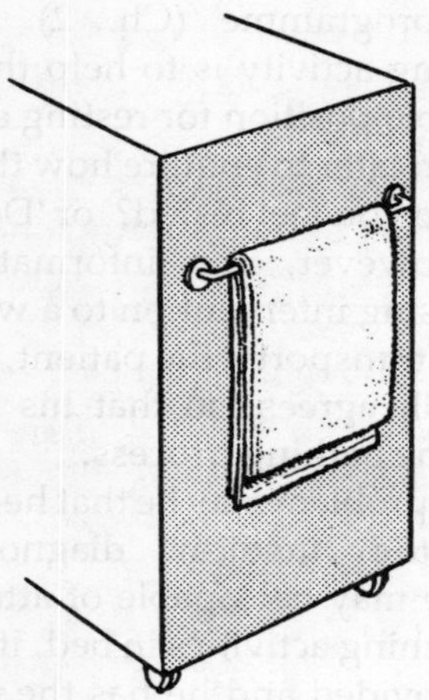

Fig. 8.5 Four thicknesses of towel only allows slow drying

silent. A nurse needs to respect this conception if the patient shows no desire to indulge in a long conversation during the bathing process. In those hospitals where it is customary for two staff members to participate in bed bathing they must refrain from talking to each other and convey to the patient by their gestures that they are not embarrassed by the lack of conversation. The extrovert patient who habitually sings in his bath will probably talk volubly throughout the procedure, ignoring the abnormal situation. The offer by the nurse to talk to the patient should be left wide open, so that the ensuing conversation can be patient-directed (p. 20).

To the nurse, bathing a patient affords an opportunity for observation of his body and estimation of his mental reactions.

To the patient a bed bath can provide the opportunity to exercise his body within the limits of his capability. He will thus be making his contribution to the prevention of pressure sores (p.116), chest infection (p.203), venous thrombosis and pulmonary embolism (p.211).

An unconscious patient needs intelligent, skilful bathing if he is to be unharmed by the process. If his body temperature has been intentionally reduced (hypothermia), the temperature of the bathing water will need to be adjusted accordingly. The limbs will probably be stiff and spastic and will need to be supported by one nurse without stretching the muscles and tendons, while the other nurse washes and dries the skin. Prevention of maceration of the skin folds and cleanliness of the genital area are temporarily the nurse's responsibility, as well as care of the nails, hair, teeth and eyes. The bath provides an opportunity for putting all joints through their full range of movement (passive movement).

The primary object of most bed-baths is cleansing and refreshment, but the procedure can be modified to:

- reduce an increased body temperature (pyrexia, hyperpyrexia) when it is called tepid sponging
- sedate a restless patient; long, soothing strokes need to be used to achieve this.

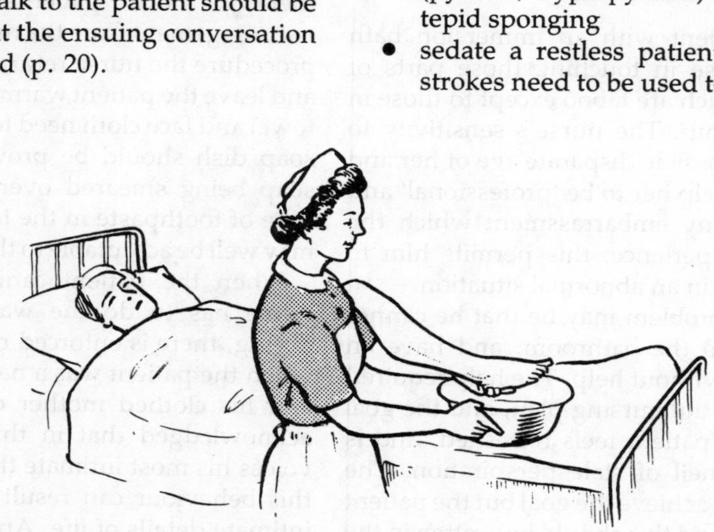

Fig. 8.6 Bed bathing

Evaluating

This chapter so far illustrates well that the four phases of the process of nursing are not carried out separately, but they can be overlapping. Evaluating depends on the goals set and these will be very different; they will be in tiny steps in a habilitating programme as might be used for those with mental handicap; or in bigger steps in a rehabilitating programme for a person who has a right hemiplegia. The goals will have been set in observable terms, such as when washing/bathing is carried out, where, how independently and so on. Whenever possible there will be detailed assessment data about such things as the level of independence a child has achieved; individual habits in relation to washing/bathing; and any problems which a patient is experiencing. The assessment data can be used as criteria for evaluating the stage of goal achievement. Evaluating is an ongoing activity and is not just carried out on the date set for it on the nursing plan; so on the date, inspection of the patient's nursing notes may reveal aspects of summative evaluation.

Included in the title of this chapter 'Helping patients to keep the body clean and well groomed' is care of nails, hair, feet, perineum, mouth and teeth and these will be discussed in that order in the context of the process of nursing.

CARE OF NAILS AND THE PROCESS OF NURSING

Nails were mentioned as part of the top to toe assessment proforma (p.9). Now that readers have had some practice in 'thinking process-wise' a few more aspects of assessing nails can be added here. Again written lists look formidable but they help nurses to 'scan' patients — almost subconsciously (professional judgement). The presence of the following will be noted on the assessment form:

- ragged cuticles
- a split in the flesh at the ends of the cuticle: hacks and keens are names used in different parts of the country
- long/medium/short nails
- neglected nails which curve over the finger end, more common with toe nails than finger nails
- honeycomb consistency on cutting nail, indicative of non-active fungal infection
- bitten nails — all/which ones?/right/left hand
- black line at the junction of the skin on the finger end and the nail: usually a collection of black grease used in some occupations: extremely difficult to remove
- blueness/cyanosis
- pale, rather than pink
- black area from pressure
- uncared for appearance
- nail varnish.

In very few instances will these observations result in identification of a problem which will be written on the nursing plan and so on. However for ragged cuticles and keens the nurse might suggest preparations like Dermidex which can be bought at the chemist's shop. The patient may or may not want the honeycomb condition of one or more nails reported to the doctor. The only advantage is that if the condition recurs, a prescription in the acute phase will prevent the honeycombing.

The planning phase of the process might need to be used if the patient has been admitted for operation on one or more nails; or if the patient has been admitted as an emergency with trauma to one or more nails.

The implementing phase is used each time a nurse helps a patient with an immersion bath or a bowl-bath in bed, or carries out bedbathing of the totally dependent patient. Should an incontinent patient get faeces under the nails it is the nurse's responsibility to remove it. People with disabled hands may be pleased to know that an emery board on a magnetic base is available from the Disabled Living Foundation. Application of coloured varnish may help to raise the flagging morale of a female patient coming to terms with loss of a part of the body; or changed self-image as in hemi/para/tetraplegia.

The evaluating phase may well be used by

people who are not nurses, including visitors to the ward. The standard of nail care in a ward conveys to visitors the value which nursing staff attach to this aspect of personal hygiene. Of course for those patients who have had nail surgery there will be 'formal' evaluation of whether or not the wound is healing and free from infection.

CARE OF HAIR AND THE PROCESS OF NURSING

Suggestions to be used when assessing the condition of a patient's hair are on page 8. Formal assessment is necessary for patients who are admitted with lacerations of the scalp and hair which is matted with blood and perhaps gravel or earth. In such an instance precise detail will be written on the patient assessment form so that the subjective and objective information can be used as criteria against which evaluation will be made. The patient's problems, identified from the assessment data, and if he is not exhausted, verified with him, are likely to be:

- experiencing pain
- feeling anxious about the amount of blood lost (the scalp is a highly vascular tissue)
- feeling frightened (remembers something about tetanus/wound/earth)

These may be written on the assessment form or the nursing plan whichever is the custom where you work.

When assessing the hair, particularly of children, nurses must be conversant with the appearance of infested hair and a scalp which is shedding dandruff. Here the nurse may encounter a situation where she perceives lice-infested hair as a problem but the patient does not. She needs to use all her creativity and ingenuity to persuade the patient to have the hair treated immediately to prevent infestation of staff and other patients. An ethical point may be involved: if the patient says he does not want the fact recorded, what should the nurse do? Another objective at the initial interview is to discover the patient's individual habits related to care of hair, and if it is relevant, it will be written on the assessment form.

The planning phase of the process of nursing related to care of hair is not necessary for the majority of patients. However for some, brushing and combing the hair may provide therapeutic movements, for example after a right mastectomy in right-handed people; after a left mastectomy in left-handed people. For the patient with scalp lacerations the nursing plan is likely to include use of a painometer; use of anxiety level scores; and teaching about tetanus innoculation.

The implementing phase (in the sense of carrying out a planned nursing intervention to achieve a goal set in relation to a problem which the patient is experiencing) is not necessary for the majority of patients. Some nurses do write the hair washing frequency on either the assessment form or the nursing plan of patients likely to stay for several weeks, so that this activity which is essential to patients' well-being does not get forgotten. Ill patients often sweat profusely, particularly at the nape of the neck. It is well known that stale perspiration is mal-odorous and to deal with this problem, the frequency of hair washing should be increased on the nursing plan.

A bed patient with two good arms and hands and a mirror can continue to look after her own hair. A bed patient with one good arm and hand can brush and comb her hair, but will need help with styling and fastening. As already mentioned, in some conditions combing the hair is a form of physiotherapy and such patients need encouragement and praise from the nursing staff. For a helpless patient a nurse has to take over the combing, brushing and arranging of hair in a becoming style. In illness the scalp often feels tender. The skill of removing tangles from the distal portion of a strand of hair while supporting the proximal portion against the scalp must be developed (Fig. 8.7). Facilities should be provided for at least weekly washing of brushes and combs.

An ambulant patient can continue to wash her hair as often as she does at home. Some hospitals provide a hairdressing salon; others arrange for a hairdresser to attend the wards. A patient requiring hair washing and confined to bed

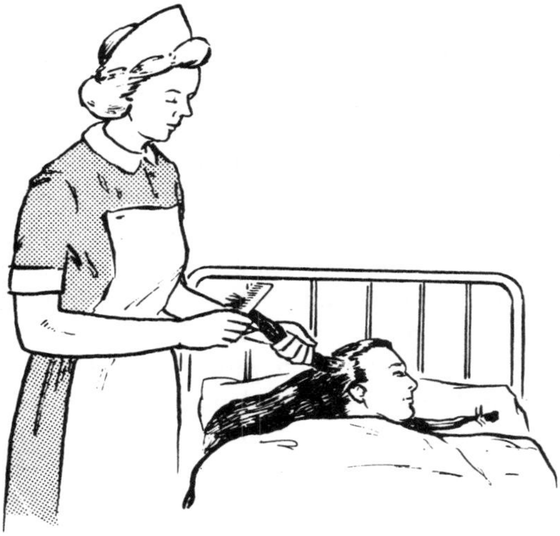

Fig. 8.7 Removing tangles from hair

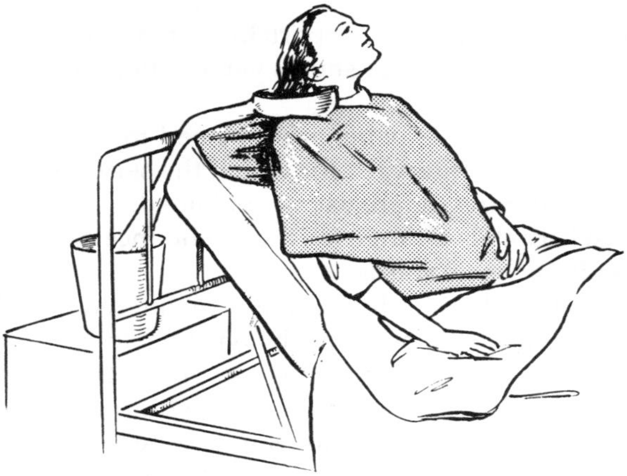

Fig. 8.9 'Back-wash' tray, mackintosh and bucket

presents a challenge to the nurse and/or hairdresser. Injury to the patient's and the nurse's back must be avoided (p. 157). A bed with a removable bed-head can be wheeled to a sink (Fig. 8.8). Some hairdressers use a 'back-wash' tray; a mackintosh funnels the water into a bucket at the back of the bed (Fig. 8.9). There is now a basin (Fig. 8.10) specially designed for this purpose. A patient rests her head backwards. The neck and shoulders are supported on the sloping contour at the front. When the shampoo

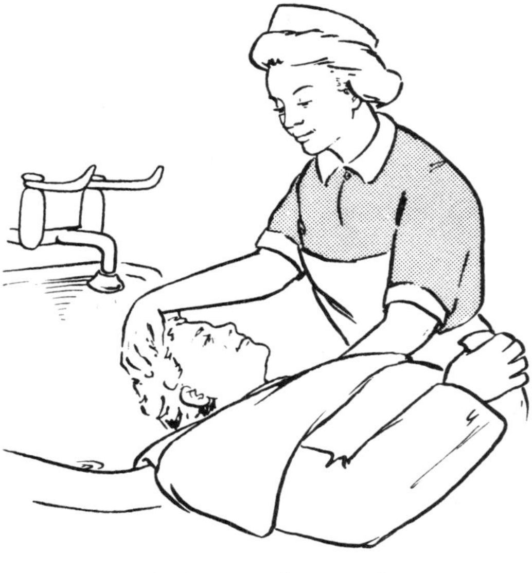

Fig. 8.8 Washing bed patient's hair at sink

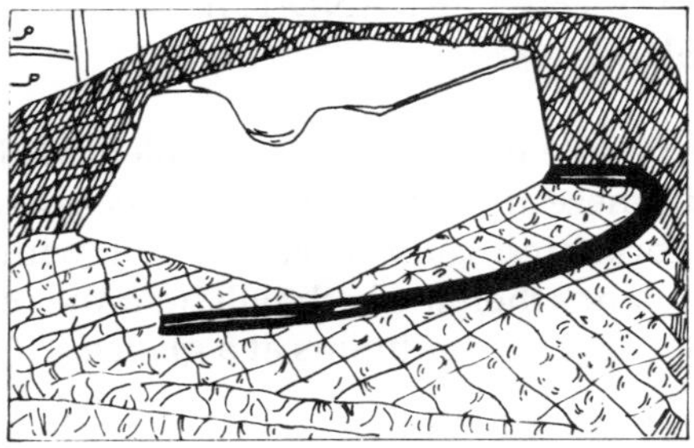

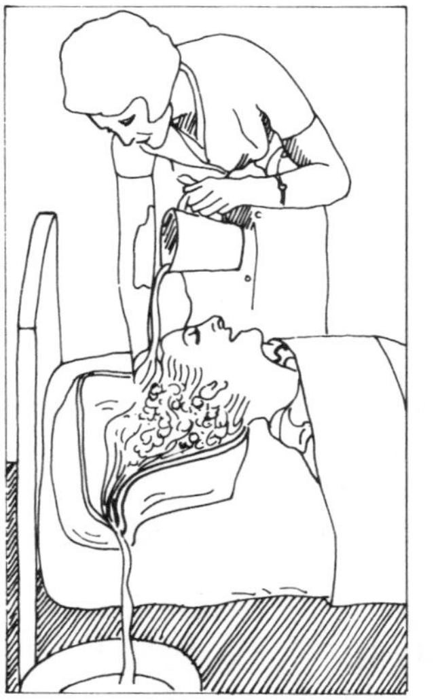

Figs. 8.10 & 8.11 Basins designed for use when washing hair in bed

is completed, the soapy water is emptied through the tubing into a portable container at the bedside. Figure 8.11 shows yet another type of basin.

Long-stay female patients may need to have their hair cut at intervals, for which the services of a local hairdresser are usually obtained.

Most hospitals arrange for the attendance of a barber in the male wards.

Evaluating the standard of hair care offered to patients may well be done by visitors to the ward, it is not difficult to recognise lank, malodorous hair on a person who is normally meticulous in caring for his hair and beard. It may involve inspecting the scalp for any remaining lice or observing a wound for stage of healing and presence of infection.

CARE OF THE FEET AND THE PROCESS OF NURSING

Many people do not have a problem with their feet but there are some who never seem to be free from corns and callosities. The following is an assessment schema which will help the nurse to rule out several conditions at a glance:

- athlete's foot
- blisters
- bruises
- bunion
- burns
- callosity
- chilblains
- cold feet
- cyanosis
- gangrene of toes
- hammer toe
- hot feet
- laceration
- lack of sensation
- malodorous shoes and stockings
- nails
- pallor
- paralysis
- perspiration
- scars
- verruca.

A patient may have one or more of these conditions even though they are not the reason for admission to hospital. Current belief among professional people is that nurses are well placed to educate and interest patients in healthy living. Whether or not the condition is written as a problem on the assessment form or nursing plan will depend on the circumstances. The patient's nursing plan may contain instructions to prepare the patient for foot surgery which means using knowledge from several chapters — 20, 21, 24. It may request that pedal pulses are taken and recorded; gangrenous toes are exposed and the rest of the body kept warm; wounds, burns and so on may be covered by a surgical dressing.

The implementing phase — putting the plan into action has already been mentioned and it serves to highlight the circulatory nature of the process of nursing. It may include helping a patient to learn about the treatment of athlete's foot and how to prevent re-infection. When implementing is concerned with carrying out a planned nursing intervention, an entry to this effect will be made on the patient's nursing notes.

Evaluation of the standard of care of feet in a ward is not as visible as that of hands! We have to go back to the patient's description of his problems with his feet, to the goals set in relation to the problems, to the nursing interventions to achieve the goals, and the date set for whether or not they are being or have been achieved. Some nurses are confused by the words evaluation and assessment; the same skills, tools and scoring systems are used in both, but evaluation is against baseline data — collected at the initial assessment interview.

CARE OF THE FEMALE PERINEUM AND THE PROCESS OF NURSING

The perineum per se is not usually 'assessed'. What is assessed concerns female urination:

- how often is urine passed, during the day/night?
- is there any scalding on passing urine?
- is there any pain on passing urine?

- is the urine cloudy?
- does the urine contain visible blood?
- if relevant, what meaning does the patient attach to the word 'cystitis'?
- is the urine malodorous? — can the malodour be described?

It is as a prevention against cystitis that care of the female perineum has been placed in this chapter about personal hygiene. Because of the short urethra and nearness of the anus through which faeces is expelled, there is ample opportunity for microorganisms from the bowel which are non-pathogenic in that organ, to enter the bladder via the urethra. Female children should be taught to carry out post micturition and defaecation toilet from front to back, and there should be separate flannels for the periurethral and perianal areas.

However there are instances when the perineum is assessed very carefully, midwifery being an example. Immediately after the birth there may be a perineal tear or an episiotomy which will be reported as factually as possible, for example length of wound, exact site — a line drawing may be useful, number of stitches, bruising and so on. Some gynaecological operations involve assessment of the perineum and occasionally people have the misfortune to fall astride a railing which results in perineal trauma. And, of course, currently, bruising and laceration from rape and incest has high publicity.

The nursing plan may have nursing interventions related to the following four broad groups:

- helping the patient to learn about the preventive aspects of perineal hygiene
- helping the patient to cope with perineal pain by using a painometer and an individualised pain programme
- providing external relief of pressure on the perineum
- helping the patient to prevent infection of a perineal wound: where relevant, teaching the use of a bidet.

Carrying out the planned nursing interventions will of course be written on the patient's nursing notes, and on the appointed date evaluating will be done, and the data compared with that from the assessment.

CARE OF MOUTH AND TEETH AND THE PROCESS OF NURSING

At the initial assessment interview the lips should be observed. A baby may be born with a hare lip and it is possible that a medical photographer will take a picture against which evaluation after surgery can be compared. Some adults still bear the scar from a repaired hare lip and note should be made of this on the assessment form. The presence of cold sores (herpes simplex), of cracks at the corners of the mouth (intertrigo), dry mouth (xerostomia) will be noted: a line drawing might be useful to inform nurses on the next shift. When admitting (assessing) children it is customary to note the presence of teeth in each quarter of a jaw on a line drawing:

5	4	3	2	1	1	2	3	4	5
5	4	3	2	1	1	2	3	4	5

20 teeth in first dentition

8	7	6	5	4	3	2	1	1	2	3	4	5	6	7	8
8	7	6	5	4	3	2	1	1	2	3	4	5	6	7	8

32 teeth in second dentition

This might be a useful schema if a patient wears a partial denture. The presence of dentures — upper/lower/both — is recorded on the assessment form and whether or not they bear the patient's name; more and more dentists are marking new dentures. Confused people can think that they brought their dentures to hospital, so this assessment information is essential. Demented patients on admission may have uncared-for dentures with soft food attached to them. This may be indicative of the fact that they are not capable of being independent in cleaning dentures. If the patient has been ill at home there may be dried brown crusts (sordes) in the mouth, on the lips and teeth. The tongue may be furred and this may interfere with appetite. The gums may bleed when even a soft brush is used and there may be an exposed nerve which is highly sensitive to hot or cold food. The breath may have a bad smell (halitosis) and if no cause can be found, such as decayed tooth or infected gum, taking a snack between meals may be helpful. A smell of acetone on the breath is indicative of diabetes. Should there be actual disease like cancer of the tongue or jaw, the sort of information to be collected by nurses is how it is affecting the person's everyday living. It may mean that the person cannot eat solids, and only drink lukewarm fluids and further questioning may reveal that inadequate calories are being taken; has the patient lost weight; if so, how much? It is a never-ending subject but enough has been said to encourage readers to think about nursing in a process context.

With the variety of possibilities outlined in the previous paragraph, beginning nurses need practice at listening to what the patient is experiencing as a problem and writing it in his words. And remember that the patient may have carious front teeth which you would expect to be a problem, but he gives no indication that he perceives them as a problem: it may not be justifiable to write it on the assessment form or nursing plan whichever is the custom, or confront him with it. It would be wise to report it verbally to the nurse in charge whose professional knowledge about the medical condition from which the patient is suffering and her clinical judgement will help her to cope with the situation.

In the implementing phase, the majority of patients in a ward will not be experiencing a problem with their teeth or mouths, but those patients confined to bed require to be given the necessary requisites for tooth cleaning at the appropriate time. The last tooth brushing before sleeping should be for 3 minutes to free the teeth from plaque which, if left, is invaded by microorganisms predisposing to dental caries. Maybe with a little humour, patients could be encouraged to develop this healthy habit.

Sometimes ill patients are unable to co-operate and the nurse is then responsible for preventing a sore mouth and dental caries. Howarth (1977) investigated the procedures (which have remained virtually unchanged over many years) to verify whether or not they were effective. She found that the mouth care procedure using swabs and forceps was ineffective at removing debris from the teeth; that an adult-size toothbrush was difficult to use in another person's mouth; that adequate hydration of the patient was all-important in preventing a dirty mouth. Those at risk of dehydration are the elderly and the drugged patients who seem to lose the protective thirst reflex. She concluded that the use of swabs on forceps was invalidated; that the use of a swabbed finger or foam applicator were more effective but that adequate brushing with a small baby toothbrush was the most effective.

Other studies (Wallace & Freeman 1978) advocate the use of battery operated automatic (oscillating not rotational) toothbrushes. Howarth (1977) found sodium bicarbonate 1 in 160 an effective cleansing agent after sordes had been softened and moistened with glycerin (glycerol) 20%. A stronger solution of glycerin (40%) is astringent! Patients with dry sore mouths found Vaseline soothing and its lubricating qualities lasted longer than glycerin as it did not get licked off as quickly. Lemon juice was the most effective salivary stimulant but excessive use can cause reflex exhaustion. Hilton (1980) found that Redoxon mouthwashes clean furred tongues and half a Redoxon tablet placed on the tongue effervesces and cleans.

Blisters around the lips are called herpes simplex or fever blisters; they are due to a virus infection and benefit from frequent dabbing with surgical spirit or spirits of camphor. Silicone cream, zinc cream and calamine lotion are also useful.

Every living person must have experienced a disinclination for food because of a nasty taste in the mouth. Anorexia and halitosis should therefore head the list of complications of a dirty mouth. Nourishment is essential for recovery from illness.

A patient with a poor appetite can sometimes be tempted to eat by cleaning his mouth before a meal.

In an attempt to help nurses to practise 'process thinking' in applying the principle of 'helping patients to keep the body clean and well groomed' there has been discussion of:

washing/bathing
care of nails
care of hair
care of feet
care of the female perineum
care of mouth and teeth

} in a process of nursing context.

APPLYING THE PRINCIPLE

A registered nurse must be capable of:

- exhibiting tolerance of, and respect for, patients' previous habits
- teaching those who are unfamiliar with the present day standard of personal hygiene
- helping patients to make maximum use of the facilities provided
- approaching the appropriate authorities for equipment which will improve the standard of personal hygiene that can be carried out by/for the patients
- ensuring privacy during these intimate procedures
- ensuring warmth, especially freedom from draughts
- ensuring that the objective for which the procedure is performed is achieved without causing fatigue of patient or nurse
- ensuring safety during the procedure, including prevention of back injury and cross infection as far as is humanly possible
- making a contribution to the hospital planning programme, whether it be modernisation of existing units, building new units or experimenting with new equipment.
- applying the principle — helping patients to keep the body clean and well groomed — in a process of nursing context.

WORKING ASSIGNMENT

Topics for discussion

- is it necessary to use a bath thermometer:

  when bed bathing
  for bathing in the bathroom
  when bathing a baby
  for washing hair in bed?

- a bed patient needs to be bathed. Only tepid water emerges from the hot water tap. What would you do?
- a patient is admitted to your ward. Her infested head is not noticed by any member of staff and is only brought to light when another patient complains of itchiness due to infestation. What steps should be taken by the staff to prevent recurrence of this situation?
- discuss the pros and cons of including a bath, in bed or in the bathroom, as part of the 'admission' of a patient
- when washing before settling for the night, a patient says, 'My towel is cold and wet, my face-cloth smells sour.'
- how would you encourage a 'dirty' patient to improve his hygiene habits? What steps can you take to help him continue these improved habits after discharge?
- there is an old lady in your ward. She has been in a month and has sweated profusely at intervals. She has not had her

hair washed. You are with the consultant when he says to the old lady, 'It looks as if it is some time since you visited your hairdresser.' What should be done?

- you visit an elderly relative in hospital. He is asleep when you arrive. When he wakens he tells you that he had a bath in the bathroom. Later he asks you to cut his finger nails.

Writing assignment

- how do the staff in your hospital cater for the cleanliness of patients' skin and appendages?
- in the rare instance of you finding a patient with an infested head, how would you treat it?
- in the rare instance of you being asked to admit a patient infested with body lice, how would you proceed?
- give the name for:

  loss of appetite
  bad breath
  brown, dried mucus on the lips and in the mouth
  blisters round the mouth
  the eggs laid by the head louse
- name an alkaline lotion which can be used for mouth cleaning
- what is the special property of an alkaline lotion with regard to a dirty mouth?
- why is glycerine used in mouth cleaning?
- name two complications of a dirty mouth
- name one preparation which will kill head lice
- name two lotions which can be used for blisters round the lips
- define the following:

  genital
  hygroscopic
  hyperpyrexia
  hypothermia
  i schaemia
  maceration
  objective information
  passive movement
  perianal
  perineum
  periurethral
  pyrexia
  spastic
  subjective information
- state the primary objective of most bed-baths
- what conditions are prevented by frequent moving of a bed-patient?
- state two objectives which can be achieved by modification of the bed-bath
- what is the average width of bath towel used by your patients?
- what is the average length of towel rail on your patients' lockers?
- is there a hook for a face-cloth on your patients' lockers?
- after use, where is the patient's tablet of soap put?
- what arrangements are made in your bathrooms and showers to prevent spread of foot infections?
- a medical diagnosis is 'laceration of the scalp'. State some possible patient's problems.

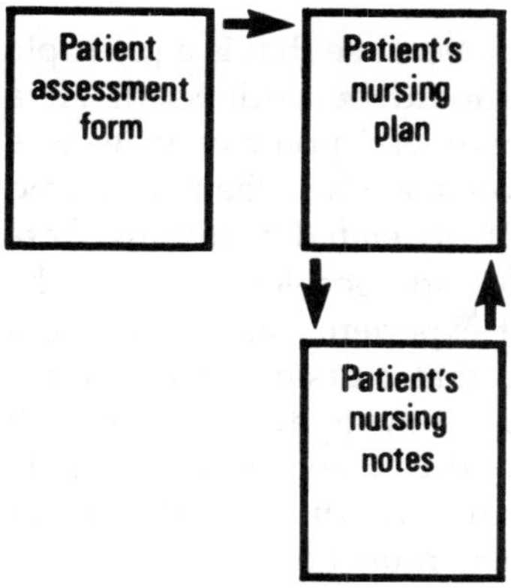

9

Helping patients to dress and undress

READING ASSIGNMENT

Disabled Living Foundation 1977 Dressing for disabled people: A manual for nurses and others. Disabled Living Foundation, London
Demonstrates not only the sorts of garments available and the modifications which can be made to ordinary clothes, but also, how with various disabilities dressing and undressing can be accomplished.

Dorado J 1980 Personal clothing for psychiatric patients: The right to one's own. Nursing Mirror 150 (15) April 10:40
Tells how a scheme to introduce personal clothes was set up; it was a success because all the people involved believed that having one's own clothes is a basic human right.

Hinks M D 1977 Clothing and the long-term patient. Nursing Mirror 144 (10) March 10: 39–41
The laundry can ruin garments; horrors of pooled underwear; statistics of mentally handicapped children and adults who have feet outside Clark's normal standard; sustained effort needed to restore patients' dignity; nursing staff had little idea of how to dress a patient.

Holland G P 1978 Clothing and the elderly. Nursing Times 74 (2) January 12: 69–70
Demoralisation from lack of personal clothing; one needs to walk into a continued care area where patients have full access to clean

clothing to feel the return of their dignity, pride and individuality.

Knight S E, Lewis J D 1978 The effect of footwear on venous pressure at the ankle. Nursing Mirror 147 (6) August 10: 22–24
Exercise sandals decrease venous pressure in the calf and thus the risk of varicose veins.

Long A 1979 Implementation of a personalised clothing policy for long stay psychiatric patients. Journal of Advanced Nursing 4 (4) July: 415–427
The evidence suggests that a change in hospital procedure needs to be accompanied by a successful information network and a change in staff attitudes.

Norton D, McLaren R, Exton-Smith A N 1975 An investigation of geriatric nursing problems in hospital. Churchill Livingstone, Edinburgh, p 162–191
Section on investigation of clothing suitable for elderly and disabled patients; illustrations of various items of clothing.

Pearce E 1980 A general textbook of nursing. Faber and Faber, London, p 19–20
Clothes associated with personality; dressing and undressing are complex activities, can be rehabilitative in nature; description of how to help disabled people to dress and undress.

Stryker R 1977 Rehabilitative aspects of acute and chronic nursing care. W B Saunders, Philadelphia, p 228–235
Dressing with quadriplegia; dressing upper trunk with one hand; lower trunk dressing; putting on hose and stockings; underclothing; problems with fastenings, jewelry; illustrated.

Thomas L 1987 Hope to preserve my dignity in old age. Nursing Standard 498 May 28:4
Poor personalised clothing systems are still a fact of life in very many hospitals. Even where personalised day clothes have been achieved, patients are still wearing underclothing from a communal supply.

It is interesting to note that though there were several articles written in the 1970s, there have since been few additions to the Reading Assignment. The title of the chapter has been changed from 'Clothing' to 'Helping patients to dress and undress' because that is a principle of nursing which should be addressed. At a conference, the consumers' point of view was expressed by a person in a wheelchair, who said that spirits could be truly elated if clothing were suitable, comfortable and good-looking. But she reported that recent experience as an inpatient had convinced her that nursing staff on the whole had little idea of how to dress a patient. If helping patients to dress and undress is to continue as a 'nursing' activity, the deficiency reported by consumers must be remedied.

BACKGROUND INFORMATION

The Municipal and Voluntary Hospitals of 50 to 100 years ago catered for the ragged poor, some of whom were infested with head and body lice. The pattern of admitting a patient was to divest him of his rags, bath him and small tooth comb his hair and then dress him in hospital attire, so there was no need of accommodation for patients' clothes. In many hospitals today there is inadequate accommodation. The relatives are asked to bring a case and take the patient's outdoor clothes away. A special carrier bag (Fig. 9.1) is manufactured for those admitted via an Accident and Emergency department, who do not have a case with them. To many people who are assuming the patient role in such an emergency, absence of their day clothes is a demoralising affront to their freedom.

Common sense tells us that we judge others by the clothes they wear. Clothes act as a medium of

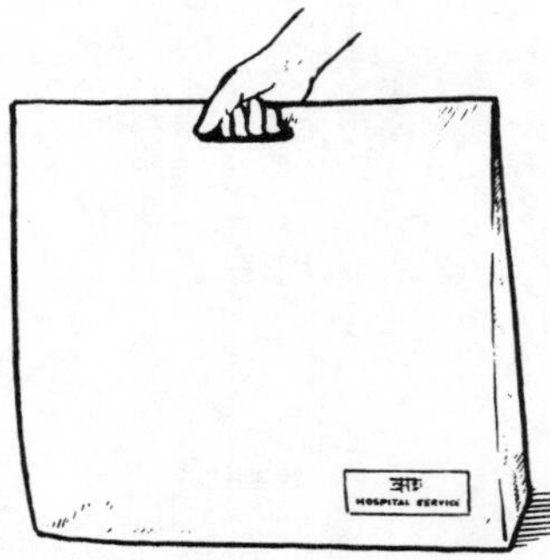

Fig. 9.1 Carrier bag for clothes

communication, just as language does. We need to think seriously if we have any right to deprive a person of a means of communication. One cannot think of one reason, other than tradition, for compelling patients to wear their pyjamas and dressing gowns when walking about. Most people would agree that having one's own clothes is a basic human right (Dorado 1980).

It is to be hoped that in any new building, a wardrobe which will lock will be considered as essential as a bed. 'Built-in' wardrobes need to be considered in rebuilding and new building schemes. As soon as a patient can be up for a couple of hours he needs the therapy of donning daytime attire. The sight of patients clad in dressing gowns, pyjamas and bedroom slippers walking in the hospital grounds ought to spur us on to seek better amenities. Figure 9.2 illustrates how one hospital solved its 'wardrobe' problem. Dorado (1980) describes how a hospital built clothing cubicles in the old hydrotherapy room; in other wards they used space which was available because of a reduction in patient numbers.

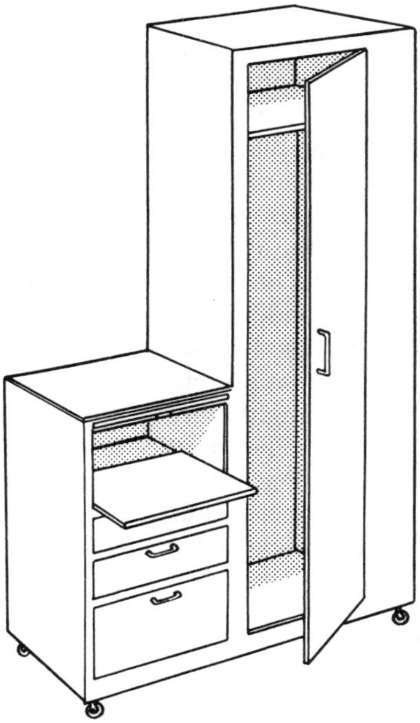

Fig. 9.2 How one hospital solved its 'wardrobe' problem

Nowadays most hospitals allow patients the pleasure of wearing their own night attire, provided they make arrangements for washing same. Nurses need to be diligent in preventing this personal clothing going to the hospital laundry. Many older patients are in the habit of sleeping in a vest. It is unkind to deny them this warmth. Perhaps one could encourage them to have a 'day' and 'night' vest.

All hospitals need to have a stock of night attire for patients admitted in an 'emergency'. Because attire from infectious patients needs special laundering, such patients are often advised to wear garments provided by the hospital. These should be as pleasing and as practical as possible.

Since fabric handkerchiefs were previously considered part of personal apparel, in these days adequate supplies of paper handkerchiefs should be given to each patient together with a disposable bag for used ones. Some beds have a metal ring to which these bags can be attached. In some hospitals the bag is attached to the bottom sheet or the locker with adhesive tape.

There is a special double-sided, self-adhesive strip (Fig. 9.3) which enables disposable bags to be fixed to any surface without damaging it. When the bag is ready for disposal, it can be sealed by folding over the top and sticking it down on to the same strip of adhesive thereby contributing to prevention of nosocomial infection (Ch. 20).

Some outpatients need to strip down to their undergarments — vest and pants, or brassiere and pants. A dressing gown is provided for modesty and warmth while waiting for the examination. Many outpatients needing X-ray are asked to remove all their clothes and put on a simple cotton gown with an over-wrap and waist tie. Over this they place a dressing gown while waiting. Both these are large garments to wash after each wearing, but have we any right to expect a patient to wear a gown that has covered someone else's naked or near naked body? The expense of sufficient gowns, storage space, adequate arrangements for worn gowns and laundering, appear to influence the recommendations in the most recent Department circular: it advocates washable material and clean gowns daily. Some hospitals are advising

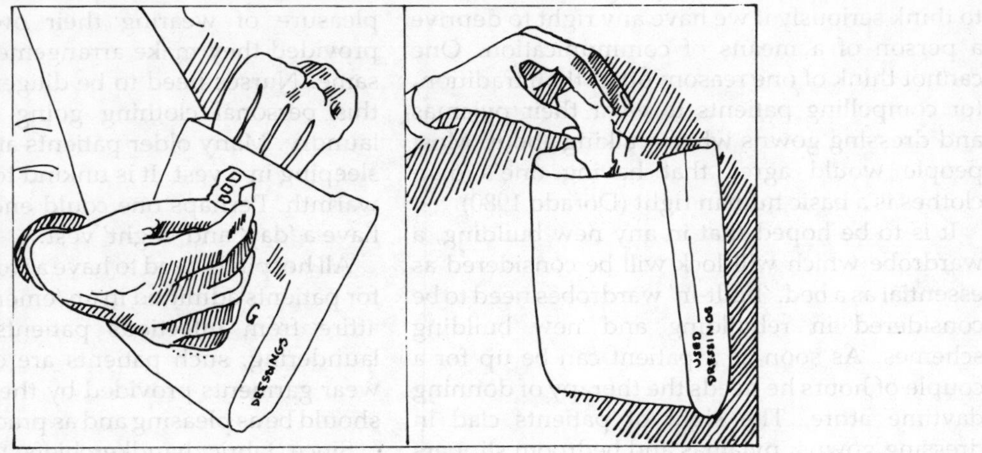

Fig. 9.3 Fixing disposable bags using double-sided self-adhesive strip

outpatients to bring a dressing gown with them.

DRESSING AND UNDRESSING AND THE PROCESS OF NURSING

There is a sense in which nurses first have to learn what it means to patients to be dressed in:

- night attire of their own choice, which means that they are dependent on visitors for collecting, laundering and returning it
- hospital night attire, either because:
  - — they were admitted in emergency
  - — there is no one to attend to private laundry requirements
  - — they have an infectious disease and the garment will require special treatment
  - — they are incontinent of urine and/or faeces and the garment will need to be laundered frequently.

Nurses should try to imagine the further indignity heaped upon a patient when clean garments are not available due to deficiencies in the hospital laundry service.

Nurses have to learn to respect the fact that individuals express their individuality and different aspects of their sexuality in both night attire and day clothes. But the main association with night attire occurs while a child, having to conform to the parents' interpretation of bedtime and thereafter for most people night clothes are associated with sleeping or relaxing about the house, whereas the donning of daytime attire, especially shoes instead of bedroom slippers, is of deep positive psychological significance. To those who have been very ill, possibly in a life threatening situation, donning daytime clothes may mean the beginning of restructuring life, even though they may have tried very hard to exercise by walking along the corridors outside the ward. There is an unreality about walking along, clothed in a dressing gown and meeting strangers. Before the illness the person was in charge of his life as he perceived it; he dressed according to his mood, or the appropriateness of the occasion; he felt that he had a measure of control over the situation, but not now when he is the one wearing night attire in the daytime.

Now to attempt some 'practice thinking' about the concept of dressing and undressing in the four phases of the process of nursing — assessing, planning, implementing and evaluating.

Assessing

Where do nurses practise skills in assessing clothing as a form of non-verbal communication? The health visitors' clients are dressed in dayclothes whether the initial assessment interview takes place in the home or at the health clinic. School nurses do not normally conduct initial assessments of every school child and the clients are unusual in that in some schools they wear uniform! Nurses working in outpatients' departments see patients in outdoor clothes, then wearing whatever gown is provided. For patients who are admitted from the waiting list, the custom in many hospitals is to escort them to the bedside and ask them to get into nightclothes in readiness for the doctor's admission examination.

Nurses need to develop a schema of questions which can be borne in mind, not necesssarily asked, when assessing clothing, such as:

- are they appropriate for the environmental temperature?
- are they socially appropriate?
- are they clean and free from:
  - blood
  - vomit
  - faeces
  - urine
  - stale odour?
- are they new/shabby?
- do they give any clue as to:
  - a religious order
  - expressing sexuality
  - culture
  - sports allegiance and so on?

If the admitting nurse observes any of the following:

- arm in a sling
- limb in plaster
- leg in caliper
- absent limb/s
- artificial limb (prosthesis)
- rheumatoid hands

she is alerted to discover what this means to the patient in relation to dressing and undressing.

Children who are not yet independent for all aspects of dressing and undressing will need a detailed initial assessment, so that nurses on each succeeding shift, after reading the assessment form, will know exactly what the child is capable of doing independently, and with which aspects he needs nursing or parental help. During a long stay, a child may acquire a greater degree of independence in some of the actions which are part of dressing and undressing skills. Observation (assessment) of increasing habilitation will be recorded on the patient's nursing notes to facilitate individualised nursing, whichever nurses are on duty.

Mentally handicapped people suffer from the same illnesses from time to time as the rest of the population and are therefore likely to be admitted to a medical or surgical ward. By virtue of the handicap the person is a slow learner; even though he may have a biographical adult age, he has a mental age, and a developmental age of a child. For these patients exact details of what can and cannot be done in relation to dressing and undressing needs to be written, so that all nurses, after reading the information on the assessment form, know what nursing help to offer. In more recent years behaviour modification programmes have helped many mentally handicapped people to be completely independent in dressing and undressing.

People who live in wheelchairs (because of such conditions as spinal injury, and neurological diseases, the best known of which is probably multiple sclerosis) usually require some form of help with dressing and undressing. This is not a new problem in the patient's life and it has been adequately coped with in the community. Exactly what sort of nursing help is needed must be written on the assessment form for use by nurses on each succeeding shift. But in the case of, for example, multiple sclerosis, there can be gradual deterioration which will probably mean that increased human help will be needed and this can be recorded on the patient's nursing notes, or, on the nursing plan because it will probably need a nursing intervention related to 'teaching relatives', or it may involve procuring an 'aid' to help the patient to dress and undress.

Another large and increasing group of people who need to have well developed rehabilitation programmes related to dressing and undressing are those who have suffered a stroke (cerebrovascular accident CVA) which has caused hemiplegia. An initial assessment, possibly with input from a physiotherapist, will reveal which of the tiny actions that make up the composite dressing and undressing skills, have to be practised by the patient with much praise and encouragement from nurses. The patient's problem 'cannot move right arm and leg' will affect several other everyday living activities.

After having discussed four groups of people — children, mentally handicapped people, wheelchair people and people who have had a stroke – in an 'assessing' context, it is pertinent to remind readers that since assessing is an ongoing activity, information on the assessment form records the patient's dependence/independence for dressing and undressing on that date, and further information will be written in the patient's nursing notes; should a new problem be revealed, it will be written on the nursing plan, together with the goal and the nursing intervention to achieve the goal.

Planning

Starting with the patients' nursing plan, the majority will not require an entry related to clothing, dressing and undressing. Where an entry is necessary, in many instances there will need to be long-term goals and it is important that these are divided into tiny measurable steps, achievement of which will serve to reinforce flagging motivation in a rehabilitation programme which can be a long haul. There is a danger that without these tiny steps, inexperienced nurses will demand the long term goal of independence long before the patient's musculature is capable of achieving it. It is therefore important that the nursing intervention is written in sufficient detail for the patient's individualised dressing plan to proceed smoothly whichever nurse, on whichever shift, carries out the plan.

In the last few decades there has been generalised planning to achieve personalised clothing for all long-term patients. To acknowledge the importance of clothing and appearance to the well-being of each individual, a meeting of representatives of a number of the caring professions and organisations is reported by Hinks (1977). Summing up she wrote:

> A long-term campaign of sustained pressure on several fronts seemed to be the answer if the aim of personalised clothing for all long-term patients is to be achieved. Such an activity would include increased emphasis on the importance of clothing and dressing of patients, with the provision of adequate practical experience in the training syllabi of all caring professions, greater interdisciplinary co-operation and understanding at all levels, the involvement of manufacturers and the relations of patients, and the introduction and establishment of the post of clothing manager at hospital level.

But the mere introduction of a personalised clothing service cannot of itself change the negative attitudes some nurses have to patients and their clothing (Long 1979). The objective of the Department circular was 'to help a patient rebuild his self-respect and enable him to return to independent life in the community'. Concluding her report Long (1979) wrote:

> There was no relationship between the change in policy and the staff's perception of helping a patient rebuild his self-respect...

Implementing

Each time a planned nursing intervention is carried out, an entry will be made in the patient's nursing notes. Physically and mentally disabled patients, the frail elderly and incontinent people may require modified clothing. The Disabled Living Foundation's publication (1977) should be essential reading for all nurses. Not only does it contain suggestions about adapting clothing but also illustrates several gadgets to help disabled people to retain their independence in dressing and undressing. Further information about clothes, dressing and undressing is contained in Norton et al (1975), Pearce (1980) and Stryker (1977). The Army and Navy Stores world-wide mail order list contains some items suitable for disabled people; this is an advantage to those who cannot, or only rarely, visit shops.

The Clothing Advisory Service of The Disabled Living Foundation will answer letters or telephone enquiries about clothing and dressing.

Evaluating

The results of nurses' and patients' efforts at dressing and undressing can be evaluated by visitors to the ward! In some wards dressing and undressing may be part of a behavioural scoring system which is used: the data gained at the initial assessment will be the baseline against which scores achieved on the date set for evaluation will be compared. As the patient is progressing towards optimal independence relevant to his capabilities and circumstances, there usually has to be judicious withdrawal of nursing help.

In the long-stay areas where personalised clothing systems are advocated, standards of achieving this will be evaluated by using procedures such as Performance Indicators and Quality Assurance Programmes.

In this chapter, wearing daytime clothes has been considered as a form of non-verbal communicating. Patients wearing their own daytime clothes was advocated, particularly in long-stay areas. The principle of helping patients to dress and undress was discussed in a process of nursing context.

APPLYING THE PRINCIPLE

A registered nurse must be capable of:

- empathising with patients when day clothes have to be sent home because of lack of space
- co-ordinating a rehabilitation programme to optimise an individual's independence for dressing and undressing relevant to his capabilities and circumstances
- teaching the skills of dressing and undressing disabled patients
- carrying out or working towards a policy whereby ambulant patients can wear their own daytime clothes.
- applying the principle — helping patients to dress and undress — in a process of nursing context.

WORKING ASSIGNMENT

Topics for discussion

- helping patients to dress and undress is a nursing activity
- the patient role
- a patient's medical diagnosis is late stage rheumatoid arthritis. You observe very deformed hands. What problems might the patient be experiencing with dressing and undressing?
- patients' rights/responsibilities in relation to their clothes
- nurses' rights/responsibilities in relation to patients' clothes.

Writing assignment

- define the following:

  caliper
  cerebrovascular accident
  CVA
  expressing sexuality
  habilitation
  hemiplegia
  multiple sclerosis
  paraplegia
  Performance Indicators
  plaster
  prosthesis
  Quality Assurance Programmes
  rehabilitation
  schema of questions for assessing clothing
  sling
  stroke
  tetraplegia

- write a short essay on the part played by clothes in non-verbal communication.

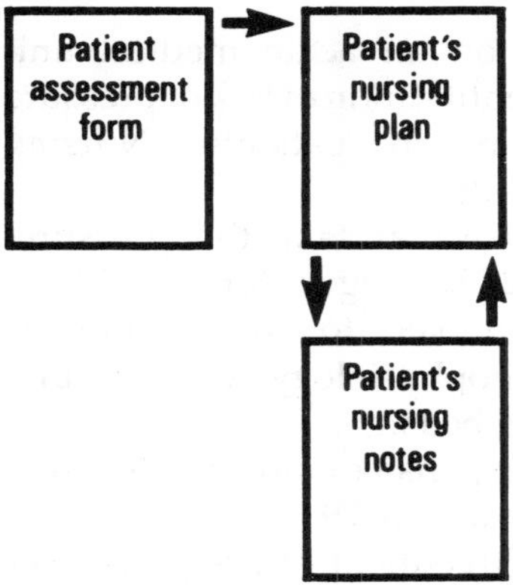

10

Helping patients to prevent pressure sores

READING ASSIGNMENT

Anthony D 1984 Measuring pressure sores accurately. Nursing Times 80 (36) September 5: 33–35
Describes the highly complex problem of measuring pressure sores — different shapes, vertically and horizontally and in depth.

Anthony D 1985 Nursing Times 81 (22) May 29: 57, 59, 61
Compares three methods to determine a procedure which provided the greatest accuracy for measuring pressure sores.

Barbenel J C, Jordan M M, Nicol S M, Clark M O 1977 Incidence of pressure sores in the Greater Glasgow Health Board. The Lancet September 10: 540–550.
Those aged 70 and over accounted for 70% of the patients with sores. Chairfast patients consistently had a higher pressure sore frequency than bedfast patients.

Barratt E 1987 Putting risk calculators in their place. Nursing Times 83 (7) February 18: 65–66, 68, 70
Reviews the various 'at risk' scales but warns that their value may be suspect, since no evaluation of their accuracy is available. However, such predictors do have a use, though they should not be substituted for clinical judgement.

Baynes V 1984 Sore point in the NHS. Nursing Mirror 159 (16) October 131: xi–xiv, xvi–xvii

The cost of pressure sores is high. The author offers a simple method of assessing 'at risk' patients.

Bliss M, Murray E 1979 The use of Ripple beds. Nursing Times 75 (7) February 15: 280–283
Detailed, illustrated account of how to use the alternating pressure mattress for prevention of, and healing of pressure sores: financially economic apparatus.

Bromley P 1985 A sore point with nurses. Nursing Times 82 (32) August 6: 65
A visitor's tale after her 90-year-old mother was admitted to hospital. We should listen to visitors — this one was a daughter!

Chapman E J, Chapman R 1986 Treatment of pressures sores: the state of the art. In: Tierney A (ed) 1986 Clinical nursing practice. Recent advances in nursing, 14. Churchill Livingstone, Edinburgh, p 105–124

David J 1986 Float like a butterfly. Community Outlook May: 19, 21– 22
Looks at the range of aids which can help to prevent pressure sores in the community.

David J, Chapman E J, Chapman R G, Lockett B 1985 A survey of prescribed nursing treatment for patients with established pressure sores. CARE The British Journal of Rehabilitation and Tissue Viability 1 (1) Spring: 18–20
Reports the most recent national survey. Recommended as essential reading.

Deacon L 1986 Does anyone read research? Nursing Times 82 (32) August 6: 57–58
Illustrates the disillusionment of a first year nurse.

Gould D 1985 Nursing Mirror 160 (1) January 2: 19–20
Advocates urgent rationalisation of methods of prevention and treatment of pressure sores.

Hibbs P 1985 Taking off the pressure. Nursing Mirror 160 (13) March 27: iii–vi
Outlines the preventive and curative methods used in the London health authority where she works.

Isles J 1986 An eradication campaign. Nursing Times 82 (32) August 6: 59–60, 62
Total commitment from all those involved in patient care is the only way the problem of pressure sores can be tackled.

Jones J 1986 An investigation of the diagnostic skills of nurses on an acute medical unit relating to the identification of risk of pressure sore development in patients. Nursing Practice 1 (4): 257–267

Livesley B 1986 Airwaves take the pressure. Nursing Times 82 (32) August 6: 67–68, 71
Explains the rationale for using airwave technology; pathophysiology of pressure; pressure relieving beds.

Livesley B 1987 An expensive epidemic. Nursing Times 83 (6) February 18: 79
With the cost of treatment of pressure sores continually rising, it is time for a national policy on their prevention.

Lowthian P 1979 Turning clock system to prevent pressure sores. Nursing Mirror 148 (21) May 24: 30–31
Principles used in designing 24-hour turning clocks; illustrated.

Lowthian P 1987 The classification and grading of pressure sores. CARE Science and Practice 5 (1) March: 5–9

Mack S 1986 Care and management of pressure sores. Nursing: The Add-On Journal of Clinical Nursing 3 (6) June: 219–221
Nursing care; pressure relief; dressings; Table of grade and treatment of sores; Illustration of a nursing care plan.

Norton D, McLaren R, Exton-Smith A N 1975 An investigation of geriatric nursing problems in hospital. Churchill Livingstone, Edinburgh
First British nursing research report; development of the Norton scoring system to identify at-risk patients, tested for reliability and validity.

Nursing Practice Committee, 1986 Pressure sores. Royal Marsden Hospital, London
Manual on the treatment of pressure sores.

Osborne S 1987 A quality circle investigation. Nursing Times 83 (16) February 18: 73, 75–76
A quality circle is a problem solving team to find ways of reducing, in this instance, pressure sores in four medical wards and it succeeded.

Pritchard V 1986 Calculating the risk. Nursing Times 82 (8) February 19: 59, 61
Describes and discusses use of the Douglas score for predicting patients at risk of developing pressure sores

Smith I.1984 Heel aids. Nursing Times 80 (36) September 5: 35–36, 39
Pressure sores on heels continue to be a major and unpredictable problem in orthopaedic wards. Heels appear to be at risk even when the patient's Norton score is relatively high.

Squibb Surgicare Limited 1986 Blueprint for the prevention and management of pressure sores. Department of Infection Control, Memorial Hospital, Darlington, Co Durham UK

Stapleton M 1986 Irish Nursing Forum and Health Services. May/June: 16, 19
A research project which compared foam, ripple pads and Spenco pads in the prevention of pressure sores.

Versluysen M 1986 Pressure sores: causes and prevention. Nursing: The Add-On Journal of Clinical Nursing 3 (6) June: 216–218
Describes the pathogenesis of pressures sores; quotes Goldstone as saying that the Norton score is the most reliable indicator for routine clinical use with the elderly.

Wade W 1984 Relieving the pressure. Nursing Times 80 (36) September 5: 41–42
Illustrates a body chart for recording presence of pressure sores: users are requested to indicate approximate size and depth.

Warner W, Hall D 1986 Pressure sores: a policy for prevention. Nursing Times 82 (16) April 16: 59–61 (Occasional Paper)
The policy which resulted from this research was to give special pressure sore preventive care to patients who would be expected to have a stay of more than 2 weeks, and who had a Norton score of less than 15.

Waterlow J 1985 A risk assessment card. Nursing Times 81 (48) November 27: 49, 51, 55
Describes the development and use of a guide which can be obtained from Dermatology and Tissue Repair Department, Pharmacia Ltd, Midsummer Boulevard, Milton Keynes MK9 3HP

Wright D, Goodman C, Hall D 1986 Pressure to act. Senior Nurse 5 (1) July: 12–13
It takes time for research knowledge to filter through to clinical practice. As a result of this survey four applications to pressure sores were withdrawn from service.

BACKGROUND INFORMATION

The rigid bony skeleton is clothed with soft tissues, composed mainly of subcutaneous tissue containing fat, and muscle tissue, all of which are richly supplied with blood and held together by the skin. These soft tissues are involved in the injury known as a pressure sore. To maintain them in a healthy condition they require:

- absence of toxins and allergens in the blood and external environment
- adequacy in volume and constituents of the blood supply
- adequate removal of waste products of metabolism
- body temperature within the range of normal
- continuity of skin surface
- intact nerve supply to receive and respond to stimuli warning of danger
- removal from the skin at intervals, of
  - dust
  - fluff from clothing
  - microorganisms
  - perspiration
  - scales
  - sebum.

Whenever people sit, lie or squat, they compress the skin and underlying tissues between the surface on which they sit, lie or squat and that portion of the skeleton which is bearing the weight — the *pressure areas* (Figs 10.1, 10.2, 10.3 & 10.4). Healthy people make frequent *spontaneous movements* in response to stimuli received by the brain even while asleep; the compression therefore is never sufficiently prolonged to cause any tissue damage.

Pressure sores

It is when there is *interference with the ability to make these movements* that the possibility of over-compression with resultant tissue damage occurs. The following conditions can result in lack of movement:

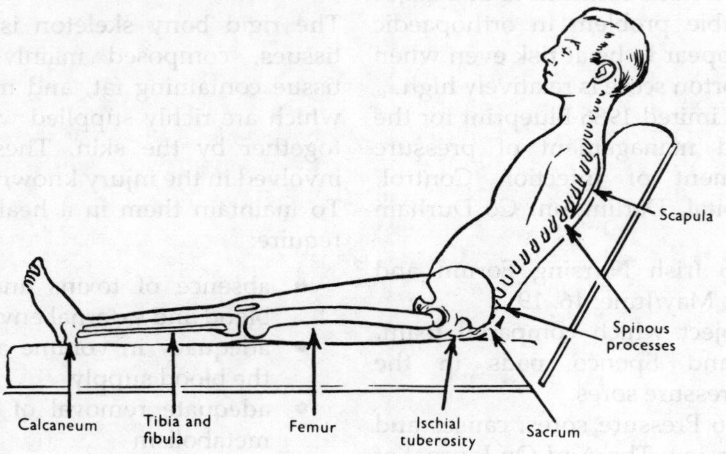

Fig. 10.1 **Pressure areas when sitting in bed**

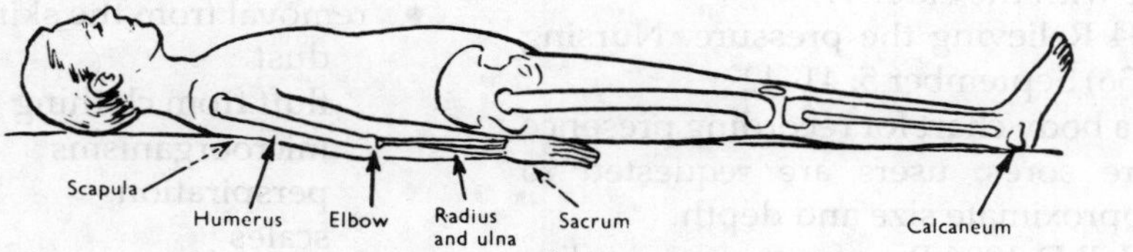

Fig. 10.2 Pressure areas when patient lying on back. The spinous processes are not shown

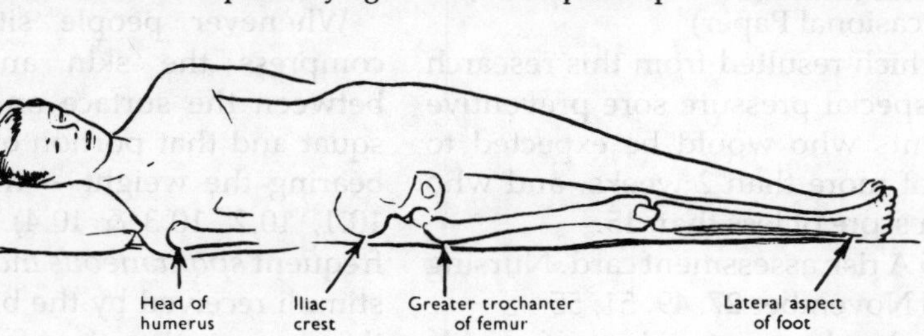

Fig. 10.3 **Pressure areas when patient lying on side**

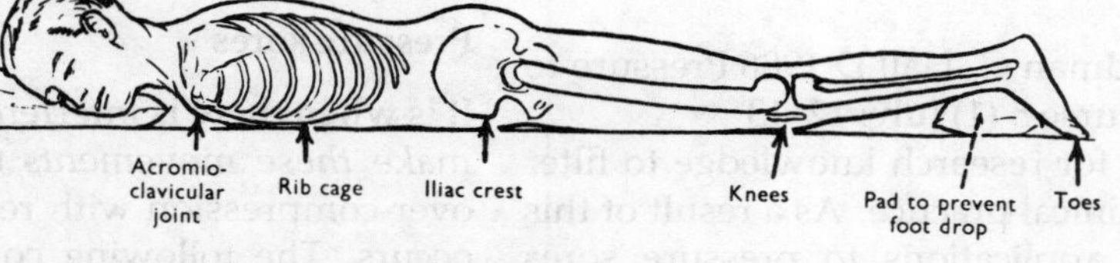

Fig. 10.4 **Pressure areas when patient in prone position**

- anaesthesia
- apathy
- changed state of consciousness due to alcohol/hard drugs/sleeping pills
- frailty
- pain on movement
- paralysis
- unconsciousness.

Over-compression of tissues for longer than the critical period, which according to research findings (Norton et al 1975) is 2 hours for those at greatest risk, reduces the blood supply; the cells receive fewer nutrients and less oxygen and there is less efficient removal of waste products. Some authors refer to what happens in the tissues as 'pathogenesis' or 'pathophysiology'. Versluysen (1986) describes the pathogenesis in terms of extrinsic and intrinsic factors. (She also gives a succinct account of the principles of prevention.) Livesley (1986) contains a very clear illustrated account of the pathophysiology of pressure sores.

Another force which can result in pressure sores is that of *shearing*. When any part of the body is on a gradient, the deeper tissues near the bone, mainly muscle with their excellent blood supply 'slide' towards the lower gradient while the skin is held at its contact surface by friction which is increased in the presence of moisture. This causes stretching and angulation of blood vessels (microcirculation) in the deep sheared area; the deep tissues become ischaemic and can become necrotic before tracking to the skin.

Before leaving the subject of pressure sores in a general context it is important to emphasise that articles in the Reading Assignment address:

- the causes of pressure sores
- assessment of patients for their risk of developing pressure sores
- changes in the tissues which are evident in established pressure sores, both superficial and deep
- the size of the problem in patients being nursed at home and in hospital
- estimated financial costs in the UK, North America, Australia, South Africa and Scandinavia
- external aids to relieve pressure which can cause pressure sores
- the variety of regimes used in treating pressure sores
- requests for rationalisation of treatment.

For those readers who already have some research knowledge, and those who want to explore the subject further, each of the articles contains references which can be obtained and read critically.

PRESSURE SORES AND THE PROCESS OF NURSING

Here it is pertinent to remind readers that 'the process' is merely a logical method of carrying out nursing and that it has to be used in an agreed context of what constitutes 'nursing'. Several nurses have published their beliefs about what constitutes nursing and have called these either 'a theory of nursing' or 'a model for nursing'. The relevant definition of theory in the Concise Oxford Dictionary is 'supposition or system of ideas explaining something', and of model is '...thing proposed for imitation'. A series of articles entitled 'Models and theories' (Aggleton & Chalmers 1984) is referenced on page 1. A quote from Livesley (1987) is appropriate here:

> Although improved use of the nursing process can go a long way to enabling every ward and hospital to produce its own information for analysis and action, two other issues are hindering this development. First, there is a widespread shortage of nursing staff which has been highlighted by seasonal factors. Second, and according to Jones (1986), 'many nurses now in clinical practice have a great deal of knowledge about the nursing process but little experience and skill in using it to bring about solutions to patient problems in an organised, systematic, and efficient manner.'

Some ideas about 'thinking in process context' — assessing, planning, implementing and evaluating — will be discussed in the following text. It has to be remembered that interpretation of the process of nursing should be greater than the sum of the four phases.

Assessing

By custom the phase of assessing is associated with the initial interview, with the prime objective of collecting the information requested by the assessment form and any other information which the interviewing nurse considers to be pertinent. We are beginning to give credence to assessing as an ongoing activity and writing the information so gained on the patient's nursing notes. The patient may have walked in and looked as if he is in reasonable general condition, but he may be scheduled for major cardiac surgery which will involve being bedfast for several days, followed by a very gradual rehabilitation to sitting out in a chair, then walking again. Consequently being at risk of developing pressure sores may not apply preoperatively but almost certainly will postoperatively.

The first scoring scale was published by Norton et al (1975). It was developed and tested on geriatric patients, and it is illustrated in Figure 10.5, with instructions for its use. Other scoring systems have been developed over the years and are included in the Reading Assignment although some prior research knowledge is needed to thoroughly understand some of them. Barratt (1987) reviews several of them but warns that their value may be suspect, since no evaluation of their accuracy is available. However she believes that such predictors still have a place, though they should not be used as substitutes for clinical judgement.

To help beginning nurses to start acquiring clinical judgement with regard to assessing those at risk of developing pressure sores the following schema is offered:

- age — over 65 at greatest risk
- mobilising — painful joints, back or shoulders can severely restrict movement, even when sitting in a chair as well as when lying in bed
- weight — over/average/under weight recent loss of weight removes 'padding' over the sacrum and ischial tuberosities
- height — tall/medium/short
- skin type — coarse/average/fine
  — greasy/normal/dry
  — looks well/under-nourished
- response to environment — alert/uninterested/apathetic/restless
- appendage next to skin — artificial limb/caliper/crutch/plaster/splint
- continence/incontinence — urine/faeces.

If the patient is 'at risk' on admission, then in 'process context' he has a potential problem of developing a pressure sore which will either be written on the assessment form or nursing plan; the goal will be 'unblemished, intact skin over pressure areas' and the preventive nursing interventions to achieve this, will be written on the nursing plan. If the intervention is 2-hourly turning, then ongoing assessment in the form of inspecting the skin will take place at that frequency, and an extra nursing record may be used — a turning clock; the one devised for general use (Lowthian 1979) is illustrated in Figure 10.6. A note of the skin condition can be made in the 'box' for signature. Use of the scoring system may only be requested at, for example, a weekly interval or if there is any change in the patient's condition in the interim. In this 'evaluation' the score will be written on the patient's nursing notes and it will be compared with that obtained at the initial assessment.

If the initial assessment reveals an actual problem, a pressure sore, then the problem has to be stated from the patient's perception — it is painful all the time/some of the time; it burns/stings when I move; I cannot lie/sit on it and so on. The actual problem has also to be stated from the nurse's perception and articles in the Reading Assignment leave no doubt about the intricacies of describing the size, shape and depth of a pressure sore. It may be useful to make a line drawing of size and shape — photographs in the articles give some idea of just how different sores can be.

If a sore develops on a patient who had not been considered to be 'at risk', immediate assessment will take place along the lines mentioned in the previous paragraph, the goal and nursing intervention to achieve it will be written on the nursing plan and theoretically we say a date will be set for evaluation of whether or not the goal is being or has been achieved. Ongoing assessment which is written on the patient's nursing note will be summative information towards goal achievement.

Name	Date	Physical Condition	Mental condition	Activity	Mobility	Incontinent	Total score
		Good 4 Fair 3 Poor 2 V. bad 1	Alert 4 Apathetic 3 Confused 2 Stuporous 1	Ambulant 4 Walk/help 3 Chairbound 2 Bedfast 1	Full 4 Sl. limited 3 V. limited 2 Immobile 1	Not 4 Occasionally 3 Usually/ur. 2 Doubly 1	

Fig. 10.5 Norton's scoring system

Instructions for use:

- identify the most appropriate description of the patient (4,3,2 or 1) under each of the five headings and total the result
- record the 'score' with its date in patient's nursing notes or on a chart
- assess weekly and whenever any change in patient's condition and/or circumstances of care.

A 'score' of 14 or below denotes need for intensive care, that is, 1–2 hourly changes of posture and the use of pressure-relieving aids. Norton, in 1987, advised an increase of score from 14 to 15 or below.
Note: when oedema of sacral region has been present, a rise of score above 14 does not indicate less risk of a lesion.

Name .... Age ....

Date chart started .... Day 2 Day 3 Day 4 Day 5 Day 6

Turning times	Sign please	Sign please	Sign please	Sign please	Sign please	Sign please	Sign please
01.00							
05.00							
07.00							
09.00							
12.30							
15.00							
17.00							
21.00							
23.00							

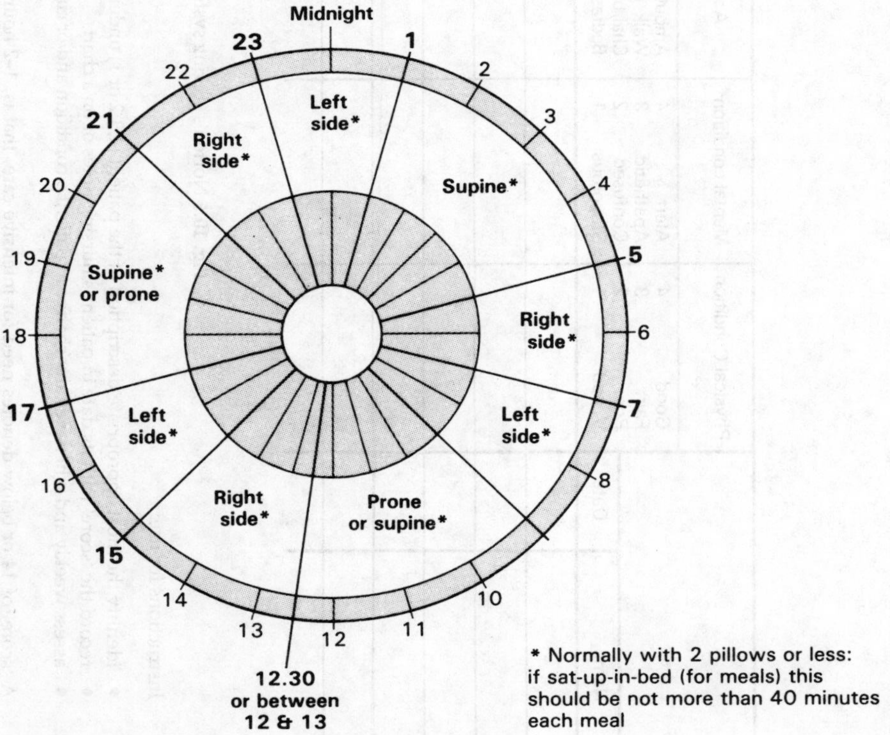

Fig. 10.6 The Lowthian 24-hour turning clock — general uses (Reproduced by kind permission of Peter Lowthian, Senior Nurse (Research), Royal National Orthopaedic Hospital, Stanmore)

Size of problem

Various estimates have been made of the size of the problem over the years which demonstrates that discussing pressure sores in a process context is greater than the sum of the four phases as applied to an individual patient. In the first large study in this country (Barbanel et al 1977) of a population of 10 751 patients in the hospital and in the community, 8.8% had at least one pressure sore. David et al (1985) report a National Survey which showed a 6.7% prevalence of sores, that is, at any one time, between 6 and 7 in every hundred hospital patients will have at least one pressure sore. With an increasingly elderly population, the prevention of pressure sores is a tremendous national challenge.

Cost of problem

Various estimates have also been made of the cost of prevention and treatment of pressure sores to the National Health Service. Waterlow (1985) gives an estimated cost of £200 million per annum!

A problem like pressure sores cannot only be considered from the perspective of financial cost. The articles in the Reading Assignment amply demonstrate the pain, discomfort and frustration of the patients; the long periods which they spent in hospital and the inordinate amount of nursing time spent dressing the sores together with time spent preventing a sore developing elsewhere on the patient. It is important that nurses put into practice the best available knowledge; it is gratifying that an increasing amount is being generated from research.

Planning: individualised

The document associated with the planning phase of the process is the patient's nursing plan and an idea of its use has already been given. The possible interventions for preventing and treating pressure sores are legion and are well described in the articles; the most comprehensive account is given by Chapman & Chapman (1986). The objective of the nursing plan (together with the assessment form) is to facilitate individualised nursing. A pertinent point to remember is that when the nursing intervention has achieved the goal of 'intact skin over...', the patient is probably still 'at risk' of developing another sore — in 'process context' he now has a potential problem of developing a pressure sore, and the appropriate nursing interventions to prevent it becoming an actual problem will be written on the plan. The nursing plan may well include the use of a painometer (p. 52) and nursing interventions to achieve pain control.

Generalised planning

Although individualised nursing plans are written and implemented at the clinical level — home, day-care facilities or hospital — a great deal of generalised planning precedes the availability of adequate resources at that level. These are listed with brief notes but they are, in the main, described in more detail in articles in the Reading Assignment.

Aids to relieve pressure

- special beds:
  - flotation
  - low air loss
  - Clinitron
  - tilting bed
  - water bed

  the number and type are ever-increasing and evermore expensive: they automatically change the pressure on successive areas of the body.
- mattresses: the main one is the ripple mattress which can be applied to an ordinary hospital bed. Bliss & Murray (1979) give a detailed account of its use and emphasise that it is financially economic. If nurses had learned about, and used ripple mattresses efficiently, would there be any need for the increasingly expensive 'special beds'?
- pillows: pillow packs which can act as a mattress to support leg/s so that heel/s are free from pressure; also used for patients sitting in bed to prevent sliding and shearing

- cushions: foam/bead/gel can be used for patients sitting up in bed, on the seat of chairs/wheelchairs
- fleeces: natural or synthetic
  large: on which all of the body can rest
  medium: for sacral area when sitting in bed
  small: for chair seat
- absorbent sheets: probably the best known is the Kylie washable sheet used for incontinent patients. It is constructed so that urine drains away from contact with the skin
- monkey poles: a chain with a handle attached via a curved tube to the head of the bed: a patient can grasp it and raise the buttocks from the bed, thereby relieving pressure
- bed cradles: strategically placed can relieve pressure from the upper bedclothes on various parts of the body
- chairs: provision of a variety of chairs so that nurses can match the chair to the patient's physique. All chairs used by patients should be covered with a non-slip material to avoid forward sliding which by friction can cause a superficial sore, or by shearing can cause a deep sore.
- wheelchairs: constructed so that the arms will bear the patient's weight while the buttocks are raised to relieve pressure.

Treatment and human resources In a national survey reported by David et al (1985) the choice of treatment for 1506 sores was made by nurses for 82% of them. However nurses may be constrained by the resources available for treatment. They can be classified as:

- drugs: to relieve pain
- medicaments: to cleanse wound
  to encourage healing
- dressings: to encourage healing
  to prevent adherence to a freshly granulating surface
- staff: to ensure that adequate nutrients are being taken
  to select appropriate pressure-relieving equipment
  to execute manual turning for relief of pressure
  to use aseptic technique when dressing wounds
  to encourage a positive attitude as some sores take a long time to heal.

Implementing

The implementing phase of the process of nursing in the context of preventing and treating pressure sores is the carrying out of the 'planned' nursing interventions at the prescribed time. Each time the intervention is carried out a note about the condition of the skin or the sore will be written on the patient's nursing notes. In the interest of economy in paperwork, if a turning clock is used, the nursing intervention does not need to be duplicated in the nursing notes. If the nursing intervention includes teaching, particularly paraplegic people who are not only paralysed but have no sensation in their lower limbs, then the nursing plan will indicate the activities to be taught. As each activity is taught and the patient becomes skilled at doing it, this will be recorded in the nursing notes, and this will be summative evidence on the date set for evaluation.

Despite the incredible difficulties in describing the shape, size and depth of a pressure sore, at each implementation, experienced nurses are able to observe and judge when a sore is clean and healing. A factual account of this ongoing assessment will be written on the patient's nursing notes and this will provide summative evidence on the date set for evaluation of whether or not the set goal is being achieved.

If, during implementation, a nurse observes that a pressure sore has become inflamed and pus is present, she will respond by taking a swab of the pus so that in the laboratory the offending microorganism can be identified. This is an example of an 'unplanned' nursing activity. The doctor may prescribe an antibiotic and the nurse will sign the medication Kardex each time she implements this delegated nursing intervention.

Evaluating

Evaluating that the potential problem of pressure sores has not become an actual one is the easiest part of this phase of the process of nursing. The difficulty in describing the size, shape and depth of an actual sore is discussed by Anthony (1985) and Lowthian (1987).

The goal when using a painometer is to have a pain-free patient but there will not be a date set for evaluation because there is 'immediate' evaluation of a pain control programme, each time the patient indicates his current experience of pain on the painometer.

The text so far has clearly demonstrated that evaluating is an ongoing process and on the date set for evaluation of whether or not the planned nurse-initiated intervention is achieving its set goal, there will be considerable information in the nursing notes which should be consulted. If the goal has been achieved this is recorded on the nursing plan and the nursing intervention/s cancelled. If the goal has not been achieved, a decision has to be made as to whether:

- to continue the nursing intervention/s and set a future date for evaluation
- to change the nursing intervention/s and set a future date for evaluation.

The Nursing Practice Committee at London's Royal Marsden Hospital has produced a manual which can be used as a resource whenever nurses require specific guidance on particular procedures and policies. An article from the manual about Pressure Sores was published in Nursing Mirror, Clinical Forum 5, 156 (23) June 8: i–vii

In this chapter the principle — helping patients to prevent pressure sores — has been discussed in a process of nursing context. The opportunity was taken in the assessing section to broaden it into what has been done to assess the size of the problem nationally, and the cost. In the generalised planning section, aids to relieve pressure, and treatment and human resources were considered.

APPLYING THE PRINCIPLE

A registered nurse must be capable of:

- accepting and instituting change for the better and discarding routines which are no longer useful
- using a reliable scoring scale to identify patients 'at risk'
- accepting the responsibility for overseeing that each patient eats adequate protein and vitamin C. Where there is no dietitian this responsibility is even greater for tube-fed patients
- procuring for the patients any equipment which will help maintain an intact skin
- relieving pressure and shearing force by skilful lifting of patients without straining her own back or injuring the patient's skin by dragging. Teaching these skills
- instructing a capable patient about the time and method of relieving pressure
- recognising the first sign of a pressure sore
- differentiating patients into:

  a. the 'at risk' group needing 2-hourly relief of pressure, day and night. This applies whatever happens to the patient, for example if he spends several hours in a chair; if he attends another department, if he goes to the operating theatre. The relief *must* be at the appointed time

  b. the 'partially at risk' group needing 4-hourly relief of pressure at the appointed time

  This involves the skill of deployment of available nursing staff, the skill of organisation whereby every member of staff knows at what time each patient has to be attended to, what attention each patient needs, including the position each patient has to be changed into.
- applying the principle — helping patients to prevent pressure sores — in a process of nursing context.

WORKING ASSIGNMENT

Topics for discussion

- factors contributing to pressure sores
- prevention of pressure sores
- the particular method of prevention of pressure sores advocated in your hospital

- the financial cost of preventing pressure sores might well be greater than that of treating them
- the article: Bromley P 1985 A sore point with nurses. Nursing Times 82 (32) August 6: 65
- A patient's additional medical diagnosis is carcinomatosis. He has a 'large, deep, infected sacral pressure sore'. State some possible patient's problems in the words which he uses to describe them.

Writing assignment

- what factors are required to maintain the skin, underlying subcutaneous and muscle tissues in a normal state?
- name the predisposing causes of interference with the ability to make spontaneous body movements
- name the factors contributing to pressure sores
- name some aids to the prevention of pressure sores
- give an estimate of the financial cost to the National Health Service in Britain of treating pressure sores
- describe the formation of a superficial pressure sore
- describe the formation of a deep pressure sore
- define:

  allergens
  eschar
  carcinomatosis
  extrinsic
  intrinsic
  ischaemic
  ischial tuberosities
  microcirculation
  necrotic
  pathogenesis
  pathophysiology
  sacrum
  shearing force
  toxins.

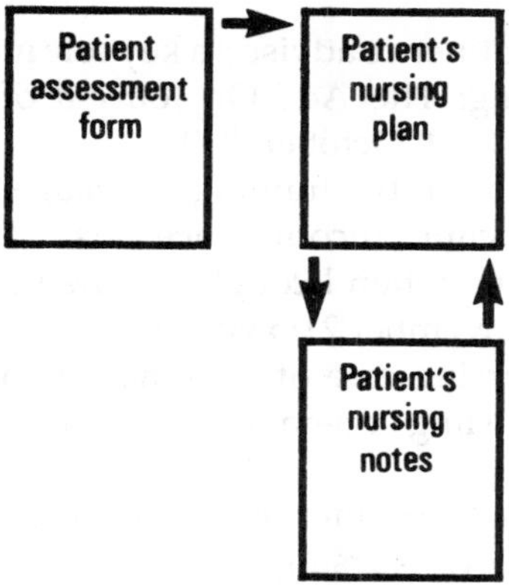

11

Helping patients to achieve continence/manage incontinence

READING ASSIGNMENT

Betts A 1984 All under control. Nursing Mirror 159 (19) November 21: viii–ix, xii–xiii
A scheme to assist district nurses in the management of patients suffering incontinence; illustration of 'habit training chart'.

Blannin J 1984 Services for the incontinent patient. Nursing: The Add-On Journal of Clinical Nursing 2 (28) August: 6–7
General practitioners; continence adviser; continence clinics; health centres; enuresis and enuretic clinics; laundry service; disposal; Aids centres; the Red Cross; pharmacies; the Health Education Council; and a list of helpful literature.

Blannin J 1984 Assessment of the incontinent patient. Nursing: The Add-On Journal of Clinical Nursing 2 (29) September: 863–865
Describes assessment of the type of incontinence and explains in detail how to set up a habit training programme to achieve continence.

Blannin J 1984 Nursing care of the incontinent patient. Nursing: The Add-On Journal of Clinical Nursing 2 (28) August: 3–5
Questions used to assess incontinent patient; factors considered when choosing an incontinence device; excellent account of available devices.

Blannin J 1986 My three D's. Nursing: The Add-

On Journal of Clinical Nursing 3 (10) October: 3
A young vivacious mother of two teenage children says that her episodes of incontinence are degrading, demoralising and debilitating.

Blannin J 1986 Incontinence and the individual. Nursing: The Add-On Journal of Clinical Nursing 3 (10) October: 1–2
Essential reading for anyone who wants to understand the person who happens to be incontinent.

Borthwick J 1985 Speaking from experience. Nursing Times 81 (14) April 3: 69
A straightforward account written by a young married man who at 20 became doubly incontinent.

Brocklehurst J 1984 The nature and problems of urinary incontinence. Nursing: The Add-On Journal of Clinical Nursing 2 (28) August: 1–2
Discusses the neurological control of micturition and the unstable bladder.

Broomhead L 1986 Incontinence. A personal account. Nursing: The Add-On Journal of Clinical Nursing 3 (10) October: 11
The writer if given the chance of walking again or regaining continence would choose the latter.

Deegan S 1985 Intermittent catheterisation for children. Nursing Times 81 (14) April 3: 72–74
Describes this technique and how it is taught to children and their families.

Glew J 1986 A woman's lot? Nursing Times 82 (15) April 9: 69
Reports a survey carried out by a women's magazine and many sad facts are highlighted.

Gooch J 1986 Care of the urinary incontinent patient. The Professional Nurse 1 (11) August: 298–300
Describes the types of incontinence; assessment of the patient's physical and emotional state. Discusses various aspects of care and the appliances available.

Hurst K 1986 Living with incontinence. The Professional Nurse 1 (12) September: 326–327
Part of the study asked incontinent people for their views of their problems; gives five situations adapted from some of the responses as a useful basis for thought or discussion.

Jones V 1986 The continence adviser: a key role in the team. Nursing: The Add-On Journal of Clinical Nursing 3 (10) October: 8–9
Explains a community training package; multidisciplinary clinic; incontinence aids.

MacLeod E 1984 Only when I cough… Nursing Mirror 159 (19) November 21: xvii–xviii, xx
Describes the nursing care of a woman who had a urethral sling operation for stress incontinence.

Mandelstam D 1984 Incontinence: re-education of the pelvic floor. Nursing: The Add-On Journal of Clinical Nursing 2 (29) September: 867–868
Describes stress incontinence; anatomy of the pelvic floor; treatment by exercise; urgency and frequency (unstable bladder).

Millard P 1986 A programme for continence. Nursing Times 82 (15) April 9: 57–58
It is essential to establish whether patients have voluntary or involuntary loss of control of urine or faeces, as the approach to control of each is different. Explains how to assist patients according to their type of incontinence.

Montgomery E 1986 Steps to regaining pelvic control. Nursing Times 82 (15) April 9: 58, 60
There is some evidence that progressive exercises to strengthen the pelvic floor muscles, combined with relaxation, assisted in the reduction of stress incontinence in a group of patients in Bristol.

Mowlam V, North K, Myers C 1986 Managing faecal incontinence. Nursing Times 82 (48) November 26: 55, 57, 59
Explains a new type of faecal collector which has a skin-protective barrier to improve hygiene for both patient and nurse.

Norton C 1986 Promoting research. Nursing Times 82 (15) April 9: 55
We need more research into the practical management of this distressing condition; sees hope in the new specialty of continence adviser.

Norton C 1984 Challenging specialty. Nursing Mirror 159 (19) November 21: xiv–xvii
Uses the headings: potential role; patient referrals; teaching and education; advisory service; supplies liaison; research; liaison

with industry.

Reader Service 1985 No 105 products for incontinence. Nursing Times 81 (14) April 3: 81–82
Illustrated round-up of what is currently available from the manufacturers to help incontinent people.

Oliver J 1985 Fresh and dry? Nursing Times 81 (30) July 24: 21
How is it that an incontinent woman is told to think twice before laughing, or a man has to buy masses of sanitary towels? Incontinence needs are clearly not being met.

Playford V 1987 Management of male incontinence using a sheath. The Professional Nurse 2 (7) April: 227–228
Detailed practical account.

Roe B, Chapman R, Crow R 1986 Checking catheter care. Nursing Times 82 (48) November 26: 61, 63
After analysing data from a research project they recommended that nurses should understand the principles of infection prevention rather than performing rote procedures.

Rooney V 1985 How would you manage? Nursing Times 81 (14) April 3: 65–66
A skill testing exercise.

RCN 1983 The problem of promoting continence. Royal College of Nursing, London (Booklet)
Report of study days held throughout the country.

Roper N, Logan W, Tierney A 1985 The elements of nursing, 2nd edn. Churchill Livingstone, Edinburgh, p 352, 355

Ryan-Woolley B 1987 Aids for the management of incontinence. King's Fund Publishing and Press Office, 2 St Andrew's Place, London NW1 4LB

Shillitoe, Reed 1986 Dry at night. Community Outlook March: 20–21, 23

Stewart M 1985 Preparing for the future. Nursing Times 81 (14) April 3: 62–63
Does the continence adviser have to be a nurse? It is a challenge which some think the nursing profession is accepting too slowly. Will other disciplines begin to respond more rapidly?

Swaffield J 1985 Nursing Times 81 (14) April 3: 77, 79
Describes how a structured team approach can promote continence in handicapped children in the community.

Swaffield J 1986 Avoiding incontinence — health education and preventive care for women. Nursing: The Add-On Journal of Clinical Nursing 3 (10) October: 6–7
Discusses stages in the lifespan where health education could be introduced.

Swaffield J 1986 How did you score? Nursing Times 82 (15) April 9: 62
Fifteen questions to test your knowledge. The answers are on the upturned page!

Tallis R, Norton C 1984 Incontinence in the elderly
1 The rehabilitative approach. Nursing Times 80 (39) September 26 Supplement
2 Treating the impairment. Nursing Times 80 (44) October 31 Supplement
3 Preventing the disability. Nursing Times 80 (48) November 28 Supplement
4 Nursing the incontinent patient. Nursing Times 81 (1) January 2 Supplement
5 Incontinence aids. Nursing Times 81 (5) January 30 Supplement
6 Summary and conclusions. Nursing Times 81 (10) February 27 Supplement

Tattersall A 1985 Getting the whole picture. Nursing Times 81 (14) April 3: 55, 57–58
A holistic approach to continence promotion including sexuality.

The professional file 1987 Biofeedback in combating stress incontinence. The Professional Nurse 2 (6) March: 162
A résumé of a research report.

Time 1986 'The last of the closet issues.' Time 40 October 6: 31
Reports the testing of a bladder pacemaker.

Turner A 1987 Childhood continence problems. The Professional Nurse 2 (4) January: 119–122

White H 1984 Aids to continence — simple and sophisticated. Nursing: The Add-On Journal of Clinical Nursing 2 (29) September: 855–858

White H 1986 Incontinence: prevent, treat or ignore? Nursing: The Add-On Journal of Clinical Nursing 3 (10) October: 4–5
Ostracized for being smelly, chastised for being dirty, accused of being lazy, yet one in

three women over the age of 35 suffers from incontinence. The time has come to make incontinence a respected subject.

Willington F, Yarnell J, Sweetman P 1981 Cleansing incontinent patients: an evaluation of the use of non-ionic detergents compared with soap. Journal of Advanced Nursing 6: 107–109

The results showed a reduced cleansing time, and evidence that the marked degree of alkalinity encountered in cleansing with soap is avoided.

Wilson M, Righing S 1986 Staying fresh. Community Outlook March: 15– 16, 18

Describes a project which replaced an unsatisfactory system of managing incontinence, with one where the emphasis was on individual care. Illustrates an incontinence checklist.

Young P 1986 Setting up an advisory service. Nursing Times 82 (48) November 26: 68, 71

A continence adviser describes a project which resulted in an assessment form and the group are in the process of testing it.

BACKGROUND INFORMATION

When thinking about the subject of incontinence, we tend to forget that there is a period in every person's life when he or she is incontinent of urine and faeces. It is a natural phenomenon before establishment of voluntary control over these reflex actions. Skin should not remain in contact with urine and/or faeces any longer than is necessary. This necessitates frequent changing and washing of the area. A simple grease such as petroleum jelly or lanolin minimises the amount of contact between skin and urine or faeces.

Faeces contain bacteria which are capable of splitting the urea contained in urine into ammonia. Should urine and faeces be left in contact with skin sufficiently long for this chemical action to occur, the ammonia so formed will irritate the skin, and give rise to a condition described as ammonia dermatitis. Some people call it 'urine rash'. Since a baby's skin is more delicate than that of an adult, the condition is seen more frequently among babies than in adults who are incontinent from any cause. The stools of a breast-fed baby are usually acid. The acid can neutralise any ammonia that is formed. The stools of a baby fed on cow's milk are usually alkaline, so that any ammonia formed is unlikely to be neutralised. Keeping both napkins and the skin acid can help. Napkins, after washing and rinsing in the usual way, should be soaked for a few seconds in a weak solution of acetic acid (vinegar: 6 ml per litre of water), followed by drying. Ointments containing benzalkonium chloride help to keep the skin sufficiently acid to counteract any ammonia formed.

In consideration of attitudes to adult incontinence, we think of that which goes into the digestive tract as 'clean', and we would refrain from putting anything which we considered 'dirty' into it. What comes out of the digestive tract is that portion of food which has not been absorbed, together with digestive juices and enzymes, some bacteria from the natural intestinal flora, and shed epithelial cells from the surface of the tract. In many people's thinking, faeces are dirty, nasty or even filthy. Certainly the smell has changed, for example, from that of an appetising beef stew, to that of faeces. The smell of the latter can be, but is not always, unpleasant. However, it is reasonable, from a health and social point of view, for society to expect those who are mentally and physically capable of co-operating, to pass urine and faeces in a specially designated place, be it latrine or lavatory. Elimination and privacy have had a long association in most adults' minds.

So when, after an episode of incontinence, urine and/or faeces become visible to others, the person naturally experiences feelings of shame and embarrassment. Should there be malodour, the carers may well have feelings of guilt and all may feel disgust. Tension can build up and the carers can display negative attitudes to the unfortunate incontinent patient.

However, the attitude of both lay people and professionals to incontinence is changing and nurses are urged to change their image of their role related to incontinence from one of negatively dealing with the results, to one of positively promoting continence.

Enuresis is the name given to urinary incontinence, usually at night (nocturnal) after the age at which continence could reasonably be expected. Shillitoe & Reed (1986) discuss what can be done to encourage continence at night. Turner (1987) discusses toilet/potty training as well as enuresis and encopresis.

PROMOTING CONTINENCE AND THE PROCESS OF NURSING

The objective in using the process is to individualise nursing and from your reading you will not be in any doubt that this is essential to help incontinent patients to achieve continence. You will also be aware that any age group can be affected. Children with congenital abnormalities such as spina bifida have benefited from developments in surgery and pharmacology, enabling them to reach adulthood in spite of incontinence. Young adults can be involved in road traffic accidents and this can result in incontinence from severe head injuries, paraplegia and tetraplegia. And from the articles you will be aware that we are an ageing population and erroneously it was thought that incontinence was an inevitable part of ageing for many people.

Excessive paperwork is one of the negative attitudes to using the process of nursing. The objective of this book is to help nurses to think about nursing in a process context. Consequently it is pertinent to remind readers that to give consistent practice in this mode of thinking three documents are used. Firstly a patient assessment form which requests biographical, health and everyday living data, inspection of which, in conjunction with the patient whenever possible, permits identification of the problems he is experiencing with everyday living activities which are amenable to nursing. The information about everyday living activities which are not problematic will be useful throughout the patient's stay and will help each nurse to individualise her interaction with the patient.

For each identified problem, a realistic, achievable, observable and measurable goal will be set, and written on the nursing plan, together with the nursing intervention to achieve it and a date for evaluation. This will be discussed in the planning section.

Each time the intervention is carried out, it will be recorded on the patient's nursing notes, with any relevant factual information, together with the date and time. Each of the phases of the process of nursing will now be discussed.

Assessing

Assessing a person's state of incontinence of urine and/or faeces is the most detailed of all the assessments. There are several assessment forms in the articles and they are easily identified either by the title or the annotation. In order to pose relevant questions and prompts while assessing, it is important that nurses have adequate background knowledge about the different types of incontinence. This information is presented in several of the articles: Figure 11.1 illustrates stress incontinence and Figure 11.2 overflow incontinence. Incontinence is one assessment in which the nurse's sense of smell can be used, especially if interviewing a person at home. It is pertinent to assess several everyday living activities other than eliminating urine and/or faeces, because they may have a bearing on incontinence:

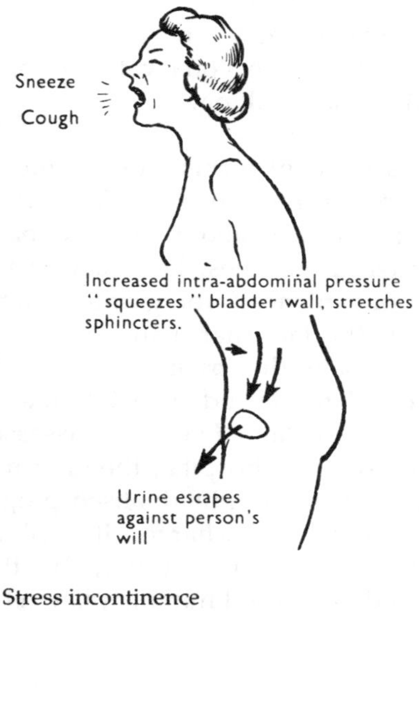

Fig. 11.1 Stress incontinence

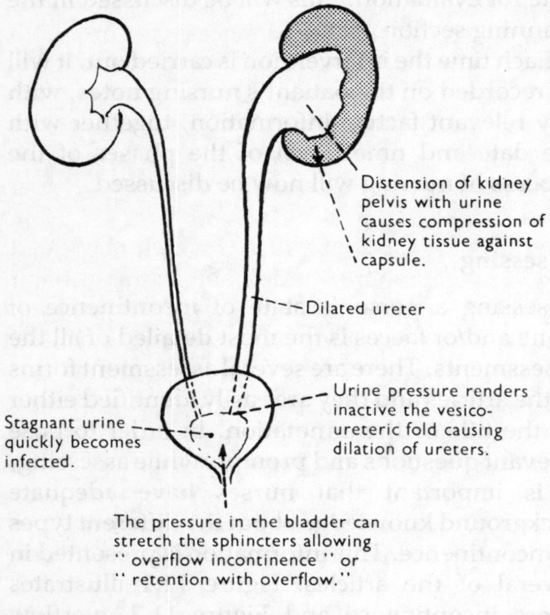
Distension of kidney pelvis with urine causes compression of kidney tissue against capsule.
Dilated ureter
Urine pressure renders inactive the vesico-ureteric fold causing dilation of ureters.
Stagnant urine quickly becomes infected.
The pressure in the bladder can stretch the sphincters allowing " overflow incontinence " or " retention with overflow."

Fig. 11.2 Overflow incontinence

- ability to rise from a chair
- ability to mobilise so that the lavatory can be reached in time
- ability to stand
- ability to sit on lavatory seat
- manual dexterity of hands to manipulate clothing and perform post micturition/defaecation toilet
- type of clothing worn
- ability to see label on lavatory door
- eating and drinking.

Many assessment forms request information about 'Type of residence' so for incontinent patients it has to be about lavatory, bathroom and laundering facilities. It is easy to take 'all modern conveniences' for granted and to be ignorant of the fact that many houses have a lavatory outside the back door, or share a lavatory on a landing and in most terrace houses the lavatory is upstairs. Even if the assessment is being carried out in hospital, the information is essential, to plan an individualised programme and the patient's discharge. If facilities are unsatisfactory at home, it may be that the patient's individualised nursing plan in hospital should be use of a commode at a particular distance from the bed, and early contact with the social services department for provision of a commode in the home.

People with neurological diseases such as spina bifida and multiple sclerosis who have managed incontinence at home, can be admitted to hospital for another reason, and it is imperative that nurses ask them about details of management, so that staff on each succeeding shift can offer the individualised nursing help required.

As much factual information as possible should be collected. Exactly how many times is the patient wet during the day? How wet? Contained in crotch of pants? Dampens outer clothing? Dampens seat of chair? Large amount runs down legs and pools on floor? During the night? At what time? Can he describe how wet he is — pants only; pants and bottom/top/both sheets? Of course it is subjective information but in a warm and accepting atmosphere, and with skilful prompting, it will be as factual as possible.

We usually think of the assessment form as being used at the initial assessment but in the case of incontinence, a chart on which every incident of micturition/defaecation is recorded is an essential assessment tool and the experts advise that it should be kept for 3 to 7 days to elucidate the pattern, frequency and amount of leakage. This information refers to the patient's biological problem and may well be used as a basis for planning medical investigations.

The purpose of collecting assessment data is identification of the patient's problem(s) related to micturition/defaecation, written in words which reflect the patient's perception of them. Nurses cannot ignore the words which patients use to describe their plight:

- degrading
- demoralising
- distasteful
- distressing
- embarrassing
- humiliating.

It is obvious that they have lost confidence, suffered a change in body image, self-esteem, self-respect, self-dignity and so on and need individualised help to rebuild these personal traits. It is unacceptable to write the problem as 'incontinent of urine/faeces'; the patient may not even know the meaning of the word; indeed many professionals have difficulty in defining the word precisely. Some patients' problems can be inferred from the questions posed previously in this section. For those living alone, it may be the feeling of having cold wet clothes until someone can come to wash and change them. For others it is the difficulty in procuring sanitary pads, in disposing of soiled pads, laundering of soiled clothes and so on. For some it is the malodour from decomposing urine/faeces and the consequent social isolation — possibly self-imposed, but it can be that friends are embarrassed at the malodour in the house.

Planning

From your reading of appropriate articles and this chapter so far, you will realise that a plan to individualise nursing is essential. Incontinence of urine/faeces gives rise to many patients' problems which in turn influence the goals which will be set for each patient. People are not going to become continent overnight; and with an already demoralised person it is necessary to set tiny achievable short-term goals so that praise can raise morale and motivation to persevere towards the long-term goal of continence.

Should any drugs be prescribed by the doctor for the patient they will be written on the medication Kardex which the nurse will sign each time a dose is given. On the plan, the nursing intervention will be to observe for signs of what the drug is expected to do, and for signs of any known side-effect. Some nursing plans (Roper, Logan & Tierney 1985) request that nursing interventions from medical prescription are recorded separately from the nurse-initiated interventions related to everyday living activities.

Implementing

Learning to think about incontinence in process context shows very clearly that the phases cannot be put into containing boxes to be carried out sequentially. For example the chart used in the assessment phase to record all incidents related to passing urine/faeces, in order to identify the patient's actual biological eliminating problems (for which nursing interventions are required) can continue to be used in the implementing phase and it will give up-to-date evaluation of whether or not the short-term goal is being achieved.

Other nursing interventions which may need to be implemented include habit training, habit retraining, condom drainage for male patients, use of a self-retaining catheter and a closed urinary drainage system, prevention of nosocomial infection, teaching and supervising self-catheterisation. For those patients who for whatever reason cannot be retrained, then management has to be by protective clothing and bedding. These are discussed in the articles.

As each planned intervention is carried out a memo to this effect is written on the patient's nursing notes. In using the process of nursing it is important that we do not abandon the art of nursing. When there has been an episode of incontinence, be it of urine or faeces, it should not be assumed that a nurse has the right to attend to the patient without asking him. Use of words such as 'make you clean' or 'clean you up', infers that he is dirty and this is not good for his self-image. It is therefore wiser to ask if one can make him comfortable, or make him ready for visitors or whatever is appropriate. The area should be as warm and draught-free as possible. Visual privacy is afforded by drawing curtains or placing screens around the bed. It has to be remembered that this does not afford auditory privacy, and conversation with the patient should be conducted in such a manner as to prevent any loss of dignity. He is adult and any temptation to converse with him as one would converse with a child must be resisted and his concept of modesty should not be infringed. On leaving, it is important to place needed articles within the patient's reach; he may want to read, write or listen to the radio. It re-inforces his self-esteem if the nurse shows interest in what he will do after she leaves the bedside.

It is customary to remove urine and faeces from the skin with a cloth and soap and water.

However Willington et al (1981) reports a trial to establish the most suitable hygienic wipe for sanitary cleansing in faecal incontinence. The results showed that when removing faeces from the skin, an initial dry Scrim wipe, followed by about 7 g Cetomacrogol 1000 BPC (a non-ionic detergent cream) on a moistened Scrim wipe achieved emulsification of faeces which was removed by another dry Scrim wipe. The data collected related to:

- allergenicity
- detergency
- ease of cleansing
- odour control.

The condition of the skin was recorded as excellent and the figures indicated a possible saving of 20% nursing time.

Evaluating

The quality of evaluation is dependent on the statement of the goal planned which, in turn, is dependent on the problems identified from the assessment data. The factual information collected at the initial assessment — number of times urine/faeces is passed involuntarily during the day and night is the baseline against which the evaluation is made. There will be some summative factual ongoing evaluation on the chart mentioned in the implementing section. Absence of malodour cannot be measured but it can be subjectively evaluated by the sense of smell. The subjective factual information about damp clothes, bedding and so on will again be the baseline against which evaluation is made. When the goal is containment then the efficiency of the pads and garments will be evaluated against no leakage. Here a realistic note must be sounded — some Health Authorities provide only a limited selection of pads and garments thus putting a constraint on the quality of nursing which can be offered to patients. Clinical nurses who would select other pads and garments, if they were available, should record this factual information so that Health Authorities can be informed about constraints to quality of nursing at clinical level — of course, this demands the personal responsibility of clinical nurses to continually update their knowledge of what is available on the market. And patient satisfaction cannot be forgotten. Using the word in a more general sense, the number of incontinent patients on a geriatric or a psychogeriatric ward may be an item in a Quality Assurance Programme.

In this chapter the wide ranging subject of incontinence in its many forms has been discussed. An attempt was then made to discuss the principle — helping incontinent patients achieve continence/manage incontinence — in a process of nursing context.

APPLYING THE PRINCIPLE

A registered nurse must be capable of:

- eliciting information about incontinence from patients
- encouraging staff to participate in retraining for continence programmes for individual patients
- procuring the most suitable articles and equipment for incontinent patients to cope with their incontinence
- applying the principle — helping incontinent patients achieve continence/ manage incontinence — in a process of nursing context.

WORKING ASSIGNMENT

Topics for discussion

- retraining for continence
- the particular policy in your educational programme for management of ambulant incontinent patients
- the particular policy in your educational programme for management of bedfast incontinent patients
- sexuality and the incontinent patient
- a patient is incontinent of urine by day and by night. Write some of the possible problems which he/she might be experiencing in the words he/she uses to describe them.

Writing assignment

- define the following

bladder drill
catheterisation
Cetomacrogol 1000 BPC
closed drainage system
clothing related to continence/incontinence
condom urinary drainage
constipation
cystitis
dribble incontinence/overflow
encopresis
enuresis
excoriation
faecal impaction
frequency
Kanga bedsheets
Kanga pants
Kylie bed sheet
maceration
manual evacuation of faeces
midstream urine collection
overflow incontinence
reflex incontinence
retention of urine
retention with overflow
Scrim wipe
self-catheterisation
stress incontinence
stress/urge incontinence
toilet training
urge incontinence
urgency.

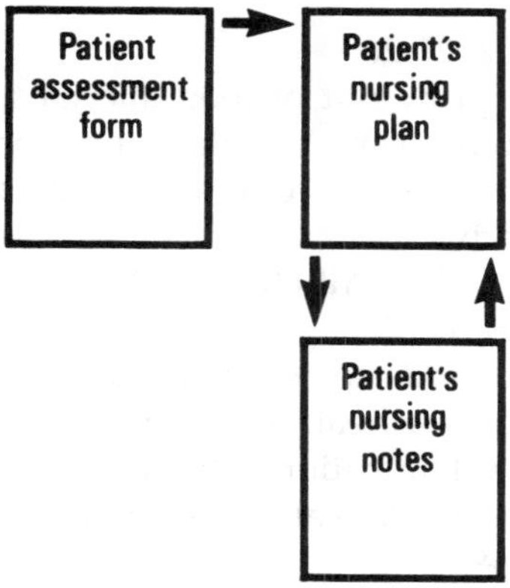

12

Helping patients to eat and drink

Reading assignment

Background information
- *Increased knowledge available to the public*
- *Nursing Times 'Care about food' campaign*
- *Malnutrition in hospital patients*

Eating and drinking in process context
- *Assessing*
- *Planning*
  - *Generalised planning*
  - *Ward planning*
  - *Individualised planning*
- *Implementing*
  - *Helping patients with particular problems*
  - *Helping patients with diet modifications*
- *Evaluating*

Applying the principle
- *A registered nurse must be capable of:*

Working assignment
- *Topics for discussion*
- *Writing assignment*

READING ASSIGNMENT

Allan D 1984 Patient care in hyperalimentation. Nursing Times 80 (18) May 2: 28–30
Malnutrition among hospital patients was once very common. Describes a new method of feeding very ill patients in detail.

Axelsson K, Norberg A, Asplund K 1986 Journal of Advanced Nursing 11 (5) September: 553–559
Using a training programme developed by Heimlich, we have attempted to train swallowing in a 78-year-old man who had been fed by nasogastric tube for 3 years after a stroke.

Beech C, Brooke O 1986 Satisfaction guaranteed? Community Outlook June: 34, 36
Investigates whether babies who are fed infant formula containing more protein and minerals cry less and appear more contented.

Bender A 1986 Slimming safely. Nursing: The Add-On Journal of Clinical Nursing 3 (7) July: 240–243
Describes the lengths to which some people will go to avoid controlling their food intake.

Bewsher C 1984 Nutritional problems in the infant. Nursing: The Add-On Journal of Clinical Nursing 2 (22) February: 640–641, 644
Discusses those problems which can occur in the western world. Malabsorption; excessive loss; excessive intake.

Biley F, Savage S 1984 Anorexia nervosa.

Nursing Times 80 (31) August 1: 28–32
Describes the condition and the interventions needed to restore and maintain weight.

Bladen L 1986 Enteral feeding. Nursing: The Add-On Journal of Clinical Nursing 3 (8) August: 281–285
Describes the various routes for tube feeding and gives the possible complications of nasogastric feeding.

Nursing Times 1985 The sugar debate. Nursing Times 81 (38) September 18: 35
Two letters about a previous article.

Bryce-Smith D 1986 Prenatal zinc deficiency. Nursing Times 82 (10) March 5: 44–46
Advocates a zinc supplement for pregnant women.

Caunter M, Penrose J 1983 Solving feeding problems. Nursing Times 79 (51) December 21: 24–26
Mentally handicapped people often have eating problems, which can be a source of tension. A physiotherapist and speech therapist outline some of the causes and suggest ways of tackling the problem. Describes in detail the acts of sucking, chewing and swallowing.

Coates V 1985 Service included. Nursing Times 81 (15) April 10: 32– 33
It can take up to 30 minutes to feed a person who cannot feed himself. Many patients were left to feed themselves. Loss of dignity, loss of substantial amounts of food, and socially unacceptable behaviour may be the result of fostering an independence of which the person is not capable.

Cockcroft G, Ray M 1985 Feeding problems in stroke patients. Nursing Mirror 160 (9) February 27: 26–29
A dietitian and a speech therapist review normal feeding mechanisms, list some of the more common eating difficulties after a stroke and suggest approaches to treatment.

Darbyshire P 1987 Fussy eaters. Nursing Times 83 (3) January 21: 57– 58
Many are the battles between parent and child over the meal table, but parents should try to regard fads as a normal part of their child's development.

David T 1985 Intolerant babies. Community Outlook March: 22, 27-28
Children usually grow out of food allergies, but the symptoms can be alarming for parents. Looks at the more common allergies and offers some advice.

Deakin J, Forrester I 1986 All change. Nursing Times 82 (14) April 2: 47
A study on four wards to see what patients thought about the new healthy menus.

deLooy A 1986 Infant nutrition. Nursing: The Add-On Journal of Clinical Nursing 3 (12) December: 446–449
Discusses bottle v. breast and supporting the mother in her decision, goes on to consider weaning.

Devlin R 1984 The great sterilising debate. Nursing Times 80 (27) Community Outlook July 12: 242
Confusion caused by changing a 35-year-old instruction 'do not rinse' to 'rinse' feeding bottles soaked in Milton to be in line with the modern idea of not introducing chemicals into the body.

Devlin R 1985 Disability: coping in the kitchen. Community Outlook March: 11–12, 14
Kitchen units; sinks; electrical and gas appliances; tin, bottle and jar openers; non-slip aids; holding aids; graters, slicers and mincers; teapot and kettle tippers; water heaters; taps, tap turners and valve; weighing scales; trays; saucepans and accessories; trolleys; kitchen stools; ironing equipment.

Dewar B 1986 Total parenteral nutrition at home. Nursing Times 82 (28) July 9: 35, 37–38
What would it be like never to be able to eat solid food again? Looks at some of the psychological problems faced by those patients who, for the rest of their lives, will have to rely on a mechanical device as a means of feeding.

Dickerson J 1986a Food intolerance: fact or fallacy? Nursing: The Add-On Journal of Clinical Nursing 3 (8) August: 276–280
A nutritionist says that there is no doubt that adverse reactions to food are a cause of considerable morbidity.

Dickerson J 1986b Nutrition in health and illness. Nursing: The Add-On Journal of Clinical Nursing 3 (8) August: 303–307

While general guidelines are possible for the healthy, the needs of patients must be assessed individually; surveys the main groups of patients who require special dietary consideration.

Dickerson J 1986c Hospital induced malnutrition: prevention and treatment. The Professional Nurse 1 (12) September: 314–316
A questionnaire completed on admission could be a useful tool; simply charting the food intake of at-risk patients is a useful procedure; assessing for protein-energy malnutrition.

Dickerson J 1986d Hospital induced malnutrition: a cause for concern. The Professional Nurse 1 (11) August: 293–296
Malnutrition is usually associated with young children in developing countries. This article suggests that it not only occurs in hospital patients but actually results from their stay in hospital in some cases.

Dowding C 1986 Nutrition in wound healing. Nursing: The Add-On Journal of Clinical Nursing 3 (5) May: 174–176
Providing good nutrition for our patients is a clinical skill, the importance of which is sometimes overlooked.

Dunning Y 1986 Feeding babies with cleft lip and palate. Nursing Times 82 (5) January 29: 46–47
Provides some useful hints.

Elliot R 1985 A healthy start. Community Outlook March: 19–20
Offers some help to health visitors who are faced with advising vegetarian, vegan and macrobiotic parents on weaning their babies.

Fine G 1987 International conference on obesity. Nursing: The Add-On Journal of Clinical Nursing 3 (16) April: 616–618
Methods of treating obesity vary from simple caloric restriction, to behaviour modification therapy, to drug therapy and surgery.

Fisher C 1985 Feeding the relationship. Nursing Times 81 (4) January 23: 51
Physical problems in breast feeding which need to be overcome.

Fisher C 1986 Successful breastfeeding. The Professional Nurse 1 (12) September: 329–331
Has a handout which can be photocopied and given to parents.

Flint C 1984 Midwives and breastfeeding. Nursing Times 80 (15) April 11: 30–31
Breastfeeding is a very private and personal experience. Midwives should be enablers rather than helpers.

Francis D 1985 Food, fats and facts for nutrition in children. Nursing: The Add-On Journal of Clinical Nursing 2 (39) July: 1149–1152
Discusses the NACME and COMA recommendations. Table of conditions which require special dietary considerations.

Francis D 1984 The infant feeding controversy. Nursing: The Add-On Journal of Clinical Nursing 2 (22) February: 635–638

Gent A 1984 Intravenous nutrition. Nursing Mirror 158 (22) May 30: 19–21

Gillett J 1984 Food for health. Senior Nurse 1 (38) December 19/26: 16–17, 19–20
Spells out the importance of dietary advice in counselling mothers.

Goodinson S 1986 Assessment of nutritional status. Nursing: The Add-On Journal of Clinical Nursing 3 (7) July: 252–258
Poor nutritional status may have an adverse effect on wound healing, resistance to infection, physical strength, psychological wellbeing and duration of hospitalisation.

Hadley A 1985 Campaign for real food. Nursing Times 80 (12) March 20: 42–43
Why do nurses have so little involvement in patients' nutrition? A mitigating factor has been the plated meals service. Involvement should begin in OPD; obese patients should be given dietary advice backed up with written instructions. Those for surgery should be advised to eat well so that the body is in the best possible condition.

Hadley A 1986 Eat to your heart's content. Nursing Times 82 (9) February 26: 18–19
Hackney's heart group has taken its campaign to the pubs, cafes and restaurants in the district. This is a progress report of Nursing Times 'Campaign for real food'.

Hadley A 1985 Vegetarianism — blowing the myths. Nursing Times 81 (42) October 16: 27–29
Can a vegetarian diet provide sufficient nutrients for people at all stages of life?

Hamilton-Smith S 1972 Nil by mouth. Royal

College of Nursing, London
Research report of nurses' and doctors' interpretation of the term 'nil by mouth'.

Harvey J 1985 Staff of life. Nursing Mirror 161 (12) September 18: 24
Good nutrition is particularly difficult to maintain for cancer patients and nurses are in the best position to offer support.

Holmes A 1986 Food additives. Nursing: The Add-On Journal of Clinical Nursing 3 (8) August: 293–295
Colouring agents; preservatives; antioxidants; buffers; emulsifiers; flavouring agents; are food additives safe?

Holmes P 1985 The indigestible facts. Nursing Times 81 (46) November 13: 46
Political factors affecting what is eaten.

Holmes S 1984 Stress and nutrition. Nursing Times 80 (38) September 19: 53–55
Despite a shortage of research, there is some general advice on diet which can be given to stress sufferers.

Holmes S 1985 The risk business. Senior Nurse 2 (2) January 16: 20–23
Analyses the COMA report on diet and cardiovascular disease and the role of nurses in implementing the findings.

Holmes S 1985 A most important duty. Nursing Mirror 160 (7) February 13: 20, 22–24
Traces the factors which influence our eating behaviour and why some people find it difficult to change their established habits. Points out that with a meals tray service no one knows what the patient has eaten.

Holmes S 1985 Drug-nutrient interactions. Nursing Mirror 160 (13) March 20: 43
Explains how the interactions between drugs and nutrients can affect drug action and nutritional status.

Holmes S 1985 Differing needs. Nursing Times 81 (13) March 27: 35–36
Patients' nutritional needs vary according to their physical age as well as their physical state.

Holmes S 1985 Catering for the patient. Nursing Times 81 (28) July 10: 27–29
Discusses nutrition in the context of the cancer patient.

Holmes S 1985 Fat modified diets. Nursing Mirror 161 (7) August 14: 31–32, 34, 36
Explains unsaturated and polyunsaturated fats and the significance of fat in food.

Holmes S 1985 Advice that's too hard to swallow? Nursing Times 81 (38) September 18: 17–18
Explains the background to the NACNE report and discusses the delay in publishing it.

Holmes S 1985 Start right with every bite. Nursing Times 81 (43) October 23: 64–66
Healthy eating begins at birth — if not before. The London Food Commission has produced guidelines for pre-school children.

Holmes S 1986 Radiotherapy. Planned nutritional support. Nursing Times 82 (16) April 6: 26–29
How many nurses realise the impact that drugs can have on the patient's nutritional status or are aware that different foods may modify a drug's efficacy?

Holmes S 1986 Nutritional needs of surgical patients. Nursing Times 82 (19) May 7: 30–32
To ensure patients are in the best state to withstand trauma of surgery it is vital they have adequate nutritional support both pre- and postoperatively. Explains the body's metabolic response to trauma and points out nurses' responsibility in seeing that adequate feeding programmes are initiated.

Holmes S 1986 Determinants of food intake. Nursing: The Add-On Journal of Clinical Nursing 3 (7) July: 260–264
An understanding of the factors influencing eating behaviour will help the nurse in helping patients to adjust to dietary change.

Holmes S 1986 Fundamentals of nutrition. Nursing: The Add-On Journal of Clinical Nursing 3 (7) July: 235–237, 239
Describes macronutrients and micronutrients; the production of energy; utilisation of nutrients; achieving good nutrition.

Holmes S 1987 The young vegetarian. Nursing Times 83 (3) January 21: 51, 54–55
Suggests possible supplements for weaning vegetarian infants.

Hunt S 1985 Below the breadline. Community Outlook October: 19, 21
Is it realistic to advise low income families on

the merits of a low fat, high fibre diet with plenty of fruit and vegetables? Explains why the NACNE diet is not feasible for those on the breadline, and explodes a few myths in the process.

Ibbotson M 1986 The Professional Nurse 1 (8) May: 219–220
Gluten-free diets — helping patients to cope. People with coeliac disease have to avoid gluten in the diet which makes it very restricted.

Ibbotson M 1986 Living with a diabetic diet. The Professional Nurse 2 (3) December: 69–72
Discusses today's diabetic diet.

Janes E 1986 Changing our eating habits. Nursing: The Add-On Journal of Clinical Nursing 3 (7) July: 268–272
Discusses the NACNE and the COMA reports and the reasons for the recommended changes.

Johnson L, Silman A 1985 Ready salted. Nursing Times 81 (32) August 7: 34–35
Looks at the background to the salt/health debate.

Jones D 1984 Breastfeeding problems. Nursing Times 80 (33) August 15: 53–54
A study of breastfeeding which suggests that common problems are not helped by antenatal advice or preparation.

Jones D 1987 Breastfeeding practices. Nursing Times 83 (3) January 21: 56–57
Do maternity units give proper encouragement?

Lask S 1986 The nurses' role in nutrition education. Nursing: The Add-On Journal of Clinical Nursing 3 (8) August: 296–300
Contains a teaching plan.

Lee B 1987 Total parenteral nutrition. Nursing Times 83 (1) January 7: 33–35
Uses a patient study to illustrate the technique.

Lewin D 1985 Hospitals can make you thin. Nursing Times 81 (19) May 8: 36–37
Table of nutritional assessment and one of nutritionally high risk patients.

Lewin D 1985 Liquid nourishment. Nursing Times 81 (20) May 15: 48– 50
Looks at the various methods of ensuring that all patients receive an adequate diet.

Margiotta P 1985 What do children eat? Nursing Mirror 161 (17) October 23: 22-23
Gives three useful techniques for finding out what they normally eat as a basis for the health visitor's further discussion.

Mathews P 1986 Fast food. Nursing Times 82 (11) March 12: 47–49
Are there more hyperactive children? Evidence which suggests that it may be connected with greater intake of food additives.

Moore J 1985 Feeding sick children. Nursing Times 81 (51) December 18/25: 29–30
Advice available on children's nutrition and what they should be encouraged to eat. Table of foods to avoid and those to encourage.

Nursing Mirror Supplement 1984 Procedures for nasogastric feeding. Nursing Mirror 158 (20) May 16.
From the Royal Marsden Hospital's Manual of clinical nursing policies and procedures.

Nursing Times 1985 Pick a plateful. Nursing Times 81 (12) March 20: 40–41
Helping patients to choose a meal from the menu cards can offer an excellent opportunity for nurses to start talking about the important links between nutrition and health.

Nursing Times 1987 WHO code on breast milk not met in UK. Nursing Times 83 (5) February 4: 7
Staff in 20 hospitals still hand out free samples of infant formula, which is expressly forbidden by the WHO code.

Sadler C 1985 New hot drinks therapy. Nursing Mirror 160 (11) March 13: 44

Savage S, Biley F 1984 Bulimia nervosa. Nursing Times 80 (32) August 8: 42–45
Although some patients with anorexia nervosa binge-eat, bulimia is an eating disorder which is described in this article together with its incidence and treatment.

Scott D 1986 Time and patience. Nursing Times 82 (32) August 6: 36– 37
Describes the case of Paul, blind and mentally handicapped, and a student nurse's struggle to teach him to feed himself.

Shircore R, Baichoo S 1985 Understanding Asian diets. Community Outlook March: 16–17
Knowledge of their cultures and dietary

patterns is vital if health visitors are to give Asian parents appropriate advice on feeding babies and young children.

Smallman S 1987 Nutritional assessment of children in hospital. Nursing Times 83 (5) February 4: 55–57

Describes how to assess children at risk by using a range of assessment tools.

Thomas M 1987 More fibre makes sense. Nursing Times 83 (3) January 21: 39

Despite an abundance of literature on the importance of high fibre diets, many doctors and nurses continue to 'treat' constipation instead of preventing it.

UKCC 2E 1984 Code of professional conduct for the nurse, midwife and health visitor. United Kingdom Central Council, 23 Portland Place, London, W1N 3AF

Wilson-Barrett J 1985 What you thought about food. Nursing Times 81 (11) March 13: 27

Nursing Times ran a questionnaire asking nurses what they thought about hospital food and the findings are analysed in this article, and contributed to the 'Care about food campaign'.

Wood S 1986 Nutritional support: an overview of general principles. Nursing: The Add-On Journal of Clinical Nursing 3 (8) August: 301–302

Dietary manipulation; liquid oral supplements; tube feeding; intravenous nutrition. Decision-making flowchart.

Wright M 1986 We're getting there. Nursing Times 82 (9) February 26: 16–19

A report of the 'Care about food' campaign launched by Nursing Times. The results were encouraging.

Wright S 1986 Altered body image in anorexia nervosa. The Professional Nurse 1 (10) July: 260–262

A disease of the West; changes in behaviour; distorted sense of appearance; inability to compromise.

Yates J, Whitehead G 1986 Aids to feeding. Nursing: The Add-On Journal of Clinical Nursing 3 (7) July: 244–248

Illustrated article of the many aids which are available to help disabled people maintain independence for feeding.

BACKGROUND INFORMATION

Eating and drinking is surely a subject which has gained high publicity. Knowledge about many aspects of the science of nutrition, as well as increasing, is at an ever higher level of sophistication. The number of articles in the professional journals has grown apace. The Reading Assignment is long, and information in some of the articles will be needed on particular clinical allocations. Either the title or the annotation will guide students to relevant articles. Before putting the activities of eating and drinking in the context of the process of nursing, a brief introduction will be given to the following:

- increased knowledge available to the public
- Nursing Times — 'Care about food' campaign
- malnutrition in hospital patients.

Increased knowledge available to the public

The media — radio, television, non-professional journals and the national press — have brought current thinking about nutrition to the notice of the general public. The food advertisements, particularly on television, have responded to the increased knowledge. But where did it come from?

A report entitled 'Proposals for nutritional guidelines for health education in Britain' was published by the Health Education Council in 1983; it is popularly known as the NACNE report. It was followed by a government (DHSS) report 'Diet and cardiovascular disease' referred to as the COMA report (Committee on Medical Aspects of Food Policy) in 1984. These were discussed at length on the radio and television; they were written about in the national press, and suggestions were made that political manoeuvring had delayed publication of the COMA report. Holmes (September 18, 1985) discussed the political aspects related to these reports, and Janes (1986) discusses both of them and suggests ways of implementing them in our daily living. A booklet is available to all from the Health Education Service entitled 'Eating for a healthy heart'.

A marked increase in the number of health food shops and the availability of wholefood produce in many towns would seem to indicate an increased interest in a healthy diet. The superstores are responding by displaying 'health' foods on the shelves and manufacturers are improving nutritional information on their products.

The inference of this for nursing is that although patients may not be able to assess nurses' technical skills, they are capable of assessing the standard of the meal service, and the standard of nursing during mealtimes, and of spreading horror stories of ill and helpless patients being left to manage, so that more food landed on night attire than actually entered the mouth.

Nursing Times — 'Care about food' campaign

In the context of increased information available to the public and an increasing number of reports identifying malnutrition in hospital patients (about which more will be said later), the Nursing Times mounted a campaign in March 1985 — 'Care about food'. It advocated that each district should set up a Hospital Food Policy Committee, and invited nurses to send in information about current practices in particular hospitals. These were published on a 'Feedback' page from time to time. A selection of them are included in the Reading Assignment. Sadler (1985) paints the background of change in serving hot drinks to patients, but it could equally be applied to serving meals.

Not all the changes in nursing have been for the better and designation of meal service as a 'non-nursing duty' has had, in some instances, a disastrous result. Holmes (February 13, 1985) says:

> ... patients' meals are distributed, and trays collected, by domestic staff, which means that nurses are not actually certain how much, if any, food is consumed and whether the food eaten is sufficient to meet the patient's needs.

Approximately 1 year after the 'Care about food' campaign was initiated, Wright (1986) reported a nationwide evaluation of it. The conclusion is that moving towards healthier and more varied menus in hospital wards and canteens seems to be gaining strength.

Malnutrition in hospital patients

In the third edition of this book (1982) there were three references to malnutrition in hospital patients, all written by doctors. The subject has since become more widely recognised and some nurses have carried out research projects which are included in the Reading Assignment. The overall message from them is loud and clear — nurses must accept the responsibility of assessing a patient's nutritional status on admission; must record on the nursing plan the type of diet prescribed, even if it is the customary 'Normal diet'; must record how much food was eaten, which in fact constitutes immediate evaluation, although weekly weighing of the patient will be another criterion of evaluation. Later in the text, eating and drinking will be considered in the context of the process of nursing.

It would seem that change in hospital policy to 'meal service' as a 'non-nursing' duty has produced a dichotomy, and nursing has abdicated its role at mealtimes. Yet many ill or frail patients and those with disabled hands require to have the heavy metal covers removed from the plates; the cling film removed — a difficult task at the best of times; and to be so positioned that the spatial track from plate to mouth is manageable.

EATING AND DRINKING IN PROCESS CONTEXT

For most people eating and drinking activities provide pleasant interludes in each day. Helping patients to continue carrying out these activities the nurse has to remember Florence Nightingale's maxim — *the hospital shall do the patient no harm*. One way of avoiding harm is by using information from the assessment form, and, if relevant, from the nursing plan, to individualise mealtimes. There follows some 'practice thinking' in process context about a principle of nursing — helping patients to eat and drink.

Assessing

It is likely that some type of assessment form will be in use in the wards. It may be called a nursing history, patient profile or another name. It is used at the initial assessment to record such things as the well established pattern of time at which the patient eats; type and quantity of food eaten. This is subjective data and it has to be remembered that people may have different perceptions of 'large' and 'small' helpings. However, by discreet observation during mealtimes, the nurse can collect ongoing assessment data which, though still subjective, should be recorded in factual terms on the nursing notes.

Some people have religious impositions on their diet; others have a self-imposed regime, for example vegetarian. Yet others have fads and fancies — cheese for supper makes them dream; eggs make them constipated; cucumber gives them indigestion; rhubarb gives them diarrhoea and so on. If the patient is capable and there is a menu choice, he can continue to be independent for these idiosyncrasies.

Most people have well established pre-meal activities such as going to the lavatory to make themselves comfortable in readiness for the meal, and it is hoped that everyone washes hands before eating. If the patient is mobile, it is courteous to show him the location of these facilities; to tell him whether or not soap and towel are provided, or toilet requisites have to be taken with him. For bed patients, personal hygiene should not be compromised and he can be advised to use a hand wipe before meals.

Disabled people are admitted to hospital for reasons other than their disablement. The nurse needs to know how eating and drinking were coped with previously. Any 'aids to independence' should continue to be used and responsibility for washing and safe keeping between meals must be clearly stated. In broad terms, the nurse is trying to discover if the patient requires any help from the nurses to continue carrying out this activity, and if he does, exactly what sort of help. This information will only be recorded once — on the assessment form — which must therefore be easily available to the nurses on each shift.

Height and weight are two objective criteria which can be used to assess nutritional status even in the outpatients' department. Is the patient gaining or losing weight? Gross loss of weight may be evidenced by ill fitting clothes. In view of what was written previously about malnutrition in hospital patients, nurses with specialist knowledge are advising that other nurses should use two objective measurements — skin calipers which are non-invasive and grasp the skin over the outer arm; they measure subcutaneous fat which is the body's main calorie reserve (Coates 1985). Mid-arm circumference, left and right gives a non-invasive means of assessing body protein, which is not a reserve, but is part of the body's structure, mainly the muscles. When insufficient nutrients are being taken, the energy store in fat will be used first and in the case of a continuing deficient diet, muscle cells will yield their protein. It is to emphasise these facts that the term 'protein calorie malnutrition' is preferred by many to the word 'malnutrition'.

Assessment data about eating and drinking are collected for the following reasons:

- to inform each nurse of the patient's previous eating and drinking habits
- to discover any help which the patient requires. (In many instances this need not be re-written, as long as nurses learn to use the information on the assessment form.)
- to discover any potential or actual problems which are amenable to nursing, the intervention for which will appear on the nursing plan
- to record basic nutrition measurements against which evaluation can be measured. Again these do not need to be written elsewhere in the patient's nursing records.

Planning

By common consent the second phase of the process of nursing is planning, and in 'process thinking' the objective of the patient's nursing plan is individualisation. The subject of this chapter however lends itself to introducing the student to the notion that planning is not the prerogative of the nursing plan; generalised planning may well dictate the resources available when making decisions about the nursing plan; and ward planning is an essential background activity to carrying out the individualised nursing plans.

Generalised planning

It may be difficult for a student of nursing to realise that to facilitate patients' eating and drinking in the wards, a great deal of planning has gone into the provision of facilities to achieve this, such as:

- a dining area which can be as different as:
  - a dining room
  - a dining area in the ward
  - tables in the day room
  - a bedtable for bed patients
  - a lowered bedtable over a chair
- food, and pharmaceutical preparations for provision of nutrients to those patients who cannot take them orally
- staff and kitchens in which to cook food, and pharmacies in which to prepare nutrients
- crockery and cutlery etc. for serving and eating food
- aids to independence in preparing food, and eating it
- equipment to move prepared food from kitchen to ward
- staff to move this equipment
- staff — nursing and/or non-nursing — to deliver food to each patient and supervise mealtime in the ward
- staff, in the majority of hospitals non-nursing, to collect trays, or crockery and cutlery in each ward
- staff to remove these to the central kitchen
- staff to deal with 'washing' even where dishwashers are provided
- hygienic storing of such equipment between meals.

Co-ordination of all these different facilities is no mean feat. However 'centralising' meal services leaves nursing staff in the wards little control over the timing of meals. Some hospitals are solving this problem by installing a microwave oven in the ward kitchen, in which to cook the meals prepared by the central kitchen. All well and good if the patients eat the meal prepared for them. Appetite is notoriously fickle during illness so arrangements should be made for procuring alternative nourishment if a patient does not eat the prepared meal.

A microwave oven would also be useful on those occasions when a patient is away from the ward in another department when the meal is served. We know that in an ideal world this should not happen, but the reality is that the various departments do have a tight working schedule. Some tests involve sequential blood and/or urine analysis; require the patient to fast, and even though started in the morning, may not be complete until after lunch time when the patient can then eat.

Generalised planning is necessary in the community so that those who are being cared for at home can eat and drink adequately. Devlin (1985) describes adaptations in the kitchen so that people can more easily prepare food. Most local authorities offer a home-help service which provides for shopping and the preparation of a meal in the person's home. The meals-on-wheels (a voluntary service) brings a hot meal to the person's home on several days of the week, so that a satisfactory nutrition status is maintained, or improved if that is the goal.

Ward planning

There is much more to helping patients to eat and drink than actually placing the food in front of each patient. Just as one prepares for a meal at home, so certain things have to be attended to in the ward before the food trolley arrives from the kitchen. All other activities should be planned so that they are finished and the patients are in a pleasant and anticipatory mood. In view of the research evidence about malnutrition in hospital patients, a policy should be worked out with medical and paramedical staff so that their visits to the ward do not coincide with meal times. Patients with a malodorous discharge require to have the dressing changed with appropriate deodorant application, so that the ward atmosphere is odour-free at meal times. Where a menu service is the policy, ward planning includes having nurses available in the evening to help patients make appropriate choices and more will be said about this later. Most people prefer to be sitting in a chair rather than in a bed, so for relevant patients their 'up' period can be planned for mealtimes. The optimum position for patients with a particular constraint, for example a hip spica, may be achieved by having an extra pillow for meal times. Some patients will need to have their particular equipment available to help them eat and drink independently. On wards where several patients need to be fed by another, planning will include the presence of these 'others'. Relatives may appreciate the contribution of feeding a terminally ill patient; or a patient on for example a neurosurgical, a ward for mentally handicapped patients, a children's ward and so on.

Individualised planning

The document associated with individualised planning is the patient's nursing plan which usually contains a planned nursing intervention related to a patient's problem, actual or potential. An example of a potential problem might be vomiting as a side-effect to a drug which the patient is taking.

As far as eating and drinking is concerned, even though the patient and the assessment data do not reveal a problem, a prescription for 'Full diet' should appear on the plan; this is recommended by the nurse researchers into malnutrition in hospital patients. But it is not the end of nursing's responsibility to the patient as will be discussed later (p. 143).

Even though the patient and the assessment data do not reveal a problem, if the patient is scheduled for surgery or investigation, then the prescriptions will be:

- a light diet for the preoperative period
- fasting: from fluid for 4 hours
  from solids for 6 hours
  pre-anaesthetic (Hunt 1987)
- light diet postoperatively
- progressing to full diet.

In this instance the plan changes quite rapidly, but not in response to a problem, which is the usual reason for changing, or adding to the nursing plan.

Analysis of the assessment data about eating and drinking may lead to a decision between patient and nurse that a light diet would better suit a delicate appetite than being deterred by the larger full diet. (Even in restaurants it is often difficult to achieve a smaller serving; the waiter thinks he is being helpful when he says — just leave what you cannot eat, missing the point that the client has already been repulsed by the large helping!) Prescription for light diet will be written on the nursing plan, and unlike the transient nature of the light diet prescription in the previous paragraph, this one will probably need to be carried out throughout the patient's stay.

The patient may not have a problem with a diet which is determined by culture or religion, or even a self-imposed one like that of a vegan. However some hospitals may have difficulty in providing it, and the message here is to ask the patient. Whether or not these dietary details are recorded on the nursing plan (do remember that the patient does not have a problem), depends on how much information is recorded on the assessment form and whether nurses on succeeding shifts will have adequate information to enable them to offer a 'different' but not a 'special' diet.

For those patients who for different medical reasons have the problem 'cannot take food by mouth' but the rest of the digestive tract is functioning, then the nursing plan will have written on it a nursing intervention for enteral (artificial) feeding. The liquid is passed into the stomach via a nasogastric tube, or through a stoma in the wall of the stomach (gastrostomy). Should the dysfunctioning part of the digestive tract be the intestine, then the nursing intervention on the plan will provide details of how to accomplish total parenteral nutrition for that patient — even to supervising a patient in his own home.

A text cannot possibly cater for the 'individuality' of the nursing plan, suffice it to say that whatever the nursing intervention, it will have been planned to achieve a particular goal which is stated on the plan, together with a date for evaluation of whether or not the goal is being or has been achieved.

Implementing

The implementing phase of the process of nursing was, in the early days of its introduction to the wards, taken to mean carrying out the nursing interventions which were prescribed to achieve a goal which was set to alleviate or solve a problem which the patient was experiencing in relation to eating and drinking. However, experience has shown that there are necessary nursing activities in the absence of patients' problems — hence the nurse/nutritionist researchers' recommendation to write 'Full diet' on the nursing plan. But it is useless writing it on the nursing plan unless nurses check that the patient receives and eats it. The 'hotel service' recommended by the work studies carried out in the '50s and '60s is not meant to replace the nursing service which continues to be responsible for knowing how much food each patient has eaten at each meal. In preparing to accept the responsibility of a registered nurse, readers are reminded, in this context, that:

> Each registered nurse...is accountable for his or her practice, and, in the exercise of professional accountability shall:
>
> 2. Ensure that no action or omission on his/her part or within his/her sphere of influence is detrimental to the condition or safety of patients/clients.
>
> UKCC 1984

In the case of a small portion mentioned earlier (p. 140) — it is too late when an uncovered tray is placed in front of the patient — the off-putting damage has already been done.

Nurses seem to have considerable difficulty in changing the nursing plan and implementing it in emergency situations when unanticipated rapid changes are essential. A suggestion was made on page 142 of a possible way of coping when the rapid changes are anticipated.

Some patients do not have a problem — they just eat a different diet and it is important to remember that non-specialist servers in the kitchen can send inappropriate dietary items. A glance at the contents of the tray will convey that you are interested in this deeply personal part of living.

The inappropriate dietary items can also apply when a patient is on a special diet! In anticipation of compliance after discharge from hospital it is important that teaching is a part of the nursing plan to be implemented.

Listening to the patient who will have to stay on a very restricted diet such as 100 g of protein daily, the nurse may see a potential problem of non-compliance in, for instance, a young mother with two young children. Discussing the possibility with the mother, it may transpire that she would welcome help. The nursing plan will therefore include teaching the patient why such a drastic reduction is necessary. Nurses need to acquire the skill of helping patients to understand how the body works by explaining it in simple, non-technical terms. And it is essential that nurses seek feedback from the patient as to what has been understood. Once-only teaching of such a complex subject is useless, as is once-only feedback of what has been understood immediately after teaching — feedback needs to be at an increasing time interval if it is to achieve the permanent memory store.

Of course we cannot leave this section on implementing without a reminder that as each planned nursing intervention is carried out it is recorded in the patient's nursing notes with the date and time, and any relevant information from ongoing assessment which summatively will be used on the date set for evaluation.

Lest the 'art' of nursing be forgotten, the following portion from the third edition is being retained.

Helping patients with particular problems

Patients can experience innumerable problems in relation to eating and drinking and nurses need to be knowledgeable and innovative in offering help so that patients can cope. Some of

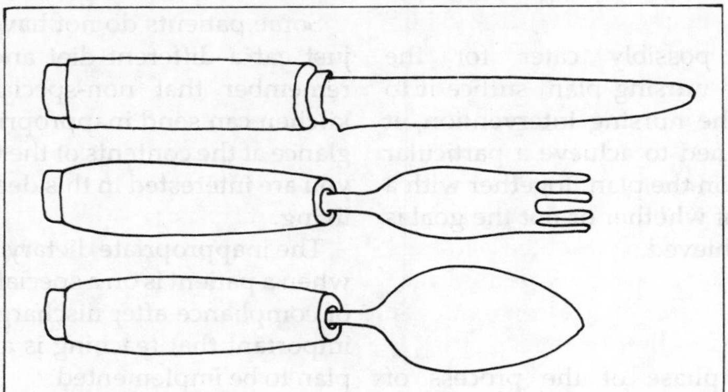

Fig. 12.1 Cutlery with foam-covered handles for easier grip

the problems in alphabetical order will now be discussed. A physiotherapist and a speech therapist (Caunter & Penrose 1983) have written an illustrated article to help nurses, to help those patients who have problems with sucking, chewing and swallowing so that they cannot feed independently. A dietitian and a speech therapist also give guidance to nurses helping patients regain independent feeding after a stroke (Cockcraft & Ray 1985).

Absence of all natural teeth renders a person 'edentulous' and for this condition most people wear dentures. Those who do not, need a soft diet, not too hot, and without scattered additional salt, pepper, acids, spices on the food, as the healed gum surface remains more sensitive than the rest of the mouth.

Anorexia means that the patient has lost his appetite, observable as his disinclination for taking food. The change of food, lessened physical activity, raised anxiety level and the illness itself can all contribute to the condition. Aperitifs may be useful in re-establishing appetite. Thin soups can be given at the beginning of a meal to act as an appetiser; beef tea comes into this category. Drugs called stomachics can induce appetite; they are bitter and are given 20 minutes before a meal, undiluted with no attempt to disguise the taste.

Several of the references refer to a particular type of anorexia — anorexia nervosa.

Coughing can present problems when eating and drinking, particularly when the cough is dry and irritating as in whooping cough. Patients are best advised not to eat dry, crumbly food such as biscuits, and to avoid sprinkling pepper and spices on food.

Disablement of the preferred hand can be overcome by expanding the handles of cutlery with tubular plastic foam (Fig. .12.1) and providing a 'tip-up' stand for teapot (Fig. 12.2). There are also looped-handled spoons and pushers for rheumatoid, geriatric and spastic hands; unbreakable plates with guards,

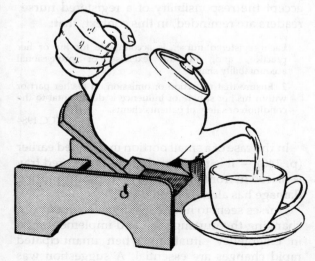

Fig 12.2 'Tip-up' stand for teapot

and mugs of non-spillable design. There are useful illustrations of many eating and drinking aids in Yates & Whitehead (1986).

When the disablement involves the problem of eating while lying flat the patient can be helped by serving his meals on a transparent plate or in a transparent bowl or dish. It may cause less disturbance to eating if a member of the family can come at meal times. Some disabled patients, particularly those who have a hand tremor from any cause, are apt to 'spill' food on its journey from plate to mouth. Soiling of their clothes is distressing to many of them. A nurse must use her judgement in each situation to solve the problem to the patient's satisfaction, so that he continues to look forward to mealtimes, and is not made to dread them because he is different from others in the ward who manage to feed themselves cleanly.

Dysphagia means that the patient's problem is difficulty in swallowing. Those with a sore mouth or throat can be helped before a meal by holding aspirin mucilage against the soreness, then swallowing the mucilage. Omission of condiments, spices and bitter things is also helpful. Sometimes semi-solids are more easily swallowed than liquids. Those with paralysis (hemiparesis) of the face (Bell's palsy, stroke) are best advised to let the food and fluid go along the unaffected side to initiate the swallowing reflex. Patients with a splinted fractured jaw usually suck food through a tube that the surgeon leaves in situ. Their food needs to be pulped sufficiently finely to go through the tube, and a good drink at the end of a meal should be encouraged.

Dyspnoea is breathlessness and it can create several problems related to eating and drinking. Breathless patients are already short of oxygen and oxygen is essential for the chemical and physical processes of digestion. They need a soft diet which does not need much chewing, and the nurse by her thoughtfulness may be able to spare them further muscular activity, for example she may feed them. Breathless patients need extra time to eat and they should be spared the effort of talking while eating; at the same time they should not be ignored. The nurse should phrase her conversation so the patients need only to nod or shake their head, or utter a monosyllable.

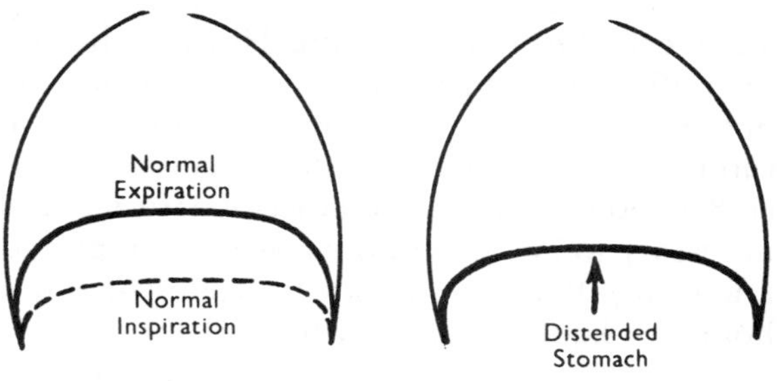

Fig. 12.3 Descent of diaphragm impeded by distended stomach

It is wise not to offer breathless patients crumbly food and not to sprinkle further condiments on their food. Coarse vegetables which can cause intestinal flatulence which in turn can interfere with diaphragmatic movement (Fig. 12.3) should be excluded from the diet of dyspnoeic patients. Smaller meals given at more frequent intervals may keep these patients more comfortable. A drink with each mouthful of food may make chewing easier but can produce flatulence which will need treatment. There may be increased difficulty if the patient feels a need to 'conform' by eating with a closed mouth; there is less breathlessness with a slightly open mouth.

Excessive fluid intake can be so severe that it interferes with the patient's daily living. It is not a common phenomenon but the nurse needs to be aware of the possibility so that she can recognise and report it. Rarely post head injury patients manifest this condition and undiagnosed young diabetics are so afflicted.

Excessive food intake over energy expenditure leads to obesity. It is now recognised that the cause may be of a complex psychological nature. Fine (1987) reports research papers which were read at an international conference on obesity. Obese patients can be encouraged to join one of the several self-help groups whose objective is the establishment of good food habits and control of body weight.

Imposed fasting before anaesthetic or investigation undoubtedly creates an anxiety problem for the patient. Hamilton-Smith (1972) discusses many different interpretations by nurses and doctors of the term 'nil by mouth'. If such a patient is conscious and able to co-operate he should understand the exact hours of fasting and the ill-effects of not fasting. He can be helped to fulfil his obligation if he is given the opportunity to be out of the ward, for example he can take a bath when breakfast is served. Hunt (1987) reports that a multidisciplinary team is necessary to implement the research-supported knowledge that pre-anaesthetic fasting of only 4 hours for liquids, and only 6 hours for solids is necessary. The majority of patients are fasted for much longer and this may be a contributory factor to malnutrition in surgical ward patients (Dickerson 1986d). It is administratively easier to have a rule on a ward — anyone for operation the next day (at whatever hour) should be fasted from midnight (which really means the previous 9 pm, the time of the last drink). Hunt (1987) describes the multidisciplinary effort necessary to convert research findings into reality.

Inadequate fluid intake or excessive output via any route causes dehydration when the patient's problems are dry mouth and skin, and loss of weight. Elderly patients are specially at risk as their thirst reflex is often diminished. The weight loss can be measured by weighing scales and it can be observed as sunken eyes and loss of skin elasticity; if the skin is gently drawn between finger and thumb it remains wrinkled and puckered. The body attempts to conserve its fluid, so that only a small amount of concentrated urine is passed and constipation may be troublesome. In a young baby there will be a sunken fontanelle.

Inadequate intake of, or absorption from, food can lead to malnutrition. The deficiency may be in one nutrient or essential element or compound, when it usually produces specific disease. A more generalised malnutrition is called emaciation or cachexia, the same signs and symptoms being present as those given for dehydration. Once the blood protein falls below its normal 6 to 8% it has not sufficient osmotic pressure to suck fluid back into the vessels at the venous end of capillary networks and oedema results. Protein concentrates may be needed by the patient taking only a small amount of food. Patients with a poor appetite do not usually eat sufficient fruit and vegetables. The problem of introducing vitamins in little bulk must be solved.

Indigestion and flatulence may result from the increased anxiety and lessened physical activity consequent on admission to hospital. After-dinner mints owe their popularity to prevention of these conditions. Peppermint water is a carminative available in most hospitals. It is most effective when given in hot water. Heartburn, waterbrash and pyrosis all refer to indigestion. Tympanism and tympanites are terms used for intestinal flatulence.

Visual handicap can be a problem when eating and drinking though many blind people are clever at eating without help and value their independence in this direction. Food should be cut into mouth-sized pieces and arranged so that the server can describe the plate clockwise, as she places it in front of the patient. Towards the end of a meal a visually-handicapped person may have difficulty in 'finding' the last remnants on the plate — usually at the edge, as they can manage food from the middle. A passing nurse can help by saying, 'There's a slice of tomato at 3 o'clock, a piece of ham at 6 o'clock and a piece of cucumber at 11 o'clock, then you've cleaned your plate' — rather than by offering to feed him.

Helping patients with diet modifications

Some patients are faced with accepting modifications of diet as part of their treatment. Each nurse must do her best to make this as easy for the patient as possible. (A low protein diet has already been mentioned — p. 143) It calls for initiative, ingenuity and resourcefulness.

The patient on '*restricted fluids*' is more likely to co-operate if the nurse discusses with him how much he normally drinks and at what time of day. Between them, nurse and patient can decide the quantity and times at which the restricted intake is most acceptable. Such patients will appreciate a pleasant tasting mouthwash (covered from dust) at hand throughout the day and night.

A patient who needs to drink '*extra fluids*' should understand why, before we can expect his co-operation. He can then protect his own kidneys from crystallisation if he is on sulphonamides, help to right his own fluid balance if he is sweating profusely or has had diarrhoea, contribute to the dilution and elimination of toxins if he has an infection, prevent constipation of his bowel and so on. Few people drink large quantities of water. The patient may manage to drink more if offered a change of flavour, for example, lime, lemon, orange, blackcurrant, pineapple, and rose-hip. Beer can act as an incentive.

Some patients are asked to accept such modifications as high or low kjoule, high or low protein, high or low dietary fibre (roughage), low fat, low animal fat, fat-free, salt-free, alcohol-free, gastric or diabetic diet, either temporarily or for life. Remembering the pleasure with which healthy people select and eat food will help those preparing diets to use imagination and enthusiasm to prevent 'sameness' in special diets. Disease, injury and operation destroy tissue; such tissues need the requisites for healing. Protein is the tissue-building food and a good supply of vitamin C facilitates its function; protein and vitamin C are therefore especially important in the diet of pre-convalescent patients.

In the last decade parenteral (tube) feeding has gained in popularity and some patients learn to feed themselves independently via the stoma. Total parenteral nutrition is feeding via a catheter usually introduced into the subclavian vein, and a few patients learn to deal with this independently and live at home. Dewar (1986) asks what would it be like never to eat solid food again? She describes some of the psychological problems such patients need to cope with. The increased importance of helping patients to eat and drink has resulted in this 'implementing' section being long. However in completing it, readers are reminded that as each planned nursing intervention is carried out it is recorded in the patient's nursing notes with the date and time, and any relevant information from ongoing assessment which summatively will be used on the date set for evaluation.

Evaluating

Already in this chapter, the word evaluating has been used, which illustrates that the four phases of the process of nursing can only be considered individually for the purpose of description. Many of the same skills are used in the assessing and evaluating phases but the data collected in the evaluating phase is compared with that collected at the initial assessment. Possible measurements are listed below:

- weight
- height — long stay children
- skin calipers
- upper arm circumference
- food can be weighed
- fluid intake can be measured
- the basal metabolic rate (BMR) can be measured
- known nutrient composition of fluid given enterally and parenterally.

In this chapter the Background information was discussed under three headings — Increased knowledge available to the public; Nursing Times 'Care about food' campaign; and Malnutrition in hospital patients. The principle — helping patients to eat and drink — was discussed in the context of the process of nursing. The opportunity was taken to widen the concept of planning to include generalised and ward planning as well as individualised planning. Implementing included discussion of Helping patients with particular problems and Helping patients with diet modifications.

APPLYING THE PRINCIPLE

A registered nurse must be capable of:

- arranging the ward routine so that at meal times the atmosphere is free from dust and offensive odours, the ward is free from unpleasant sights and no patient has just had a distressing treatment done
- applying her knowledge of 'a well-balanced diet' when feeding the majority of patients and modifying this diet according to the disease from which each patient is suffering
- helping patients to accept diet modifications
- lifting and assisting patients into the most natural position for eating, without harm to herself or the patient. Communicating these skills to others

- communicating the times of patients' meals to consultants, registrars, housemen, clergy and staff of other departments in such a way that they will not deny a patient the pleasure of meal times
- encouraging the staff to take a pride in serving meals well. Praising them when they display initiative, ingenuity and resourcefulness
- encouraging the staff to observe and report how much food and fluid each patient has taken
- using every opportunity for teaching nutrition to staff and patients
- organising so that there is as little waste of food as possible
- organising the environment and teaching the staff a reliable routine to prevent food poisoning
- keeping accurate weight charts and graphs, intake and output charts and inspiring others to do the same
- asking the appropriate authority for anything that will ease the serving of meals for the staff, increase the pleasure of meals for the patient and raise the standard of food hygiene
- helping with the planning of a new ward with adequate arrangements for patients to eat and drink
- administering, supervising and teaching enteral administration of nutrients when a patient is unable to take by mouth
- administering, supervising and teaching parenteral administration of nutrients
- applying the principle — helping patients to eat and drink — in a process of nursing context

WORKING ASSIGNMENT

Topics for discussion

- should a spoon be used when assisting a helpless patient with a savoury course?
- should a nurse sit or stand when assisting a helpless patient with feeding?
- a helpless patient requires some assistance with feeding. Should the nurse be at the patient's right or left side?
- it is sister's day off. You are in charge of the ward and are in the middle of serving lunches. A consultant comes in and wants to examine Mrs Jones who is enjoying fish soufflé and potatoes mashed with butter. What would you do?
- re skills of communication: you are asked to serve lunch to a dyspnoeic patient. Discuss suitable speech which will only require a monosyllabic contribution from the patient, or a shake or nod of his head
- re serving meals: nursing personnel v. non-nursing personnel
- the pros and cons of patients filling in the 'choice of menu' card on the previous evening.

Writing assignment

- describe the posture a tray-carrier should adopt to prevent strain and fatigue
- define the following

anorectic
anorexia
anorexia nervosa
aperitif
aromatic
artificial feeding
bacteriostatic
basal metabolic rate
Bell's palsy
cachexia
carminative
compound
diabetes insipidus
diabetes mellitus
dehydration
diarrhoea
dysphagia
dyspnoea
edentulous
emaciation
enteral
extra-oral
flatulence
fontanelle
fracture
gastrostomy

heartburn
hemiparesis
in situ
indigestion
malnutrition
mucilage
nephritis
obesity
oedema
parenteral
polydipsia
protein calorie malnutrition
pyrosis
reflex
stomachic
stroke
sulphonamides
total parenteral nutrition
tube feeding
toxins
tympanites
waterbrash
whooping cough

- give the technical term for indigestion
- name four carminatives
- give two other names for heartburn
- give the signs and symptoms of dehydration
- write the flavours for a patient on 'extra fluids'
- take half an hour to write what you understand by 'a well-balanced diet'
- name the extra-oral routes via which fluid and nourishment can be introduced into a patient unable to take by mouth
- the medical diagnosis is gastric ulcer. Give some possible patient's problems in his words — a nursing diagnosis (see p. 10).

13

Helping patients to mobilise

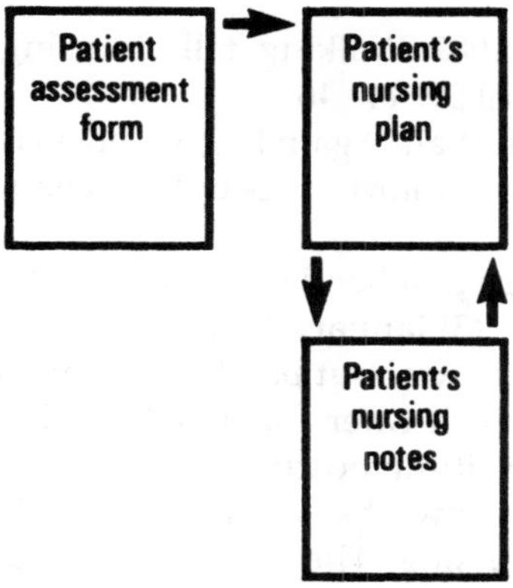

Reading assignment

Background information
- *Early ambulation*
- *Hazards of enforced immobility*
- *Multidisciplinary mobilising team*

Mobilising in a process of nursing context
- *Assessing patients' ability to mobilise*
- *Planning*
- *Implementing*
- *Evaluating*
- *Focusing the four phases to the nurse in a general context*
- *Focusing the four phases to the nurse in a particular context — bedmaking*

Applying the principle
- *A registered nurse must be capable of:*

Working assignment
- *Topics for discussion*
- *Writing assignment*

READING ASSIGNMENT

Atkinson D 1984 Mobility in the armed forces. Nursing: The Add-On Journal of Clinical Nursing 2 (32) December : 955–957
Describes the task of restoring military personnel to full mobility in the shortest possible time.

Boyle A 1984 The adult hemiplegic patient. Nursing: The Add-On Journal of Clinical Nursing 2 (32) December: 952–954
Patients should be encouraged to make the best use of returning sensation and perceptual ability. Nurses will seek to inhibit the development of any unwanted patterns of spasticity and to facilitate patterns of movement which are as near normal as possible. The special handling techniques which incorporate the Bobath approach are illustrated.

Community Outlook 1984 Back savers. October: 362, 364, 366
With the help of the Disabled Living Foundation information service offers a guide to choosing a hoist, plus suggestions for further reading and information. Illustrated.

David J 1986 Additions to the bed. Nursing: The Add-On Journal of Clinical Nursing 3 (3) March: 112–114
Uses the following headings — materials used for support; equipment made of foam;

air-filled systems; water-filled systems; polystyrene beads; fibres and gels.

Devlin R 1985 Making life easier round the house for disabled people. Community Outlook October: 27–28
Choosing the right sling is as important as choosing the right hoist. Also discusses baths, showers, basins and personal toilet.

Goldthorpe A 1984 Mobility problems for the disabled — a traveller's tale.
The philosophy of travelling with disabled people has to be — prepare for the worst, but hope for the best.

Goodlad J 1986 How to claim. National Association of Health Authorities in England and Wales, Garth House, 47 Edgebaston Park Road, Birmingham B15 2RS
If you ask for help with lifting, make a note of who was asked, especially if it is not forthcoming, and ensure a safety representative is aware of the situation.

Hayne C 1984 Safe patient movement — an alternative approach. Nursing: The Add-On Journal of Clinical Nursing 2 32 December: 931–934
Discusses some of the reasons why injuries from patient handling persist, and gives further illustration of how they can be avoided.

Hayne C 1985 Safe patient movement — an alternative approach. Nursing: The Add-On Journal of Clinical Nursing 2 (33) January: 960–965
Discusses patient transfer from bed to chair; chair to chair; chair to toilet; and lifts from the floor. Illustrated.

Henderson R 1981 A new aid to geriatric nursing. Nursing Times 77 1 January 1: 27–29
Describes the evolution of a duvet complying with DHSS standards for fire hazard, laundering, bacteriological hazards, which can be used in 'wet areas' — for incontinent patients.

Henry N 1984 Handle with care. Senior Nurse 1 (37) December: 22–23
Staff at ward level should be given the opportunity to explain their needs when alterations are being planned, or equipment ordered.

Heywood Jones I 1987 Walking tall. Nursing Times 83 (17) April 29: 44–46
The WALK Fund (Walk Again Leg Kinetics) is helping spinally injured people regain mobility.

Holmes P 1985 Shops that bend over backwards. Nursing Times 81 (3) January 16: 29
With all the publicity about bad backs, shops are appearing which cater for furniture that encourages good sitting posture.

Horgan M 1985 Low back pain and its management. Nursing: The Add-On Journal of Clinical Nursing 2 (44) December: 1298–1300
Causes; clinical assessment; investigations; conservative hospital management; surgery; rehabilitation.

Howie C 1986 Back to basics. Nursing Times 82 (39) September 24: 18–19
Reviews a research report from Surrey University — Ergonomics Research Unit. Back pain in nurses. Summary and recommendations. Besides teaching and learning handling skills and the importance of keeping the back straight nurses must be consulted before plans are drawn up for new equipment and buildings.

Hudson M 1986 Lifting and back pain. Nursing Times 82 (22) May 28: 13
A letter making an additional point that to avoid bent posture in nursing work, postural stress should be reduced by using good ergonomic principles of design.

Johnston M 1987 Handle with care. Senior Nurse 6 (5) May: 20–22
Most student nurses in a survey lifted patients without assessment or planning, and many of the lifts were unsafe.

Kaur B, Pedersen H 1986 Mind your backs! Nursing Times 82 (16) April 16: 45–47
A postural examination of 100 nurses revealed certain factors which may cause low back pain.

Lloyd P 1986 Nursing Times 82 (47) November 19: 33–35
What is the manager's responsibility towards preventing staff injuring themselves through lifting patients?

Love C 1986 Do you roll or lift? Nursing Times 82

(29) July 16: 44– 46
After total hip replacement, medically prescribed positional restrictions can affect the way in which nurses work.
McCall J 1985 Back pain: a preventive programme for nurses. Nurse Education Today 5: 78–80
Works on the principle of developing good basic movement patterns.

NT News 1986 Staff put on winter warmers. Nursing Times 82 (9) February 26: 8
One hospital persuaded its health authority to drop the traditional uniform in favour of trouser suits which are ergonomically better for nursing work.

NT News 1984 Back injuries cost health service millions. Nursing Times 80 (48) November 28: 5
Back pain causes misery to one in six nurses and costs the health service £52 million a year.

Peake G 1984 Assisting the disabled worker. Nursing: The Add-On Journal of Clinical Nursing 2 (32) December: 939–941
Gives a good account of the occupational health nurse's role in this context.

Rodgers S 1985 Shouldering the load. Nursing Times 81 (3) January 16: 24–26
Project looked at lifting as taught in the school, and how it was carried out in two general medical and surgical wards.

Rodgers S 1985 Positive lifting. Nursing Times 81 (4) January 23: 43–45
Emphasises the importance of the ward sister in creating a positive environment for safe lifting practice.

RCN 1987 The handling of patients. Royal College of Nursing London. Booklet. Details how effective training, ergonomics and lifting techniques can reduce the scale of back pain among nurses.

Scholey M 1984 Patient handling skills. 80 (26) June 27: 25–27
The phases of the process are applied to training programmes which should be taught in every ward.

Stallard J 1981 The disabled: Walk on! Nursing Mirror 153 (16) October 14: xviii, xix, xxii
Describes one of the early swivel walkers — an orthosis to help paraplegic people to walk again.

Stevens T 1985 Aids centres and the Disabled Living Foundation. Nursing: The Add-On Journal of Clinical Nursing 2 (33) January: 968, 970–971
Describes the work of these centres and gives the addresses throughout the country.

Stubbs D, Buckle P 1984 The epidemiology of back pain in nurses. Nursing: The Add-On Journal of Clinical Nursing 2 (32) December: 935– 938
Written by two researchers who led the research which was carried out at the University of Surrey.

Swaffield L 1985 Out of court, out of mind. Nursing Times 81 (3) January 16: 27–28
One in six nurses will suffer a back injury this year. Hours or years of strain at work can add up invisibly. The final trigger can be as trivial as a sneeze. To gain compensation, the nurse has to prove that management knew of the hazard, and could have taken steps to prevent it.

Tarling C 1984 Assessing the mobility needs of the dependent person. Nursing: The Add-On Journal of Clinical Nursing 2 (32) December: 974– 950
In the assessment of mobility every opportunity should be taken to give the disabled person the choice of movement rather than to leave them in a position where mobility is thrust upon them by others.

Tarling C 1985 Let the aids take the strain. Community Outlook December: 15–16
Looks at some of the products available, and their use in the community.

Tarling C 1985 Aids to patient mobility. Nursing: The Add-On Journal of Clinical Nursing 2 (33) January: 974–975, 977, 979
The ambulant person indoors; beds; toilets; baths; personal mobility aids; household tasks; outdoor mobility; the wheelchair bound person; lifting slings or lifting sheets; turntable; electrically controlled beds; hoists.

Wright B 1985 Learning to walk again — how to help the elderly. Nursing: The Add-On Journal of Clinical Nursing 2 (33) January: 982– 984
Pivoting to a sitting position on the edge of the

bed; standing from a sitting position; taking steps; moving the patient to the back of a chair; spasm and rigidity; backward leaning; frail patients require a less vigorous programme; the transfer belt; the Sunderland lifting frame; improving aids; teaching relatives.

BACKGROUND INFORMATION

Good posture, for those who have the physical ability to achieve it, is a prerequisite for mobilising. It is accomplished by alternate contraction and relaxation of opposing groups of muscles, which, being attached to bone, produce movement. Firm muscles, kept in this condition by regular exercise are much more likely to achieve good posture with its attendant feeling of well-being, than muscles in poor tone which become soft and flabby with consequent inability to achieve good posture, and this is not conducive to a feeling of well-being.

Plato said that the most beautiful motion is also that which gives the maximum result with minimum effort. It looks easy when the expert does it! But gracefulness and efficiency in posture and movement are only acquired with much thought, practice and perseverance. Nurses act as role models for good standing, sitting and walking postures which are illustrated in Figures 13.1, 13.2 and 13.3

Non-restrictive clothing and good, supporting footwear need to be considered, especially in conjunction with movement and lifting. A raglan, as opposed to a 'set-in' sleeve, looseness at the waist as opposed to waist-fitting and belted garments, are advocated by the health and beauty experts for those whose work necessitates a lot of movement and lifting. Howie (1986) reporting on research carried out at the University of Surrey said that trousers and tunics were ergonomically better than the traditional national nursing uniform.

Knowledge about helping patients to mobilise has increased considerably in the last few decades, for several reasons, one of which was recognition of the fact that prolonged bedrest resulted in serious complications (p. 155). Early ambulation was introduced to prevent these. In

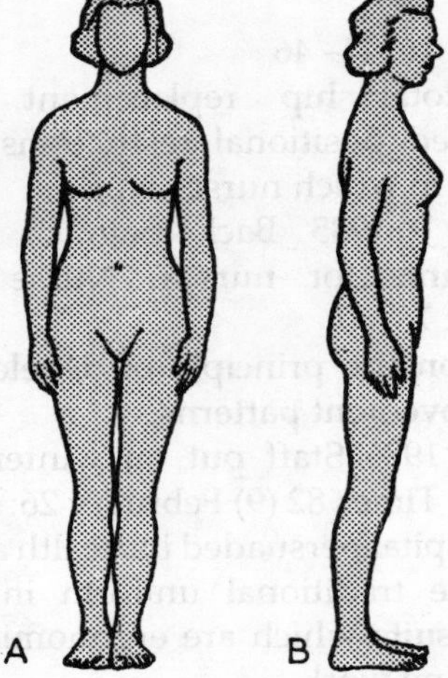

Fig. 13.1 Good standing posture (A) Anterior view (B) Lateral view

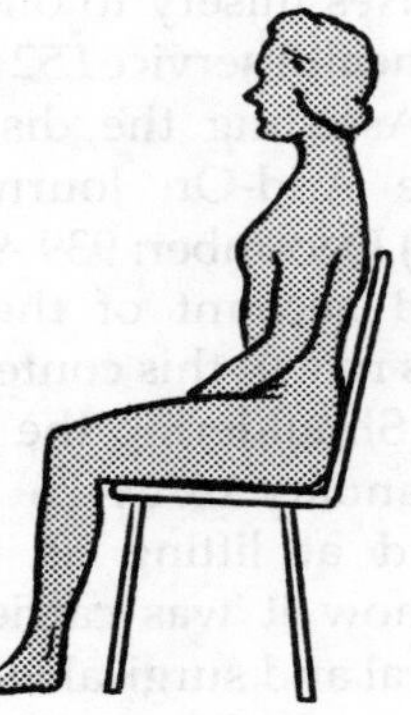

Fig. 13.2 Good sitting posture

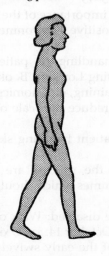

Fig. 13.3 Good walking posture

the last decade there has been increasing emphasis on people accepting responsibility for their own health and this included disabled people achieving the maximal independence for mobilising, congruent with their condition and circumstances. Staff from many disciplines contribute to people achieving their maximum mobilising potential and these different concepts will be discussed before considering mobilising in a process of nursing context.

Early ambulation

Twenty years ago most postoperative patients, after recovery from the anaesthetic, were raised into the sitting position, supported on a backrest and three or four pillows. A mackintosh-covered pillow was rolled in a drawsheet and placed under the knees, the ends of the drawsheet being tucked under the mattress. These 'donkeys' were removed when the patient used a bedpan. Every patient used a bedpan; commodes were not part of hospital equipment.

Under this régime some patients developed phlebitis. Glycerine and ichthyol dressings or kaolin poultices were applied to the afflicted leg. It was kept at rest, raised on a protected pillow. Sudden death from massive pulmonary embolism occurred in some patients so treated. Then it was decided that the leg condition was not primarily an inflammatory one, but a blood clotting one, so the term phlebothrombosis was preferred, currently the term 'deep vein thrombosis', with its abbreviation DVT, is in use. The donkeys were blamed for creating venous stasis leading to this condition, so out they came — very gradually over the whole country. But still some patients developed thrombosis and a few progressed to pulmonary embolism.

Patients were then taught to do deep breathing and toe and foot movements (see Figs 15.1, 15.2, p. 203; 15.3, p.205). Nurses were encouraged to leave the upper bedclothes sufficiently loose to allow for this. At about the same time 'early ambulation' came into vogue. This met with various interpretations. At first many patients were helped out of bed on to a hard chair, sat there for an hour or two and were then helped back to bed. There they lay like a log recovering from the exhaustion. Some patients exhausted themselves by the amount of exercise they took while 'up', and likewise lay like a log on return to bed. Some were helped to walk to the lavatory once a day which was much appreciated.

Ward furniture has improved considerably and there is now a variety of chairs in most wards — necessary because of the number of anatomical differences, fat thighs, thin thighs, long legs, short legs, long backs, short backs and so on. The use of commodes has crept in during the last three decades, and they have become increasingly popular. They are preferred to sanichairs by many people. All these factors make their contribution to the effectiveness of early ambulation.

The traffic in most wards is not conducive to the gentle, unhurried *exercise* implied in the term 'early ambulation'. In an attempt to overcome this deficiency in new buildings, no patient is far from a day room with comfortable chairs. Several lavatories need to be near the day room.

When a person thinks of himself taking exercise, involving good posture and movement, he thinks of himself as clothed in his daytime attire. A dressing gown, night attire and bedroom slippers are conducive to lounging and relaxing. So how are our patients going to get 'toned up' and in the best possible state for discharge? Some hospitals are being built with separate areas for patients needing intensive, medium and self care. In many open wards the ill patients are near sister's desk or the nurses' station; those recovering are in the intermediate beds and the preconvalescent patients occupy the beds farthest from the desk or station. It is the facilities for the latter being up and about independently that are often lacking in the older hospitals.

Hazards of enforced immobility

Early ambulation was introduced to prevent the hazards of enforced immobility, some of which were described in the foregoing paragraphs; they are summarised in Figure 2.1 (p. 40). Nursing activities related to maintaining integrity of patients' posture and movement are obviously important. Nurses need to remember that exercise helps muscles to maintain 'tone', evidenced by firmness on palpation. An adequate diet, especially with regard to protein and vitamin C, will help to keep muscle tissue in good condition. Unused muscles on the other hand lose 'tone' and feel soft and flabby; they become incapable of the contraction necessary to produce normal movement and this can cause deformity such as footdrop.

Positioning of a patient's limbs in the optimum (neutral) position, and active and passive movement of all joints twice daily help to prevent muscle atrophy with possible consequent deformity. Where physiotherapists and occupational therapists are available they will help with these preventive measures.

Multidisciplinary mobilising team

The concept of mobilising had its origins in that of early ambulation but it has enlarged considerably over the years. It now includes the complex biomechanics of:

- standing
- sitting
- transferring from one surface to another such as
  - bed to chair
  - chair to commode
  - wheelchair to lavatory seat
  - floor to chair/bed
- rising from being seated
- walking: aided walking:
  - calipers
  - special shoes
  - splints
  - artificial limbs
  - swizel walker (Stallard 1981)
  - hip guidance orthosis (Stallard 1981)
  - reciprocating gait orthosis (Heywood Jones 1987)
- moving trunk, shoulders, arms and hands in the hundred and one actions to:
  - dress and undress
  - attend to personal hygiene
  - carry out domestic activities, etc.
- physical exercising
- transporting a person mechanically:
  - buggies for children: self-operating
    - electrically operated
  - wheelchairs: pushed by another
    - self-propelling
    - electrically operated
  - cars: adapted to particular disability

This is not an exhaustive list but it is sufficient to demonstrate that helping patients to mobilise requires a contribution from more than one professional group.

The concept of a multidisciplinary team to help people who have different sorts of problems related to mobilising has enlarged over the last few decades. This is partly due to the fact that members of other disciplines, and the public at large, have become more aware of the problems which disabled people have to solve or cope with. Several agencies can contribute to disabled people achieving maximal mobilising and they are referred to by Atkinson (1984), Stallard (1981), Stevens (1985), Stubbs & Buckle (1984) and Tarling (1985). The following list, though not exhaustive, conveys the range of possible helping agencies:

- nurses
- doctors
- physiotherapists
- occupational therapists
- occupational health nurses
- remedial gymnasts
- clinical psychologists
- rehabilitation officers
- Disablement Resettlement Officer
- Disabled Living Foundation
- architects
- builders
- bioengineers
- prosthesis technicians.

Of course, there are various industries which manufacture different pieces of equipment to help disabled people to be as stable and as independent as possible when mobilising. These are illustrated in advertisements in the nursing journals and exhibited at the various nursing conferences.

MOBILISING IN A PROCESS OF NURSING CONTEXT

Mobilising is yet another example of a concept being greater than the sum of the four phases of the process of nursing. Focusing the process to the patient cannot be accomplished without considering application of the 'method' to nurses' work: there has to be dovetailing of patients' and nurses' mobilising.

Originally nurses concentrated on focusing the phases of the process to the patient and his mobilising activities, and this continues to be necessary in order to produce a patient's individualised nursing plan. However, experience is revealing that the phases of the process can be focused to the nurse in relation to:

- the mobilising aspects of many nursing activities which are carried out
- acting as a role model of good standing, sitting and walking postures (p. 154) as well as lifting and moving both people and various objects
- teaching patients good standing, sitting, walking and lying postures; as well as how to protect their backs from injury by keeping the back straight during waking hours, especially when lifting heavy weights.

A Chinese proverb says that a picture is worth a thousand words, so on this ground, Figures 13.4–13.13 are included to illustrate the points in the foregoing list. Much more can be learned about them from articles in the Reading Assignment: the message is loud and clear:

- do not overstretch back muscles
- keep the back as straight as possible throughout waking hours
- avoid stooping
- bend knees instead of back.

It is patently clear that not everyone is aware of, and carries out these principles. Low back pain results from compromising the complex structures of the 'back' and this complaint is the reason for many people attending their doctor's

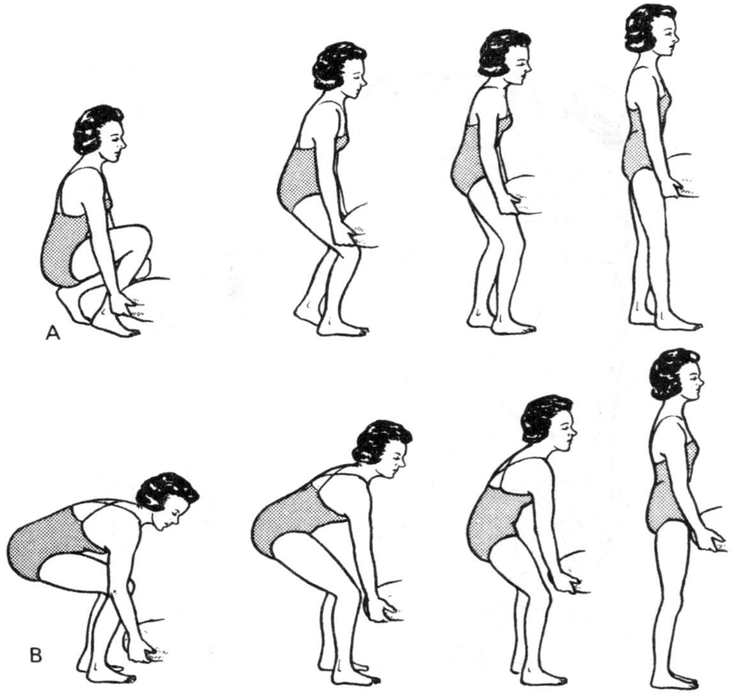

Fig. 13.4 Mechanics of lifting a heavy weight from the floor (A) Correct method (B) Incorrect method

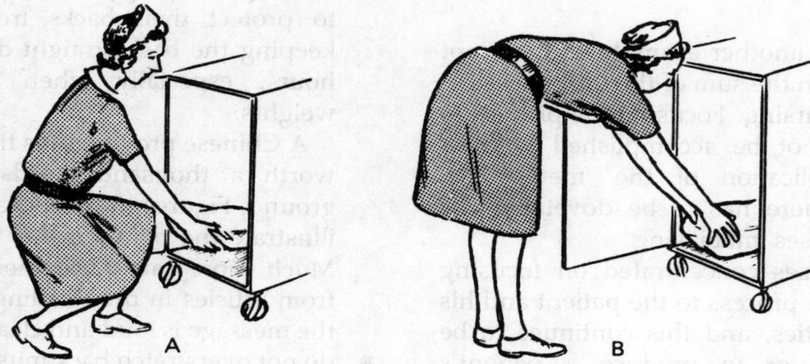

Fig. 13.5 Mechanics of lifting an article from a low level (A) Correct method (B) Incorrect method

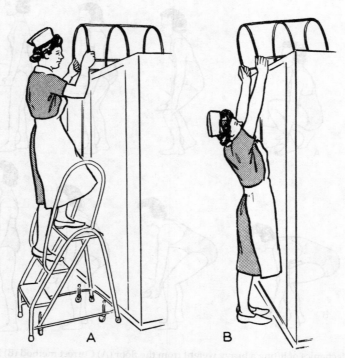

Fig. 13.6 Mechanics of lifting an article from a shelf above shoulder level (A) Correct method (B) Incorrect method

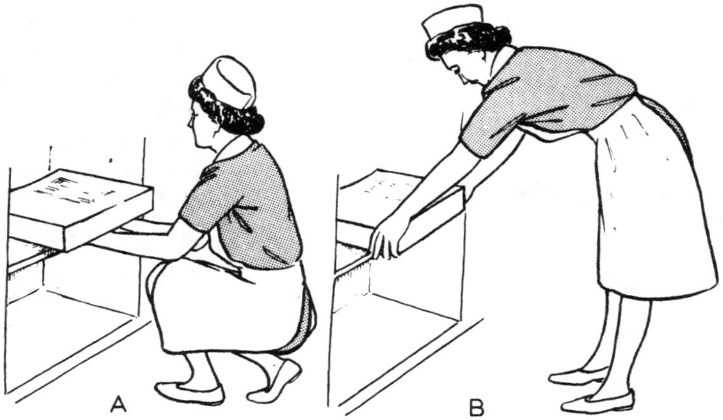

Fig. 13.7 Mechanics of lifting an article from shelf below waist level (A) Correct method (B) Incorrect method

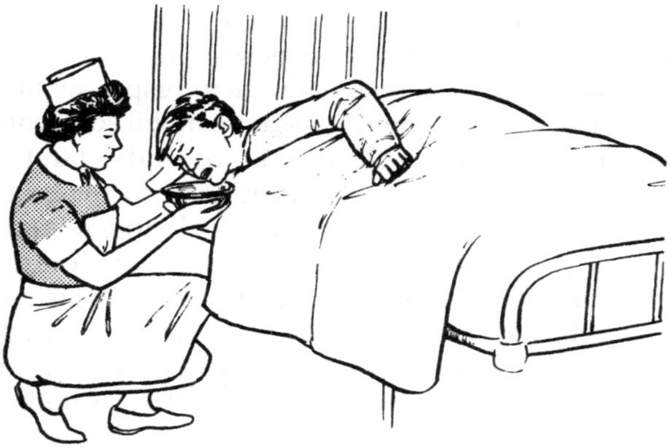

Fig. 13.8 Nurse maintaining good posture while offering assistance to recumbent patient

surgery/health clinic. Precise information of the numbers suffering low back pain is impossible as some people do not report it. Horgan (1985) states that 1 in 20 adults will see their GP each year with low back pain and gives the causes as:

- soft tissue rheumatism
- degenerative disease of the spine
- prolapsed intervertebral disc
- nerve entrapment syndrome.

She states that low back pain costs the health service between 1 and 2 million pounds annually, and it is responsible for over 30 million lost working days each year. Howie (1986) summarises a 5-year project carried out at the University of Surrey's Ergonomics Department into back pain in nurses, and states that every year nearly one-tenth of the UK's 470 000 practising nurses suffer some degree of back pain, and that 764 000 working days are lost to the NHS as a result. Another report (Nursing Times 1984) states that 1 in 6 nurses has back pain.

With a problem of this magnitude in the general population, and the nursing population in particular, nurses require detailed knowledge of how to prevent back pain, and a majority of items in the Reading Assignment discuss these preventive measures. Nurses require opportunity to practise the psychomotor skills under supervision and an opportunity to update their knowledge and skills at regular intervals. Application of the principle of helping patients to mobilise will now be discussed in the four phases of the process of nursing.

Assessing patients' ability to mobilise

To introduce the beginning nurse to the wide range of medical conditions which can afflict patients in different parts of the health service who require to have their ability to mobilise assessed, the conditions will be listed in three groups — the structures required; are these normal at birth?; and, if normal at birth, what can thereafter render disability? The lists are not exhaustive and are merely meant to alert the student to the breadth of the subject before discussing assessing a particular patient.

- structures required:

  shoulders upper limbs
  spine
  lower limbs
  (included in the assessing schema, pages 8 and 9)

- are these normal at birth?:

  absence of one or more limbs
  webbed fingers
  congenital dislocation of hip
  wry neck
  club foot/feet
  spina bifida

  at birth midwives will be involved
  during childhood, health visitors, community nurses and school nurses will be involved
  hospital nurses become involved as these children require surgery, possibly on more than one occasion
  children with spina bifida may achieve varying degrees of 'aided' independence by using calipers, crutches and so on

- if normal at birth, what can render disability, temporarily or permanently?:

  housemaid's knee
  strains of ligaments
  miners' elbow } types of bursitis
  tennis elbow } types of bursitis
  sprains of elbow } types of bursitis
  burns resulting in keloids which may produce contraction deformity
  fractures, particularly of long bones
  fracture of a vertebra which can result in paraplegia or tetraplegia
  prolapsed intervertebral disc
  sciatica
  lumbago
  arthritis, rheumatoid, small joints
  osteo, large joints
  softening of bone, osteomalacia
  loss of bone density, osteoporosis
  neurological disease such as the muscular dystrophies, one of which is multiple sclerosis; stroke (cerebrovascular accident CVA) which can result in hemiplegia; a range of medical conditions which render a person breathless thereby interfering with ability to mobilise (chronic obstructive airways disease)
  breathlessness from pulmonary oedema as a consequence of chronic heart failure
  narrowing of blood vessels (atherosclerosis) in lower limbs resulting in pain on walking (intermittent claudication).

These seem formidable lists; they are presented for three purposes: firstly that nurses will not underestimate their responsibility in assessing a patient's ability to mobilise; secondly that nurses will begin to understand the complexity of their contribution to total health care; and thirdly that nurses will understand the legion medical diagnoses (and more will be given later) which can affect a patient's mobilising for which nursing interventions will be required. In other words, it is in a nursing context that students are being introduced to the notion of medical diagnoses.

When a patient is admitted from the waiting list, the nurse who greets him and shows him to the bed which he will occupy, has an opportunity to assess any apparent non-verbal communication such as:

- use of walking stick/crutches/walking frame
- increased 'platform' on sole of one shoe
- sling
- bandage
- splint
- caliper
- bow legs
- knock knees
- curvature of the spine
- any limp
- any other abnormal gait
- own wheelchair.

A minority of patients are admitted as an 'emergency' from an outpatients' clinic. The patient probably went to the clinic expecting to return home. The medical diagnosis may or may not be directly related to the patient's ability to mobilise, but the urgency of the condition is likely to affect mobilising indirectly, and the patient will probably arrive on the ward in a wheelchair, so the nurse who greets him and shows him to his bed does not have the opportunity of assessing any non-verbal communication about his ability to mobilise as mentioned in the previous paragraph. The reason for the patient being admitted in a wheelchair may not be because of an inability to mobilise, but because mobilising is not congruent with the medical diagnosis.

The reasons are legion for 'emergency' admission of patients from the Accident and Emergency department, but all are likely to place severe, possibly temporary, limitations on the patient's ability to mobilise. Examples are:

- accident: lacerations
  fractures
  stove-in chests
  head injuries
  trauma to abdominal organs

- emergency: heart attacks
  strokes
  self-poisoning
  acute abdominal conditions.

These examples are not exhaustive; their inclusion is to help students begin to appreciate the complexity of 'nursing'. The majority of patients admitted from Accident and Emergency departments will arrive on the ward on a stretcher placed on a trolley, and again, the nurse is deprived of the non-verbal communication about assessing ability to mobilise discussed on page 160.

Having discussed the main routes by which patients arrive in the ward, it is time to practise thinking in process context to produce an individualised nursing plan. The assessing phase usually involves an initial interview with the patient. It is helpful to collect as much biographical information as possible from other records, for instance the medical notes, for several reasons:

- it helps to create a more relaxed atmosphere encouraging a positive nurse/patient relationship
- it prevents the patient feeling that he is on a conveyor belt answering the same questions asked by different people
- it helps to avoid the patient thinking that there is no co-operation between those members of staff asking the questions, which is likely to increase anxiety, and is not likely to engender a feeling of trust.

The patient's name, address, marital status, previous medical history and current diagnosis are suitable items for this exercise and during the interview, the facts can be verified. If the medical diagnosis gives a clue as to possible problems with mobilising, the conversation can be directed to discover what they are, and the patient's words used to describe them. Some aspects of non-verbal communication were mentioned previously; others include muscle spasms, purposeless movements, uncontrollable tremor, flaccid or spastic limbs. Using the assessing schema on pages 8–9, and the suggestions earlier in this chapter will give an idea of how the interview should proceed. Because the ability to mobilise involves widespread body structures it is pertinent to discover whether or not there is pain (pp. 8–9) in any of them. Useful prompts will be generated if the nurse remembers the relatedness of everyday living activities. Does the patient have any difficulty with other essential activities such as shopping, eating, eliminating, bathing, dressing and undressing? Is there any problem carrying out domestic tasks? — assuming comfortable posture for sleep? Because of mobilising status:

- are there any problems at work?
- is there any curtailment of hobbies?
- have any new hobbies been developed, congruent with current ability to mobilise?

A person's impaired ability to mobilise may not have changed, but admission to hospital because of, for instance, an acute appendicitis necessitates the nurse discovering just what the impaired mobility meant to the patient. Exactly what sort of nursing help is required should be recorded in detail, so that nurses on succeeding shifts will offer consistent help.

Any impaired ability to mobilise should be recorded in factual terms. Is there inability to raise the arm/s? Can the arm/s be raised at 45 degrees? Can the deformed hands grasp a cup? Can the cup be raised to the lips? Can the toe be pointed downwards/upwards? Can the knee be extended in a straight line with the thigh? Can the knee be bent at an angle with the thigh? Readers can continue this line of thinking so that adequate skills are developed in assessing impaired ability to mobilise.

Given the complexity of assessing a patient's ability to mobilise, readers will be reassured by the knowledge that the majority of patients will have maximum ability to mobilise; will not have a problem, but need an encouraging atmosphere and an environment in which they can continue their day to day mobilising activities. However, some may have a problem such as 'sore feet' totally unrelated to the reason for admission. There may be athlete's foot which causes excessive layers of dead skin between the toes. It can be itchy and a fissure may be formed which is difficult to heal. The nurse can discover what the patient knows about the condition. How long has it been there? Has it been treated? With what? Does any other member of the family have it? Does the patient know that it is infectious? What precautions have been taken to prevent its spread to others? Does he know that it is a fungal infection? That it can be treated by local application of an antifungal (antimycotic) powder which can be bought at the chemist's? Does he know that there are antifungal substances which can be taken orally but they have to be medically prescribed? Will the patient report the condition to the doctor? Would the patient prefer it to be reported by the nurse? This detail of a nursing assessment is included as an illustration of an opportunity to teach people about their health status. To avoid double standards it is imperative that there is an agreed plan for the bath to be cleaned between bathers, and either each ambulant patient keeps a washable or disposable bathmat for use throughout his stay, or a fresh washable or disposable one is provided each time he has a bath.

Here it is necessary to look back at the complex biomechanics included in the concept of mobilising (p. 156) and to realise that the real meaning of early ambulation (p. 155) was *gradual* return to the patient's previous level of mobilising to prevent the possible complication of pulmonary embolism. The majority of patients spend some part of each day in bed and will require to be lifted or turned into various positions and to be helped out onto a chair or helped to walk to the lavatory and so on. The possibilities are legion but articles in the Reading Assignment give a sufficiently wide selection to prepare beginning nurses for practice in the clinical areas under supervision. Johnston (1987) discusses the results of her research using the following questions:

- do nurses assess patients' mobility potential before helping to lift/move them?
- are students given help to assess?
- do students plan accurately before helping patients?
- is there a clear statement on the plan, written or verbal?

The notion of nurses assessing patients' ability to mobilise is gaining ground, and the result of the initial assessment is a nursing plan. Henry (1984) advises:

> Nursing plans should state whether there is any problem with moving a patient and, if so, which methods should be used.

It is heartening to know that the foregoing text will only act as background information to guide the nurse who is carrying out the initial assessment of a particular patient. Nurse and patient explore together the meaning of mobilising and if it is agreed that there is not a problem, the ambulant patient should be informed about where he can and cannot go, and what he can and cannot do. If there is likely to be a change in mobilising, for example, confinement to bed on the day of, and for a few days following operations, investigations and so on, this should be discussed with the patient.

This is an example of the interrelatedness of nursing knowledge — the two Franklin references, and the two Wilson-Barnett references in the chapter on Helping patients to communicate (p. 13) show quite clearly that well-informed patients experience less anxiety. This is also an example of there not being a problem to record on the assessment form, but the problem of being 'bedfast' and the consequent nursing interventions because of this, will be added to the nursing plan on the appropriate day.

Should any of the possible non-verbal communications mentioned on page 160 be present, it would alert the nurse to a possible problem directly related to the musculoskeletal system. Likewise any of the paralyses already mentioned in this chapter would alert the nurse to possible mobilising problems related to neurological conditions. And patients with severe breathlessness caused by cardiopulmonary conditions are likely to have problems with mobilising. One has also to remember the many dimensions of the current concept of mobilising mentioned on page 154. This leaves no doubt about the importance of assessing a patient's ability to mobilise. The admitting nurse requires to record details on the assessment form of how the patient has managed the many aspects of mobilising at home, so that an enabling environment can be provided for the patient to continue his mobilising activities. Should human help be required, exact details need to be written so that nurses on ensuing shifts can offer appropriate help. The 'problem/s' are not new to the patient; he has probably learned to cope with them and it is important that nurses do not create new problems by not listening to the patient. It really is the case that the patient knows best!

Not all 'assessing ability to mobilise' is done in hospital. It is carried out by community nurses in the patient's home where there may well be a low divan-type double bed against a wall, and most domestic baths have access from one side only. There can be dimly lit or unlit stairs in awkward places and so on. The four phases of the process will need to be applied to the immediate environment in these instances. Assessing may be carried out by practice nurses working from a doctor's surgery, and by occupational health nurses at their place of work. Midwives assess newborn babies for conditions which will influence ability to mobilise, some of which are mentioned on page 160. Health visitors assess habilitation related to mobilising either in the home or at the clinic, and school nurses continue this surveillance. And at the other end of the lifespan, assessing ability to mobilise is an important part of the work carried out by nurses in day hospitals and nursing homes.

Information relevant to this first phase of the process of nursing has been discussed in more detail than in other chapters because it is becoming increasingly evident that nurses need a wide range of knowledge related to this part of their work and more will be said about this later.

However, before leaving this phase it is pertinent to remind readers that initial and ongoing assessment data are collected with the objective of identifying with the patient whenever possible, any problems which he is experiencing in relation to mobilising. These are written in the patient's words, either on the assessment form or on the nursing plan, whichever is the custom, but they do not need to be written twice.

Planning

Planning, the second phase of the process of nursing is customarily carried out in relation to the patient, but it can be focused to the nurse, and also to discreet nursing activities which will be discussed later. For each agreed, identified problem, a desired goal will be discussed with the patient. For example the medical diagnosis might be intermittent claudication, but the patient's problems (nursing diagnosis) might be:

- experiences pain in both calves climbing the 12 stairs at home
- embarrassed by using a urinal downstairs which his wife then empties into upstairs lavatory
- embarrassed by having to walk so slowly, and keep stopping to get to the corner shop 100 yards away to collect a morning paper.

Writing problems in the patient's words helps the nurse and patient to formulate goals. This patient might agree, for example, to count six on each step which may enable him to get to the top without pain. When he has gained confidence he may well agree to count five and so on. It could be that with a return of confidence he may agree to go upstairs to pass urine once during the day, then increase to twice and so on. He may well have to be helped to come to terms with walking slowly, but encouragement should be given for this to continue, as it encourages collateral circulation. He can be encouraged to develop the perspective that to be able to walk slowly is much better than not being able to walk at all. The pleasure which he gets from reading the morning paper can be used to reinforce motivation for walking to the corner shop.

The preceding paragraph is just one example and when one considers the numerous medical diagnoses (p. 160) which can interfere with a patient's ability to mobilise, the need for individualised nursing plans is obvious. To give practice in process thinking readers are reminded that the plan should state the goal agreed by nurse and patient whenever possible, and the nursing intervention to achieve the goal; it should be written in sufficient detail so that whichever nurse carries it out, it will be the same intervention. With mobilising, probably more than with any of the other everyday living activities, many of the goals will be long term; they need to be broken down into tiny steps, so that achievement will encourage the patient on the long haul to, for instance, re-learning to walk after a cerebrovascular accident causing hemiplegia. The patient's previous life-style, age and particular circumstances will all be taken into consideration regarding the distance to be walked. Theoretically a date is set for evaluation of whether or not the short term goals are being or have been achieved; when this is so the goal will be increased and another date set, so the nursing plan is likely to change fairly frequently. Reference to Henry's and Johnston's articles on page 152 will be useful in this planning context.

Even though the nursing plan tells the nurse about the nursing intervention, she must 'plan' so that for instance the area is uncluttered and suitable for the patient's mobilising activity; the necessary equipment is to hand, such as a sling or a hoist for transferring the patient; any aids to walking are available such as a stick (Fig. 13.9), elbow crutches (Fig. 13.10), axillary crutches (Fig. 13.11), a walking frame (Fig. 13.12), a folding walking aid (Fig. 13.13) or a Harris re-education belt (Fig. 13.14).

Mobilising is an activity which illustrates well, that while selecting nursing interventions, nurses have to take into account available resources at ward level. Firstly these resources can be broadly classified as equipment which includes:

- dressings, external applications
- aids to mobilising
- aids to lifting and turning.

The Code of Professional Conduct published by the United Kingdom Central Council for Nursing, Midwifery and Health Visiting and that published by the Royal College of Nursing make it clear that nurses have a responsibility to keep their knowledge up to date. This includes knowing what is available on the market and this is easily achieved by glancing through the

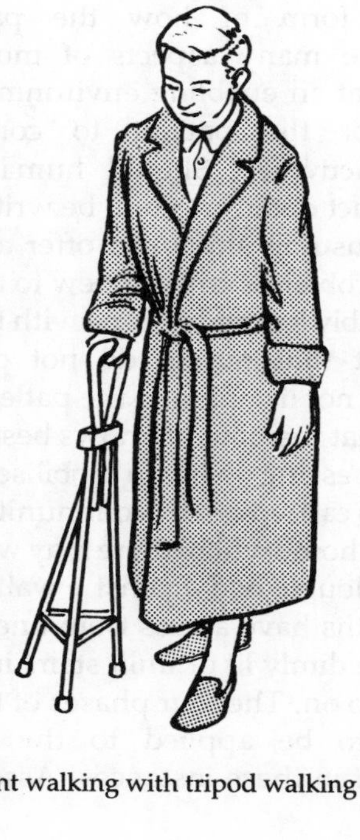

Fig. 13.9 Patient walking with tripod walking stick

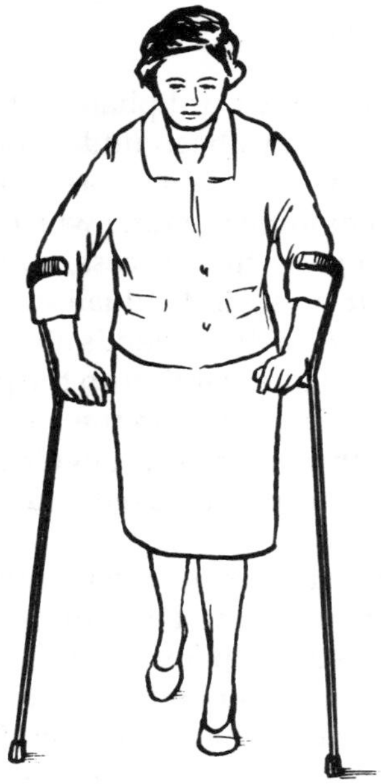

Fig. 13.10 Patient walking with elbow crutches

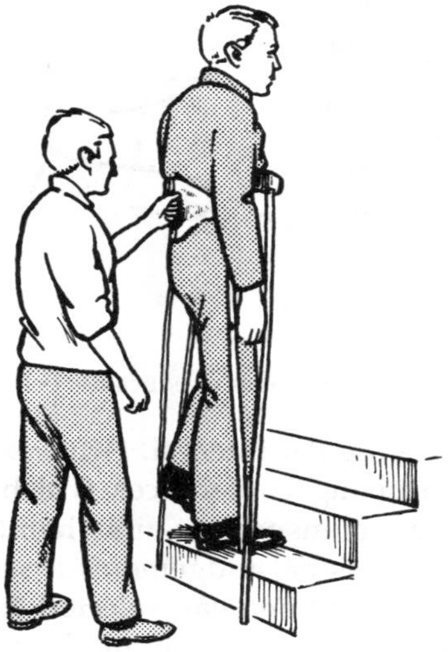

Fig. 13.11 Patient learning to go up and down steps using axillary crutches

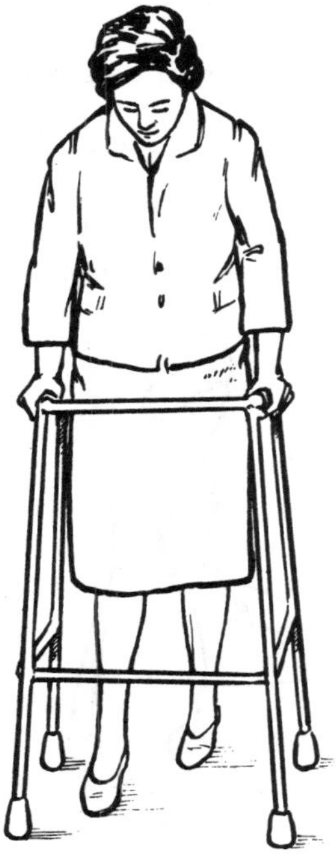

Fig. 13.12 Patient walking in a frame

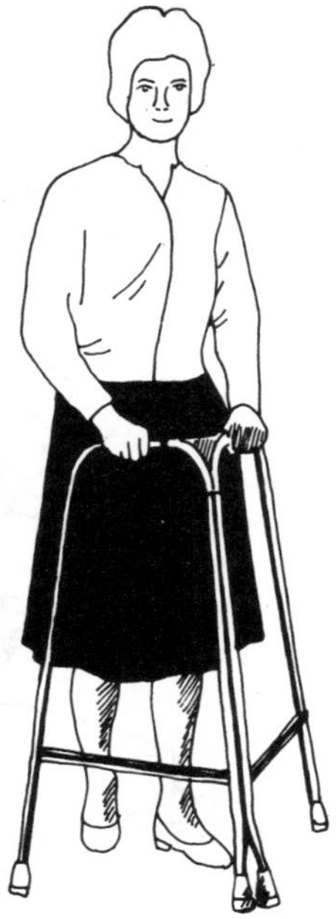

Fig. 13.13 Folding walking aid

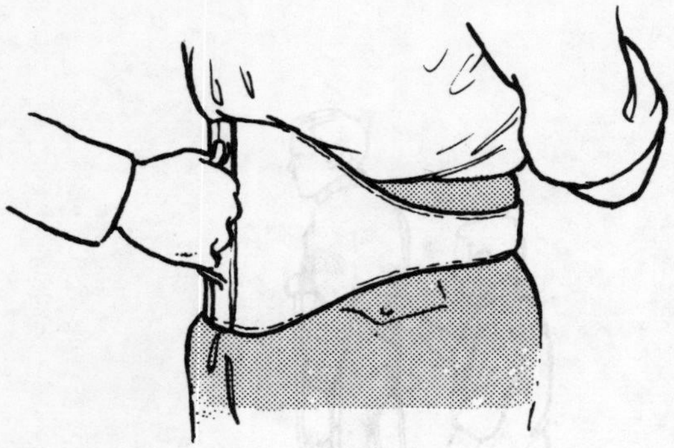

Fig. 13.14 Patient with Harris re-education belt

journals at a regular interval. Firms exhibit their goods at nursing conferences which gives an opportunity to inspect at first hand. If, in a nurse's professional judgement, a second best nursing intervention was selected because of equipment constraints, it should be recorded in writing and the nursing officer informed.

Secondly staffing resources have to be considered when planning nursing interventions. How many? To which work group do they belong? How long have they been on the ward? How much have they been taught about helping patients to mobilise? How much do they know? How much practice have they had? If the mobilising part of a patient's nursing plan cannot be carried out at the stated time because of staffing inadequacies, a record should be made each time it occurs. There will then be facts to support the statement 'we're short of nurses'.

Implementing

Implementing, the third phase of the process of nursing has always been understood by nurses as they carry out their work. However, the subconcept of implementing which is part of the larger concept of the process, now means the carrying out of an individualised plan, in this section related to the patient's ability/inability to mobilise. Each intervention on the plan, after it is carried out, is recorded on the patient's nursing notes, together with any ongoing assessment data which can be used summatively at evaluation.

The sorts of nursing interventions required to help patients to mobilise are well discussed and illustrated in many of the articles in the Reading Assignment and they can be identified by the title and/or the annotation. From reading the articles you will realise the very skilled nursing help which is required to:

- lift and turn patients in bed
- transfer patients from one surface to another
- help patients to walk
- lift a patient from a trolley to a bed (Fig. 13.15)
- lift a patient from bed to chair (Fig.13.16, p.167)
- lift a patient from chair to bed (Fig.13.17, p.167)
- lift a patient from the floor using the shoulder lift (Hayne 1985)

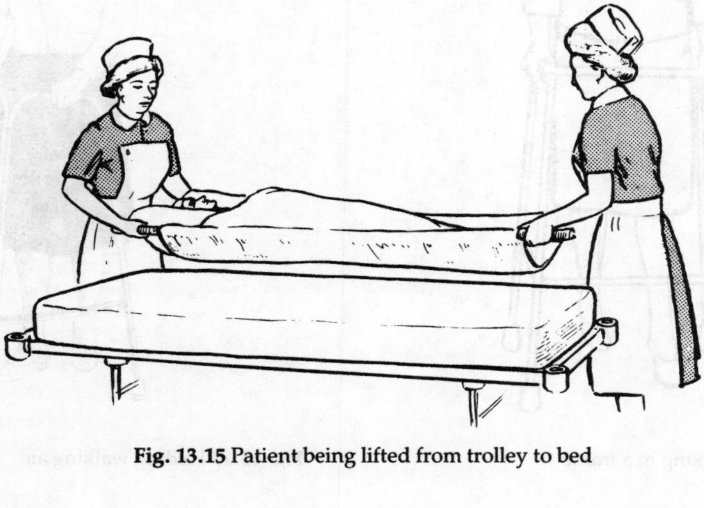

Fig. 13.15 Patient being lifted from trolley to bed

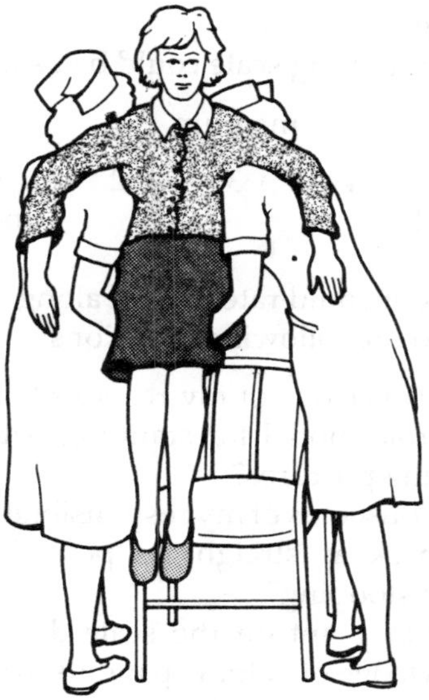

Fig. 13.16 Two nurses lifting patient from bed to chair using the shoulder lift

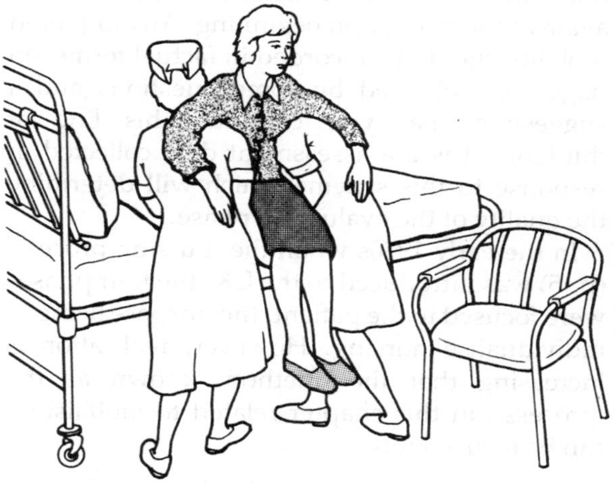

Fig. 13.17 Two nurses lifting patient from chair to bed using the shoulder lift

- mobilise patients for evacuation from a ward in an emergency.

The focus of this chapter is helping patients to mobilise but it cannot be stressed too strongly that there is a mobilising dimension to many of the other everyday living activities, which makes that of mobilising so important.

Evaluating

Evaluating is the fourth phase of the process of nursing. It is entirely dependent on the assessment data; the more factual it is, the better the quality of evaluating! Assessing patients' ability to mobilise was previously considered in some detail (pp.159 to 163).

Because of the complexity of mobilising and the multitude of possible patients' problems it is impossible to capture in a text, the specifics of evaluating. However one hypothetical suggestion follows.

Patient's problem	Goal	Evaluation
1 Jan Can only raise left arm to 45 degrees from trunk so that dressing and undressing takes ages	Long-term: will raise L arm to a functional 135 degrees by Short-term: will raise L arm	1 March
	50 degrees	6 Jan NR
	55 degrees	11 Jan NR
	60 degrees	16 Jan NR
	70 degrees	21 Jan NR
	80 degrees	26 Jan NR
	90 degrees	31 Jan Raised to 100° NR

This is an example of a greater recovery than the set goal, alerting the nurse to the fact that the long-term goal may well be achieved earlier than the set date. In our present state of knowledge it would be reasonable to increase the degree of arm lifting in the steps in less time, for example just two more steps in raising from 100 to 135 degrees by 3 days hence, instead of 5.

To help readers to get further 'practice thinking' about nursing in a process context the following is offered. Readers are advised to look again at the paragraph beginning 'Any impaired mobility should be recorded in factual terms' on page 162, followed by some questions and a suggestion that you continue this line of thinking. It is the assessment data collected in response to this schema which will determine the quality of the evaluating phase.

In the early 1970s when the 'nursing process' (p. 5) was introduced to the UK, the four phases were focused to the patient, the purpose being to individualise nursing. However, realisation is increasing that the 'method' known as the 'process', in this chapter related to mobilising, can be focused to:

- training programmes for the acquisition of patient handling skills
- the nurse in a general context
- the nurse in a particular context

Scholey (1984) gives a reminder that back pain is the most common physical complaint among nurses: it could be reduced by learning to lift correctly. She devised a teaching programme to be carried out in each ward; for this she used the four phases of the process. An introduction will now be given to the other two ideas in the preceding list.

Focusing the four phases to the nurse in a general context

It has already been mentioned that the patient's ability/inability to mobilise has to be dovetailed with the nurses' ability. Focusing the four phases to the nurse can be done in two ways:

- by use of a self-assessment/evaluation plan
- by another person assessing/evaluating the nurse's mobilising activities.

Use of a self-assessment/evaluation plan

As students' participation in, and acceptance of responsibility for their own learning is gaining ground, a nurse self-assessment/evaluation plan is proposed.

Assessing

A five point rating scale could be used:

5	4	3	2	1
very good		medium		poor

The student could rate herself along this scale according to the following questions:

- am I conscious of my responsibility to act as a role model for standing, sitting and walking postures?
- am I conscious of my responsibility to keep my back as straight as possible and to avoid stooping?
- at what point on the scale do I rate my knowledge of helping patients to mobilise?
- at what point on the scale do I rate my practical ability to help patients to mobilise?

This list can be added to, for second, and then for third year students and could include teaching the techniques of mobilising to patients and other members of staff to reduce the high incidence of back pain (p. 159).

Planning

- my goal is to increase my consciousness of acting as a role model for standing, sitting and walking postures
- my goal is to keep my back as straight as possible and avoid stooping during waking hours
- my goal is to increase (update when I become a registered nurse) my knowledge of helping patients to mobilise
- my goal is to become more skilled in helping patients to mobilise

Implementing

- practising awareness of my standing, sitting and walking postures
- practising awareness of maintaining a straight back and avoiding stooping
- increasing my knowledge of helping patients to mobilise
- practising the skills involved in helping patients to mobilise.

Evaluating
Evaluating can only be done by consulting the assessment data and using the five point scale.

- am I more/just as/less aware of acting as a role model for standing, sitting and walking postures?
- am I more/just as/less aware of maintaining a straight back and avoiding stooping?
- do I have more/just as much/less knowledge of helping patients to mobilise?
- am I more/just as/less skilled in helping patients to mobilise?

To avoid boring repetition (though repetition is necessary for learning) readers are advised to re-word this schema to make it applicable to the second item in 'Focusing the four phases to the nurse in a general context' — that is, for use by another person assessing/evaluating a nurse's mobilising activities.

And finally to apply the four phases to the nurse in a particular context, bedmaking has been selected, as making even an empty bed is intimately concerned with the nurse maintaining integrity of the musculoskeletal system, as well as another principle of nursing — helping patients to avoid hospital-acquired infection. It is yet another example of the relatedness of nursing knowledge.

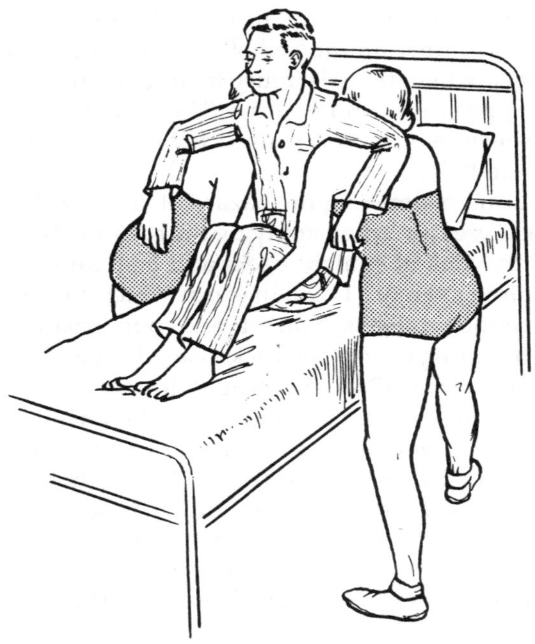

Fig. 13.18 Starting the shoulder lift

Focusing the four phases to the nurse in a particular context — bedmaking

Bedmaking undoubtedly involves posture, movement and lifting. Nowadays many ill patients can be lifted from bed to chair for bedmaking. Figure 13.16 shows this manoeuvre using the shoulder lift, and Figure 13.17 illustrates the reverse technique.

The shoulder (Australian) lift for lifting a patient up the bed is illustrated in Figures 13.18 and 13.19. The lifters, with their feet apart, stand near the bed on a level with the patient's hips. The lifters' arms encircle the upper third of the patient's thighs. They then place the corresponding shoulder in the patient's axilla. The patient places his arms on the lifters' backs. The lifters' other arms hold either the mattress or

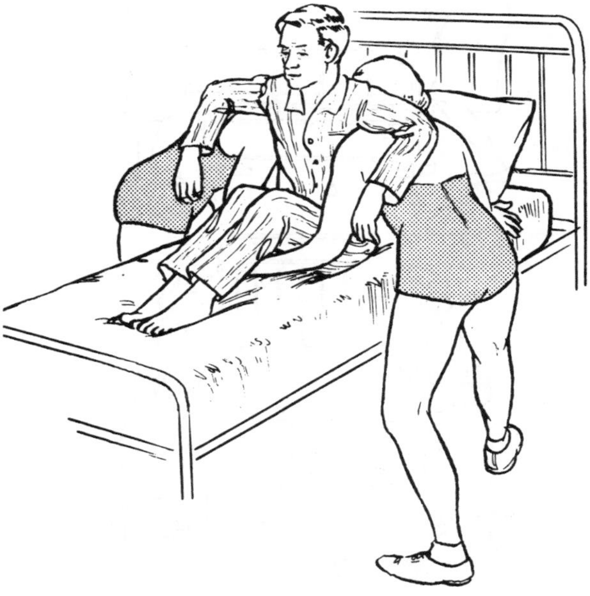

Fig. 13.19 Lifting by the shoulder method

the head of the bed. As they straighten their legs the patient is raised. As they transfer their weight to the leg nearest the head of the bed, the patient is lifted up the bed. This method cannot be used where there is injury to, or operation on the upper trunk and/or arms. There are various lift sheets which can be used for such patients (Hayne 1984).

During bedmaking the hazard of 'arching' the back is greatest when applying the bottom sheet, and the idea of straight backs and bent knees is captured in Figure 13.20. In wards which still use conventional sheets, blankets and counterpanes, it is tempting to arch the back instead of bending the knees (Fig. 13.21) when applying them.

After this general introduction to bedmaking, it is time to practise thinking about this complex activity in process context (remembering that it is closely associated with preventing nosocomial infection because microorganisms adhere to the scales of the skin's outer layer which is constantly being shed onto the sheets. Thinking

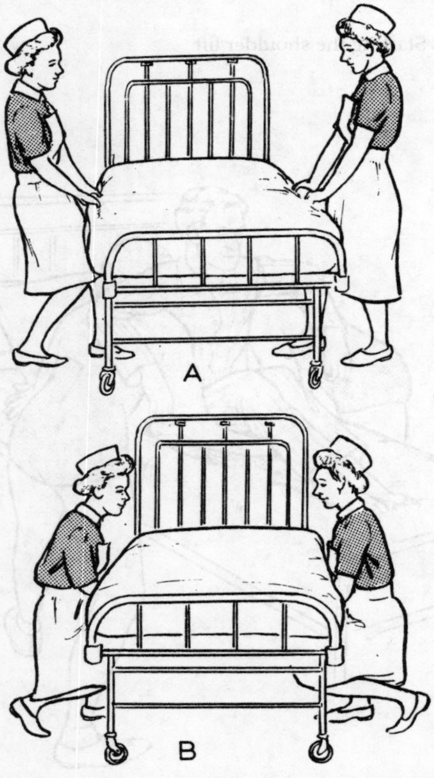

Fig. 13.20 Two stages in application of a bottom sheet

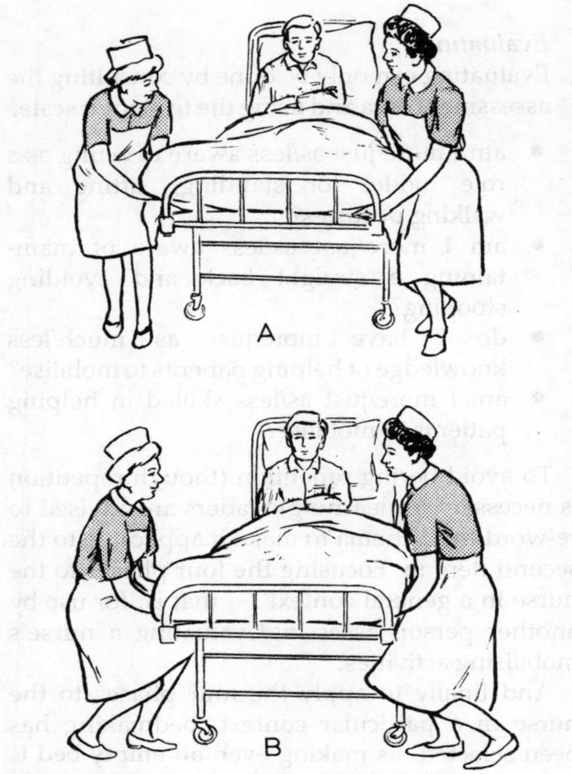

Fig. 13.21 Two stages when applying a counterpane

in process context does not detract from the art of nursing.

Assessing the nurse who is bedmaking

This section is offered, not as yet another paper/writing exercise — not a word needs to be written — but as an exercise in creative thinking to help us to develop confidence in the tasks of nursing, so that we can counter the criticism that such a task is 'basic' in a negative way, or even in a 'non-nursing' way. Taking assessing, in this context, to mean collection of relevant information, against which evaluation can be carried out, it is pertinent to think about the following:

- did the nurse consult the patient's nursing plan to discover whether or not there are any instructions about:
  - method/s to be used for turning and lifting patient
  - accessory equipment to be used for turning and lifting the patient

whether or not the patient can sit out of bed during bedmaking
the patient being scheduled for any investigations, X-rays and so on, which would preclude choice of these times for bedmaking.

Planning

'The plan' in this context is not a written one, it is 'in the mind', the result of cognitive activity. Items to be attended to might be:

- plan the time of day when it can be done in a calm and unhurried way
- plan that the necessary linen and equipment will be available at that time
- plan that the patient will be available at that time
- plan that the bed-stripper to be used will accommodate pillows to prevent less hygienic placing on lockers, bedtables and chair seats
- plan to avoid patient fatigue.

Implementing

For some patients there will need to be implementation of nursing interventions from the written nursing plan, but in the main it is a case of implementing the abstract/unwritten plan. To maintain rational sequence they are not given separately in the following list:

- collect necessary linen, equipment and used linen skip (Figs 13.22 and 13.23)
- note patient's reaction to proposed bedmaking
- provide privacy, warmth and lack of haste
- provide uncluttered area round bed to facilitate safe handling and lifting of patient
- remove upper bedclothes with gentle (as opposed to flapping) movements to minimise dust dispersal in the interest of prevention of nosocomial infection
- if relevant, implement the methods prescribed in the nursing plan for lifting and turning the patient
- if relevant, implement use of accessory equipment for lifting and turning the patient

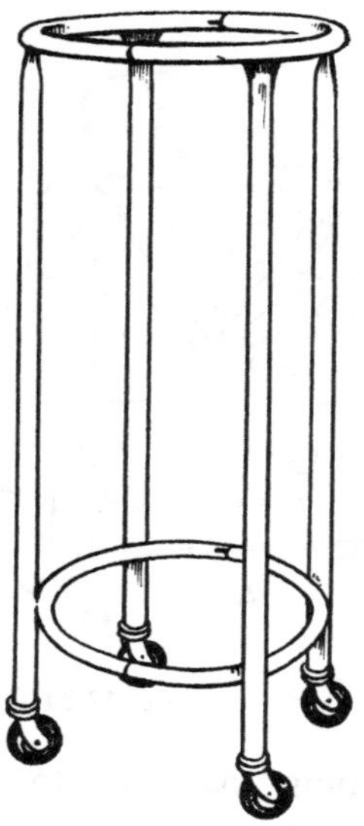

Fig. 13.22 'Closed' linen skip

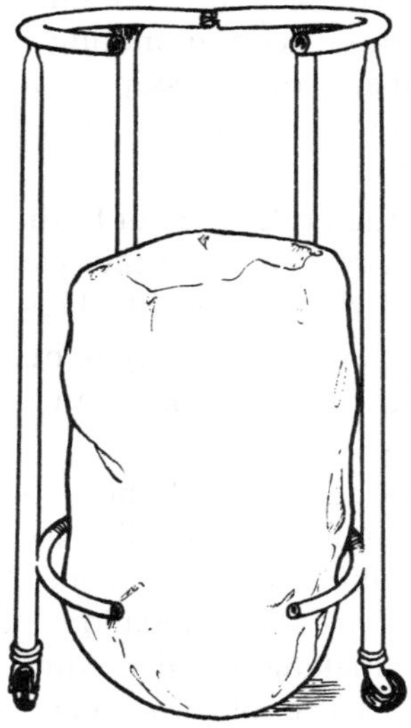

Fig. 13.23 'Open' linen skip

- if relevant, lift the patient from bed to chair and ensure that he will be sufficiently warm and comfortable while sitting out (Fig. 14.5, p.181)
- when lifting and moving patients avoid bruising and abrasion of skin thereby implementing another principle of nursing

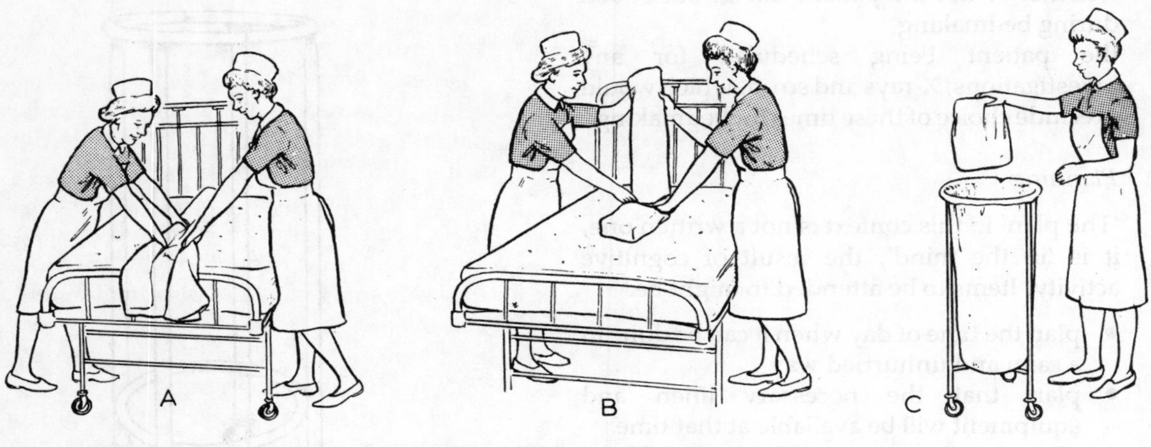

Fig. 13.24 Minimising dust dissemination during removal of a bottom sheet

'Helping patients to prevent pressure sores'.

- when removing the bottom sheet roll it from both sides into the middle (Fig. 13.24A); fold roll into three (Fig. 13.24B) and place it in the linen skip (Fig. 13.24C) without contaminating uniform or the outside of the skip as a contribution to minimising the incidence of nosocomial infection
- fit the bottom sheet to the contours of the mattress; make it taut from top to bottom and from side to side (Figs 13.20 and 13.21)
- if relevant, return patient from chair to bed (Fig. 13.16; helping him into a comfortable position
- replace top bedclothes loosely; they should be as light as possible to give the warmth required by the patient (Henderson 1981 describes the evaluation of a new concept in bedmaking (duvets) which reaches the fire and bacteriological safety standards set by the Department of Health and Social Security related to fire and infection)
- replace the furniture and place any articles within comfortable reach
- maintain integrity of nurses' and the patient's musculoskeletal system throughout the whole procedure
- note patient's reaction to the procedure.

Evaluating the nurse who is bedmaking

Our thinking about the evaluating phase of the process has been mainly concerned with comparing it to the assessment data. But in this instance the evaluating schema will also contain items from the preceding planning and implementing proformas. Readers might practise going through the first three phases translating them into question form, Did the nurse ...?

In this section the four phases of the process have been focused to the nurse while bedmaking. It could equally well be applied to other nursing activities mentioned in this chapter and throughout the book. Such detailed application might help us to:

- give credence to such phrases as 'a high standard of nursing'
- a better understanding of the relatedness of nursing knowledge
- pride in being able to articulate the cognitive complexity of what appears to the uninitiated, to be a simple task.

In this chapter the concepts of early ambulation, hazards of enforced immobility, and the multidisciplinary mobilising team were discussed before consideration of the principle — helping patients to mobilise — in a process of nursing context. The four phases were then focused to the nurse in a general context, and then to the nurse in a particular context — bedmaking.

APPLYING THE PRINCIPLE

A registered nurse must be capable of:

- acting as a role model in all aspects related to the complex activity of mobilising
- teaching staff and patients about good posture, lifting and handling techniques
- creating good body alignment in whatever position she assists the patient into, including positions necessary for examination, investigation and operation
- keeping the environment as hazard free as possible, so that the results of patients falling out of bed, sprains and broken bones, do not add to the problems of patients' ability to mobilise
- instituting that amount of movement (active and passive) in each patient, which will help to prevent deformity, venous stasis, pressure sores and pulmonary infection. Making beds so that there is room for such movement
- making the best use of facilities available for ambulant patients. Recognising deficient facilities and taking what steps lie within her power to improve these.
- using safely and effectively equipment which contributes to good posture and movement of patients and staff
- liaising effectively with other departments to procure more suitable and effective equipment as it comes on to the market; this entails updating knowledge at regular intervals
- using a maintenance policy so that equipment is in good working order
- applying the principle — helping patients to mobilise — in a process of nursing context

WORKING ASSIGNMENT

Topics for discussion

- you hear a bump. You see a frail, elderly woman lying on the floor beside her bed. What will you do?
- I don't think that it can be very comfortable sitting up in bed with nothing to prevent one slipping down
- a nurse's uniform in relation to safe mobilising
- you are the only member of the nursing staff on a ward which has no mechanical lifting apparatus. Mrs Jones, a helpless patient weighing 95 kg, wants to pass urine. What should be done?
- what should be done when nurses who have been taught the correct methods of lifting are found using incorrect methods?
- the advantages and disadvantages of variable height beds
- the contribution which can be made by nurses to management's selection of equipment for maintaining good posture and movement of patients and staff.

Writing assignment

- define the following:

active movement
allergy
antifungal
antimycotic
apoplexy
arthritis
atherosclerosis
athlete's foot
atrophy
atonic
Balkan beam
bioengineer
bow legs
bursitis
calipers
contracture
cardiac
causes of low back pain
cerebrovascular accident
chronic heart failure
chronic obstructive airways disease
clinical psychologist
club foot
collateral circulation
conjunctiva
congenital dislocation of the hip
contracture
decubitis

deep vein thrombosis
degenerative disease of spine
Disablement Resettlement Officer
disseminated sclerosis
dyspnoea
ergonomics
evaporating dressing
fatigue
fissure
flaccid
flatus tube
fractures
fungal
gait
gangrene
head injury
health and safety representatives
heart attack
hemiplegia
hernia
hip guidance orthosis
hip replacement surgery
hydrocephalus
hypertrophy
hypostatic pneumonia
intermittent claudication
keloid
knock knees
laceration
locomotor
lumbago
monoplegia
multiple sclerosis
muscle tone
muscular dystrophies
nerve entrapment syndrome
neuritis
occupational therapy
occupational health nurses
oedema
orthosis
osteomalacia
osteoporosis
paralysis
paraplegia
passive movement
phlebitis
phlebothrombosis
physiotherapy
poliomyelitis
practice nurses
prolapsed intervertebral disc
prosthesis
pulmonary embolism
pulmonary oedema
rehabilitation
remedial gymnast
retention enema
sciatica
shock
soft tissue rheumatism
spastic
spina bifida
sprain
stove-in chest
strain
stroke
torticollis
varicose ulcer
varicose vein
webbed finger
wry neck

- a patient's medical diagnosis is osteoarthritis of the right and left hips. Write out possible patient's problems in his words (nursing diagnosis)

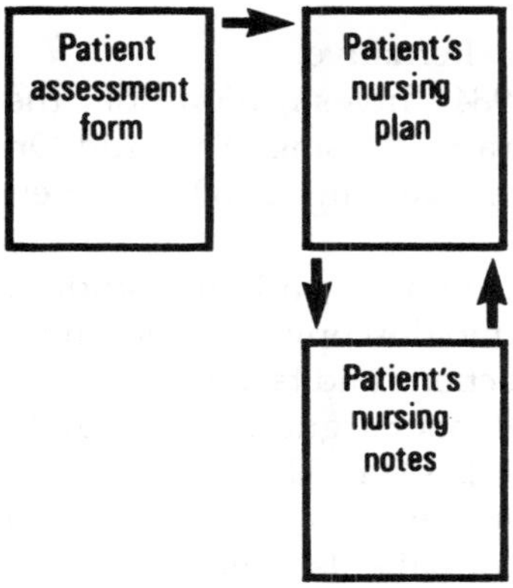

14

Helping patients to eliminate

Reading assignment

Background information
- *Elimination from bladder and bowel*
- *Equipment for bowel and bladder elimination*
  - *Commode*
  - *Sanichair*
  - *Clos-o-mat: bidet*
  - *Bedpans and urinals*

Defaecating in a process of nursing context
- *Assessing a patient's defaecating habits*
  - *Constipation*
  - *Diarrhoea*
  - *Discomfort*
  - *Pain*
  - *Paraplegia*
  - *Tetraplegia*
  - *Stoma/ostomy*
- *Planning — individualised*
  - *Ward planning*
  - *Generalised planning*
- *Implementing*
  - *Helping a patient to use a commode*
  - *Helping a patient to use a bedpan*
- *Evaluating*

Micturating in a process of nursing context
- *Assessing a patient's micturating habits*
- *Planning, implementing, evaluating*

Catheterisation and bladder infection

Applying the principle
- *A registered nurse must be capable of:*
- *Working assignment*
- *Topics for discussion*
- *Writing assignment*

READING ASSIGNMENT

Bowel elimination

Anderson J 1984 Bowel function in the elderly. Nursing Times 80 (33) August 15:52
Describes a small study to evaluate a bran pill as a bowel-bulking agent. 'The development of a science of nursing practice depends upon training nurses to become 'conscious thinkers'!

Booth B, Booth S 1986 Aperients can be deceptive. Nursing Times 82 (39) September 24: 38–39
A Table gives oral aperients, suppositories and enema: how they act and their side-effects. Deviations in bowel elimination.

Brooks S L 1984 Disturbances of bowel function. Nursing: The Add-On Journal of Clinical Nursing 2 (30) October: 870, 872, 873, 875
Contains Tables, of problem solving in constipation; preparations for alleviating constipation; problem solving in hasty elimination.

Burkitt D 1983 Don't forget fibre in your diet. Positive Health Guide, Martin Dunitz, London

Couchman M 1984 A softer option. Nursing Mirror 159 (7) August 29: 39
Fletcher's Enemette is an efficient and more comfortable microenema.

Drayton S, Rees C 1984 'They know what they're doing.' Nursing Mirror 159 (5) August 15: iv–vii

Do nurses know why they give pregnant women enemas?
Reports a study to discover how women in labour really felt about enemas.

Goodinson S M 1986 The nurse as an inventor. The Professional Nurse 2 (3) December: 87–90
A research project necessitated collecting urine samples from babies up to 6 weeks old. She developed a reusable urine collector which has been patented.

Goodinson S M 1984 Renal function: an overview. Nursing: The Add-On Journal of Clinical Nursing 2 (29) September: 843, 845–846, 848, 851
Also describes the commonly used diuretics.

Kharib H 1986 Acute gastroenteritis in infants. Nursing Times 82 (17) April 23: 31–32
Between 5 and 18 million children die every year from diarrhoeal diseases, and it is still a cause of mortality and morbidity in the Western world. Describes how 'correct care and management can aid recovery'.

Molitor P 1985 Constipation. Nursing Mirror 160 (19) May 8: 18–20
Discusses causes, symptoms, complications and treatment.

Nursing Mirror Supplementary booklet 1984 Constipation — a professional guide. Nursing Mirror 159 (12) July 18: 51–511
Gives an account of bowel physiology, causes of constipation and treatment. Does not mention Burkitt's work.

Nursing Times Supplement 1986. Focus on urinalysis
Part 1 Nursing Times 82 (17) April 23: 1–6
Part 2 Nursing Times 82 (20) May 14: 1–6
Part 3 Nursing Times 82 (23) June 4: 1–6
Part 4 Nursing Times 82 (26) June 25: 1–6
Part 5 Nursing Times 82 (29) July 16: 1–6
Part 6 Nursing Times 82 (32) August 6: 1–6

N T Directory 1986 Clinical notes. Nursing Times 82 (4) January 22: 62
The conventional wisdom which decrees that patients on bedrest must use bedpans rather than commodes has been overturned.

Shreeve C 1985 Bowel habits in the elderly. Nursing Mirror 160 (19) May8: 20–21
For those elderly people who are unable to alter their lifestyle to avoid constipation, the microenema is an alternative.

Silvester G A 1984 Investigation of the gastrointestinal tract. Nursing: The Add-On Journal of Clinical Nursing 2 (30) October: 896–897
Explains plain films, barium studies, proctoscopy, sigmoidoscopy, colonoscopy, biopsy, stool collections and testing.

Smith S 1984 A beginner's guide to research. Nursing Times 80 (22) May 30: 64–65
An account of how a ward sister investigated the fibre content of patients' diet — at home and in hospital.

Stringer M 1984 Fibre drink for diabetics. Nursing Mirror 159 (7) August 29: 48
Finnish scientists have developed a form of guar derived from natural sources which makes a highly palatable drink.

Swaffield L 1979 Dietary fibre. Any questions? Nursing Times Community Outlook 75 (15) April 12: 94–95
Records an interview between the author and Denis Burkitt a researcher who recommends sufficient dietary fibre to produce at least 150g of faeces daily.

Wallis M C 1984 The collection and testing of urine. Nursing: The Add-On Journal of Clinical Nursng 2 (29) September: 853–854
Describes the significance of abnormal values, and the colour variations in urine.

Williams G 1987 Simple solution. Nursing Times 83 (17) April 29: 41
Diarrhoea is the biggest killer of children in the world. It can be treated economically and effectively by oral rehydration therapy (ORT).

Willington F L, Yarnell J, Sweetman P 1981 Cleansing incontinent patients: an evaluation of the use of non-ionic detergents compared with soap. Journal of Advanced Nursing 6: 107–109
The results showed a reduced cleansing time and evidence that the marked degree of alkalinity encountered in cleansing with soap is avoided.

Wilson M 1987 Elimination. Nursing: The Add-On Journal of Clinical Nursing 3 (16) April: 612, 614, 615
Describes the importance of the skills required in helping patients to eliminate, and makes

several suggestions about assessing this activity.
Wilson-Barnett 1978 Patients' emotional responses to barium X-rays.
Journal of Advanced Nursing 3 (1) January: 37–46
Wright D 1984 Constipation. The researcher's view. Nursing Times 80 (22) May 30: 65–67
An attempt to estimate the extent of constipation among patients in one hospital.
Wright L 1974 Bowel function in hospital patients. Royal College of Nursing, London Research report

Stoma

Allen S 1984 Stoma management. Nursing: The Add-On Journal of Clinical Nursing 2 (30) October: 877-881
Discusses the daily management which the stoma patient has to learn; return to work; holidays; recreational and sporting activities; contraception; pregnancy; constipation and diarrhoea.
Black P 1985 The right appliance. Nursing Mirror 161 (10) September 4: 34–35
Patients should select appliances which they can wear and handle comfortably: they need guidance on disposal at home and at work.
Black P 1985 Stoma care in youth and old age. Nursing Mirror 161 (14) October 2: 23–24
Gives a further reading list and useful contact addresses.
Bridges J 1987 Restorative proctocolectomy to avoid a stoma. Nursing Times 83 (4) January 28: 63, 65, 66
After excision of a large part of the colon, necessary because of ulcerative colitis, an anastomosis was made between the cut end of the remaining colon and rectum.
Cunningham S C 1984 The cosmetics of stoma care. Nursing: The Add-on Journal of Clinical Nursing 2 (30) October: 890, 892, 895
Discusses the essential requirements of stoma bags, their attachment and gives a list of stoma care aids.
Fryer S 1985 Smiles hide the truth. Nursing Times 81 (7) February 13: 31, 32, 34
A sensitive nursing study of stoma formation in a patient with advanced cancer of the rectum; his daughters' decision was that he should not be told that he had cancer
Harocopos C 1986 Choosing the right appliance. Nursing Times 82 (4) January 22: 54, 57, 58
Jeffries E 1987 Down to basics. Nursing Times 83 (4) January 28: 59, 61–63
A practical account of the problems created by a fistula
Jones H 1985 Maintaining an active life. Nursing Times 81 (7) February 13: 36, 38
Written by the director of the Colostomy Welfare Group, London; he says that there is still a place for more research into what ostomists require.
Molitor P 1985 The continent ileostomy. Nursing Mirror 160 (20) May 15: 27–28
Describes the operation of proctocolectomy and gives a list of problems which may be caused by an ileostomy.
North K 1987 Preparing for life after a stoma. Nursing Times 83 (18) May 6: 32
Assess patient's knowledge about a stoma. Correct misinformation. Give additional information in a supportive manner as required.
Nursing Mirror (Pull-out supplement) 1984 Life with a stoma. Nursing Mirror 159 (9) September 12: Contains five articles including the psychological and sexual aspects of a stoma.
Rossiter M C 1984 Diverting the flow. Nursing: The Add-On Journal of Clinical Nursing 2 (30) October: 883–886
Contains a chart of conditions generally requiring stoma formation.
Salter M 1986 Quality above quantity. Senior Nurse 5 (3) September: 12–13
Discusses the care of patients with advanced cancer who face stoma surgery.
Snow B 1984 Ileostomy — sexual problems and self-image. Nursing: The Add-On Journal of Clinical Nursing 2 (30) October 888–889
Gives several vignettes of enquiries about these problems to the Sexual Advisory Service of the Ileostomy Association.
Stewart L 1984 Stoma care: preoperative preparation of the patient. Nursing: The Add-On Journal of Clinical Nursing 2 (30) October:

886–887
Uses the headings Physical preparation and Psychological preparation and gives a list of stoma sites to avoid.

Swan E 1986 Emergency surgery for ulcerative colitis. Nursing Times 82 (4) January 22: 49, 51, 53
Having a stoma does not preclude a normal family life as Mr Potter discovered after undergoing emergency surgery for ulcerative colitis.

Urinary elimination

Crummy V 1985 Hospital-acquired urinary tract infection. Journal of Infection Control Nursing 28 Nursing Times 81 (23) June 5: Supplement 7, 11–12
Describes the results of a study into the infection risks from catheters.

Dore D 1987 The five second flow test in urinary assessment: The Professional Nurse 2 (6) March: 171
A reduced flow rate indicates impaired voiding, common in prostatism and urethral stricture.

Fader M 1986 New thoughts on male catheterisation. Nursing Times 82 (15) April 9: 64–66
Previously female nurses did not catheterise male patients. This article proposed that catheterisation of men by female nurses should become part of standard nursing practice.

Fay J 1978 Intermittent non-sterile catheterisation of children. Nursing Mirror Supplement 146 (14) April 6: xiii, xv
Incontinence from the neurogenic bladder is chiefly from overflow; self-catheterisation at intervals empties the bladder, period of continence follows until the bladder fills again.

Fernandez J, Moore S 1986 Dry at night. Nursing Times 82 (48) November 26: 74–76
The techniques of behaviour therapy, with his parents as teachers, resulted in Robert being dry at night.

Gibbs H 1986 Catheter toilet and urinary tract infection. Nursing Times 82 (23) June 4: 75–76
Reports a small study to determine the effectiveness of a catheter toilet regime. Has a Table of principles of aseptic technique.

Gooch J 1986 Catheter care. The Professional Nurse 1 (8) May: 207–208
Contains three useful Tables — Factors which increase the risks of urinary infection — Routes for bacterial entry into the bladder if a catheter is in use — Possible causes of urine bypassing the catheter

Gould D 1985 Management of indwelling urethral catheters. Nursing Mirror 161 (10) September 4: 17, 18–20
Discusses the theory and practice of catheterisation.

Gurevich I 1985 Nurse knows best. Journal of Infection Control Nursing Supplement 8, 10, 11
Describes a points system for the selection of a urinary drainage bag.

Hamilton B 1985 Have catheter, will travel. Community Outlook October: 16–17
Modern drainage bags are designed to keep patients up and about; gives some hints on choosing the most appropriate type.

Infection Control Department 1984 Guidelines for the management of the catheterised patient. Bard Ltd. Pennywell Industrial Estate, Sunderland, SR4 9EW
An A to Z, step-by-step process.

Jacques L, McKie S, Harries C 1986 Effects of short-term catheterisation. Nursing Times 82 (25) June 18: 59, 61, 62
A study of the problem of re-establishing micturition and suggestions of some ways to help.

Johnson A 1986 Urinary tract infection. Nursing: The Add-On Journal of Clinical Nursing 3 (3) March: 102–105
Collection of mid-stream urine, specimen collection, cost of nosocomial infection, illustration of potential entry points for infection in a closed drainage system.

Kennedy A 1984 An extra hot water bottle. Nursing Times 80 (17) April 25: 57, 59
An investigation of the problems associated with catheter drainage at night and the solutions.

Kennedy A 1984 Catheter concepts. Nursing

Mirror 159 (15) October 24: 42–44, 46
Explains the development of a new indwelling urethral catheter.

Kennedy A 1984 Trial of a new bladder washout system. Nursing Times 80 (46) November 14: 48–51
Report of a trial which showed that Uro-Tainer was more effective than conventional saline bladder washouts in improving nursing management of catheter-related problems.

Meers P 1981 A dangerous place to be ill (Risk of infection in hospital). The Times Health Supplement November 13: 18

O'Neil G 1986 A drain on resources. Nursing Times 82 (38) September 17: 89
Urethral catheterisation can cause hospital-acquired infection which is estimated to cost £60 million annually.

Ringham S 1984 The ambulant catheterised patient. Journal of Infection Control, Nursing Times 80 (37) September 12: Supplement 11–12
Looks at ways of improving the quality of life for these patients.

Roper N, Logan W, Tierney 1985 The elements of nursing, 2nd edn. Churchill Livingstone, Edinburgh

Shillitoe R, Reed S 1986 Dry at night. Community Outlook March: 20, 21, 23
Discusses the methods of treatment which work best in encouraging children to be continent at night.

Turner A F 1987 Childhood continence problems. The Professional Nurse 2 (4) January: 119–122
Toilet/potty training, nocturnal enuresis, the handicapped child, encopresis and the management of bowels.

U and I Club Self-help in cystitis. U and I Club, 9e Compton Road, London N1

Even in 5 years, the health emphasis on dietary fibre and its effect on the amount of faeces eliminated has come very much to the fore. The methods of tackling prevention of the serious problem of nosocomial urinary tract infection have been pursued diligently. The role of specialist nurses participating in the care of patients with an ostomy has become even more sophisticated. As in other chapters the background information gives a general introduction to the subject of elimination.

BACKGROUND INFORMATION

Most people coming into hospital have been capable of voiding when necessary. Some have been in the habit of passing urine *before* a meal and taking advantage of the gastrocolic reflex to pass faeces *after* a meal (breakfast, lunch or evening). Each person has a varying frequency of passing urine and faeces which is the norm for him. Some people have beliefs about the ills of suppressing the passage of urine, and of constipation.

People have various attitudes to elimination. Where there are several adjoining lavatories, some people pull the chain so that the noise of the discharging cistern will drown that of urine splashing into the pan or flatus escaping from the bowel. (When asked to use a bedpan the bedclothes will help to muffle some of these sounds. When asked to use a commode some of this 'muffling' is lost.)

People have various beliefs about using a public lavatory, and this will be transferred to the hospital lavatory. Many people, especially females, have been taught not to sit on the seat! Paper seat covers are provided in some lavatories, more on the Continent than in this country. Many ward domestics take a delight in lavatories which reek of disinfectant. A few people are very sensitive to such smells which can linger in their nostrils and impair appetite.

Elimination from bladder and bowel

Most people experience some sort of emotional reaction to admission to hospital. This can affect elimination from the bladder and bowel, and produce the same sort of effect as that experienced before an interview or examination. In some areas people have to travel a considerable distance to the hospital. It is a kindness to show them as soon as possible where the lavatories are. For bed-patients this means explaining about commodes, sanichairs, Clos-o-mat:bidets where relevant, bedpans and urinals.

Equipment for bowel and bladder elimination

Commode

It is now generally agreed throughout the world that, wherever possible, even ill patients can be lifted on to a commode (Figs 14.1, 14.2). Some patients can be helped out on to a commode or sanichair (Fig. 14.3). The Renray turntable lessens the expenditure of energy and creates confidence in a patient as his feet are moved through the 90 degrees between the front of the commode and the bedside (Fig. 14.4). The patient is usually warm enough with socks and slippers and his dressing gown round his legs and over his hips. The gown should not touch the bacteria-laden floor (Fig. 14.5), thereby applying another principle of nursing 'Helping patients to prevent nosocomial infection'.

Sanichair

One stage between using a commode at the bedside and walking to the lavatory with assistance is being wheeled to the lavatory. Getting in and out of the wheelchair twice for each visit can be a tiring experience and someone had the bright idea of having a lavatory-seat type of chair which would wheel over the normal lavatory pan with its seat upturned in readiness. Lavatories and doors were widened to accommodate the 'sanichair'. But alas, nurses and patients found it was nearly as tiring freeing the buttocks of clothing whilst in the sitting position, as standing down from the chair at the door and taking two or three steps to the lavatory pan. Some patients just could not believe that they were safely over the lavatory pan and could perform without mishap!

Clos-o-mat: Bidet

The intimate care needed in midwifery and gynaecology can be made much more acceptable to each patient by installation of a Clos-o-mat (Fig. 14.6). This is a water-closet combined with an electrically operated warm water bidet and warm air drier, foot or hand controlled. The douche is started by depression of the button. When released, a warm air supply is automatically turned on for 2 minutes. The pan is then flushed by cistern release in the conventional way. The Clos-o-mat was originally designed for those people with the double disablement of blindness and absence of hands.

Midwifery units in the UK have fared best where the provision of bidets is concerned, in spite of their benefit for those who find it difficult or impossible to bath without help. Mini-clens is

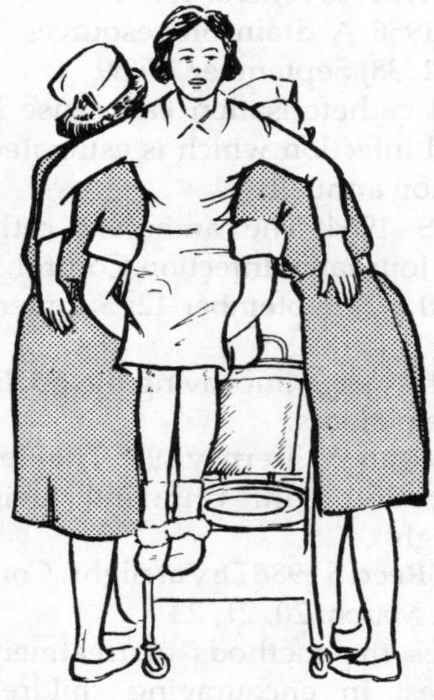

Fig. 14.1 Two nurses lifting patient from bed to commode

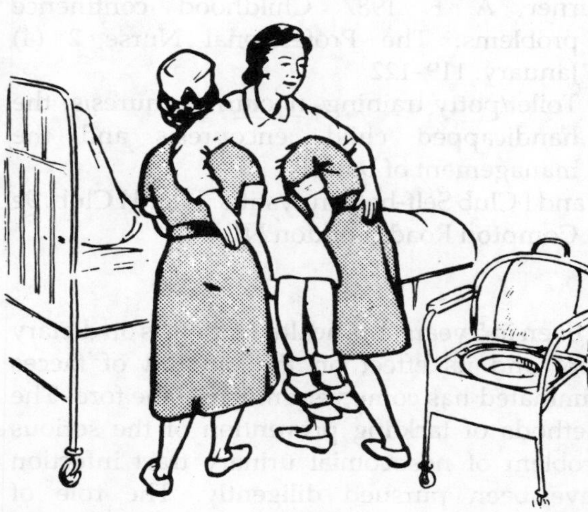

Fig. 14.2 Two nurses lifting patient from commode to bed

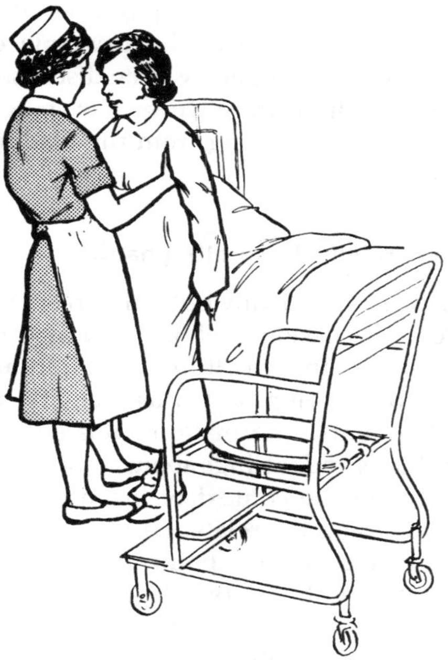

Fig. 14.3 Nurse helping patient from bed

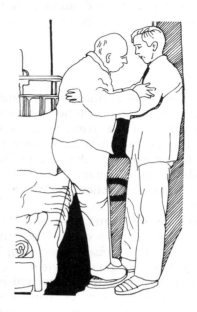

Fig. 14.4 Nurse helping patient to turn on the Renray turntable

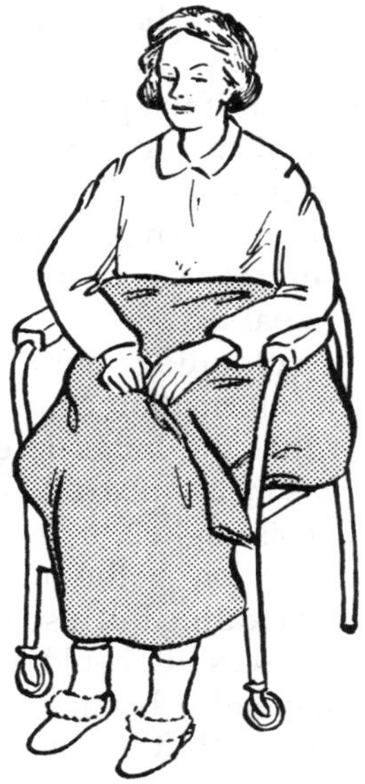

Fig. 14.5 Patient's gown free from bacteria-laden floor

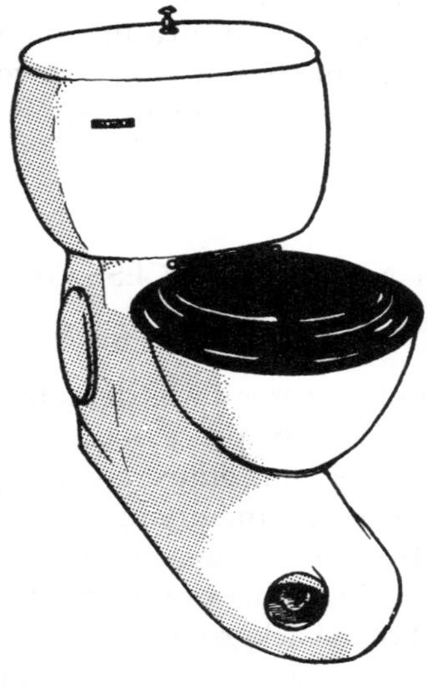

Fig. 14.6 Clos-o-mat

a portable bidet which does not have to be plumbed in, has a plugged outlet in the base so that it does not have to be lifted when full of water.

Bedpans and urinals

We now come to the minority of bed patients for whom there is no other solution but a bedpan. The Department of Health and Social Security in its Report on the organisation of the inpatient's day (1976) recommends that routine sanitary rounds should be eliminated; a bedpan should be given when the patient feels the urge to eliminate.

Stainless steel bedpans have been the most popular in the last two decades but they can create considerable noise. Some people now prefer lightweight polypropylene bedpans. There are disposable bedpan liners which can be used with these types of bedpan. There are papier mâché disposable bedpans which are used on a plastic mould; hospital policy must be followed regarding treatment of this mould between removal from one patient and giving to another. A special unit grinds the disposable bedpan and its contents to pulp before passing them into the drainage system. Disposable bedpan covers are more hygienic than cotton ones, though some people find the crackling of the paper annoying and many drains are inadequate to flush away an article of this size. In the sluice an incinerator or a large, covered, foot-operated bin may have to be provided for used covers.

DEFAECATING IN A PROCESS OF NURSING CONTEXT

In the previous chapter it was demonstrated that the four phases of 'the process' can be focused to the nurse in a general context and in a particular context. 'The process of nursing' is focused to the patient with the prime objective of individualising nursing. This cannot be the case in a text, only a broad background of information can be given to help nurses in the clinical areas to individualise nursing. It will become evident to readers that the process of nursing is more than the sum of its four phases. The principle of 'Helping patients to eliminate' will be discussed in two parts — eliminating from the bowel (defaecation) and eliminating from the bladder (micturition).

Assessing a patient's defaecating habits

Not all adults are sufficiently outgoing to enable comfortable discussion about individual eliminating habits. In all cultures, children are socialised into carrying out this activity in privacy. Pertinent information related to patients' attitudes and feelings about elimination is on page 128 in the context of incontinence, again demonstrating the relatedness of nursing knowledge. However, at a point in the initial assessment, when the nurse deems it to be appropriate, she might say something like 'to help us look after you properly is there anything you want to tell me about your bowel habits?' Judging by the number of aperients bought in chemists' shops it would appear that many people are troubled with constipation and such people will probably welcome an opportunity to discuss it with a nurse (Booth & Booth 1986).

Should the patient be elderly careful questioning will elicit whether at any time there has been 'leaking' from the bowel. Leakage from a bowel distended by faecal impaction is discussed on page 184. If the patient is a baby or a child, then detailed information will be collected from the parent. A baby can be born with an imperforate anus which the midwife will suspect by observing (assessing) that no meconium is being passed.

Of course the admitting nurse will have collected as much information as possible from other sources so that the initial interview will take place in a reasonably relaxed atmosphere. The medical diagnosis might be a clue to the need for detailed information gathering, not only about the act of defaecating but also the product of defaecation — faeces. It could be that the patient has a stoma and is being admitted for a reason unconnected with it. Or he may have a long-standing debilitating illness, for example ulcerative colitis. Or he may be admitted with an acute or chronic constipation because of an intestinal obstruction. Should this be the case, immediate surgery will be the priority to prevent gangrene of the gut; the nursing assessment will take place in gradual steps as the patient becomes able to participate; it will probably be a case of 'sequential' assessment.

Long lists can be threatening to learners, but all of the following questions only rarely need to be asked. They act as a schema held in the 'human computer', use of which, together with practical experience helps to give credence to the concept of 'clinical judgement'. The following are points to be borne in mind; where appropriate they can be used as prompts to get a complete picture of the patient's defaecating habits.

- what words does the patient use for this activity and the products?
  Some people are familiar with the term 'bowels open'; others use the word 'stool'.
- how often is faeces passed? For the majority of patients the answer to this question will establish their norm. Should the answer reveal constipation or diarrhoea questions about these deviations will be asked at this point, but in this text they will be included later.
- at what time of day? Most people defaecate after a meal, and which one should be recorded.
- is an aperient ever taken?
- how often is an aperient taken? Some people brought up with the idea that a 'weekly dose is good for you' go through life believing this. People prone to overweight may abuse aperients in the hope that less 'calories' will be absorbed.
- which one? Booth & Booth (1986) give a comprehensive list of oral aperients, suppositories and enemata.
- is any other medication being taken? Wilson (1987) gives five groups of other medications which can affect normal bowel habit.

More detailed assessment information will be required if the patient has mentioned constipation, diarrhoea, discomfort or pain; and medical diagnoses such as paraplegia, tetraplegia, colostomy or ileostomy would alert the nurse to collect information about how these conditions were managed at home. Another relevant condition, incontinence of faeces was discussed in Chapter 11.

Constipation

Has constipation been mentioned during the initial asessment? Which word does the patient use? Costive is a lay term for constipation. What notion does the patient have of this word? Some people believe that toxins (poisons) are absorbed from the bowel and cause such things as spots on the skin, lethargy, headache, furred tongue, bad breath (halitosis). What is the nurse's perception of 'constipation'? Knowledge gained from consulting the literature is that during the first half of this century it was firmly believed by most people that a daily evacuation of the bowel was essential for health, and that failure to achieve this could have dire effects. Around the middle of this century various research projects revealed that the individual norm for bowel evacuation varied widely from three evacuations per day to three per week (Wright 1974 p.18). As a result, obsession with accomplishing a daily bowel movement was to be discouraged. Wright (1974 p. 17) states that the normal weight of faeces produced in one day is from 100 to 150 g: the statement is made in the context of 'Normal physiology of colon and rectum'. Burkitt in conversation with Swaffield (1979) advised:

> 150 grams as minimum, and encourages up to 250 grams daily for several reasons other than prevention of constipation

So now we are back to advising a daily evacuation of 150–250 g of soft but well formed faeces based on extensive epidemiological data collected and analysed by Burkitt (1983).

Because output is so closely related to input, questions relevant to assessing a patient's ability to eat and drink may well be appropriate here. A list of what has to be assessed is useful as an aide memoire but should not dictate the order in which information is collected. When assessing a patient's eliminating habits it also has to be remembered that information about any impediment in the patient's ability to mobilise has to be taken into consideration as it may interfere with getting to the lavatory. And the patient's ability to dress and undress is also pertinent to eliminating.

Diarrhoea

Has diarrhoea been mentioned during the initial assessment? What notion does the patient have of this word? How long has the diarrhoea lasted? How many times a day is faeces passed? Any idea of how much? Has the diet been altered because of the diarrhoea? Is it associated with vomiting? Have there been any previous episodes of diarrhoea/vomiting? Previous episodes could alert the nurse to the possibility of food poisoning and the need for teaching personal hygiene related to eliminating and the preparation of food. Acute diarrhoeal diseases of infancy and childhood kill millions (5 to 18, Kharib 1986) of babies and children annually. When assessing such patients it is pertinent to collect information from the parents about weight loss and lethargy. It is relevant to examine skin turgor, dryness of skin and mouth: if the patient is a young baby, is there a sunken fontanelle? Is less urine being passed? Is it concentrated? These are all signs of dehydration. The medical diagnosis might suggest chronic diarrhoea, when the foregoing information would also be applicable. Rather than pain, there is likely to be soreness around the back passage (perianal region). Many nurses come from upwardly socially mobile families and many patients come from disadvantaged families. It is therefore important that we listen to the words they use and write down their problems in their words. When assessing elderly patients, do try to get information which is as factual as possible. Diarrhoea may be reported, instead of the reality which might be faecal staining of underpants: this would lead the nurse to consider the possibility of faecal impaction with leakage of faecal fluid around the solid mass.

Discomfort

Normally food/faeces is propelled along the intestine by peristalsis and segmentation described in Nursing Mirror (1984). Bacterial activity produces a little gas which is passed naturally during defaecation and/or micturition. All this activity for most of the time does not reach 'consciousness', but when constipation, diarrhoea or irritable bowel syndrome is troubling the patient, he becomes 'conscious' of abdominal discomfort which he may describe as 'feeling bloated', 'blown up' or 'distended'. There may be a feeling of fullness in the rectum, a constant desire to defaecate. 'It is uncomfortable around the back passage' probably means redness of the skin; whereas 'it is sore...' probably means excoriation of the skin. It is important to find out what meaning the patient attaches to the words he uses. Nursing's greatest use of the word 'sore' is in combination form, as for example 'pressure sore'. But the condition of 'soreness' does not appear to have been investigated.

Pain

Chapter 4 deals with the principle of nursing, 'helping patients to cope with pain'. In this portion, pain will be discussed in relation to assessing a patient's defaecating habits. Is there abdominal pain? If the patient uses any of the words — abdomen, stomach or belly, the nurse must explore what it means to him. Is it present all/most/some of the time? Are there any periods free from pain? For how long has this pattern of pain been emerging? Can the pain be described? — niggle, gripe, spasm, colic are some words which patients use to describe their pain. Is the pain confined to the back passage? Is it present only at defaecation? Is the medical diagnosis any help in guiding questions to gain nursing information about the pain?

It could be argued that knowing the medical diagnosis might introduce bias into the nurse's information-collecting, but the nurse's objective is to discover how the patient is interpreting the pain he is experiencing related to defaecating. And we have to remember that pain is a subjective experience and most researchers' definition is that 'pain is what the patient says it is'.

Paraplegia

It may be that during a 3-year nursing programme a student will encounter a patient who has only recently become paraplegic and the implementation of a plan for independent management of defaecation will be in its early stages. However, here the instance of a paraplegic person being admitted for another reason will be considered. At the initial assessment, the nurse will discover whether or not any nursing help is needed. If so, it has to be described exactly to enable nurses on succeeding shifts to offer appropriate help so that the patient is spared — explaining to each nurse; — feeling that nursing is a haphazard activity; — thinking that nurses do not communicate with each other and so on.

Many paraplegic patients learn to attend to faecal elimination independently; for some it involves manual evacuation, for others insertion of suppositories. Nurses should know what facilities they need to provide, to enable continuance of independence. Where? At what hour of the day? There may need to be a prescription for suppositories on the medication Kardex and although it is usual for the nurse to sign the Kardex when the medication is given, either the patient will sign, or he may agree to the nurse signing it after checking that the procedure has been carried out. If the patient is satisfied with the result, it may therefore be the custom to record this on the nursing notes.

Tetraplegia

The first paragraph under the heading 'Paraplegia' applies equally to the tetraplegic person. However, he cannot be independent for defaecation. Careful exploration will elicit how this has been managed at home. It could have been managed by a daily visit from the community nurse, or a family 'helper/carer' may have managed to carry out the appropriate procedure. Information from these sources would be helpful; and it may be that the patient would prefer existing family arrangements to continue. The notion of family members caring for their loved one in hospital is gaining acceptance and it could be that such arrangements would best suit solving the patient's problem of requiring another person to attend to his everyday activity of defaecating.

Stoma/ostomy

In a 3-year nursing programme students are likely to encounter patients in surgical wards or in specialist gastroenterology wards who are about to undergo surgery which will create an ileostomy or a colostomy. Some nurses specialise as stomatherapists and they interview such patients preoperatively; it may be the custom that the admitting nurse does not collect information about defaecating habits at the initial assessment. Stewart (1984) discusses the physical and psychological preparation, from which one can deduce factors to be borne in mind when assessing these patients where a specialist nurse is unavailable.

Sometimes patients who have cared independently for a well established stoma are admitted to hospital for another reason. At the initial interview the nurse needs to discuss with the patient whether or not any nursing help will be required, and if so, it must be written so that nurses on succeeding shifts can offer the same sort of help. What appliance is used; how often is the bag changed? Does the patient have a stoma kit with him? Where does he usually place it when dealing with the stoma at home? Does he sit on a chair to empty the contents of the bag into the lavatory pan? Will a prescription be required for appliances/bags? Other ideas will be gained by reading the appropriate articles in the Reading Assignment.

A wide range of conditions have been considered in this section on assessing a patient's defaecating habits in an attempt to demonstrate the complexity of nursing. At the same time readers have been introduced to several medical diagnoses — but in a nursing context. As the nursing course progresses students will need to learn much more about the medical conditions, to understand which, a good knowledge of the biological sciences is needed. The objective when the nurse collects assessment information is to identify, with the patient whenever possible, the problems being experienced with this everyday living activity, and when stated clearly, in the words used by the patient, they are the nursing diagnosis, not the medical diagnosis. For example:

Medical diagnosis: Salmonella food poisoning
Patient's problems in his words: (nursing diagnosis)

- embarrassed by passing foul-smelling gas and faeces
- no appetite
- no energy
- sore around back passage
- anxious unless near lavatory
- needs 'to go' immediately.

Planning — individualised

The planning phase of the process of nursing results in the patient's nursing plan. From published plans it seems to be the custom to state on them the identified problems which are amenable to nursing intervention, so, going through the preceding list of possible patient's problems:

- the goal would be to deodorise foul smell. The nursing intervention might be to give an oral preparation of charcoal — and/or spray a deodorant into the vessel which will receive the faeces
- the goal would be to increase appetite. Bad odour can interfere with appetite so success of the previously mentioned intervention may help to increase appetite. The nursing intervention could be 'offer small quantities of nourishing liquids acceptable to patient hourly'. 'Liquid of patient's choice on locker' (so that he can drink when thirsty) — which may well be part of the syndrome if there is dehydration. If, and when food can be tolerated, the plan will change: 'offer small quantities of low residue food with appetising appearance'.

The ongoing assessment information about bowel activity will guide changing the nursing plan to 'gradually increase food intake' until return to previous dietary habits is achieved.

- the goal would be to conserve/increase energy. The nursing intervention, 'rest in bed between incidents of defaecation' would conserve energy. Success of the previously mentioned dietary interventions would increase energy.
- the goal would be absence of soreness. The nursing intervention might be provision of a barrier cream which the patient agrees to apply after post-defaecation toilet, details of which should be written on the nursing plan, so that the patient is not confused by only some nurses offering facilities for post-defaecation toilet.
- the goal would be reduced anxiety. The nursing intervention might be to allocate to the patient a bed nearest to the lavatory. Or it may be to place a commode by the bedside if available staff permit offering post-defaecation toilet facilities. Or if a bedpan has to be resorted to — details of where the bedpan can be kept (hygienically) near the bed for immediate use should be written on the nursing plan. All staff should know of this arrangement, so that in the interest of 'tidiness' it is not removed.
- the goal would be — does not need to go immediately. Inflammation of the gastro-intestinal tract is mainly responsible for the intestinal hurry resulting in diarrhoea which in some instances is accompanied by 'urgency'. The dietary interventions would help to 'rest' the tract and reduce urgency. Lessened anxiety from the interventions to reduce odour and soreness; being near and in control of using the vessel for defaecation would also help to 'rest' the tract (which is well known to respond to excesses of emotion) and reduce urgency.

It may well be that there will be a prescription for medication written in the Kardex to reduce the inflammation. The corresponding nursing activity will be to sign the medication Kardex as each dose is given. The nursing plan will contain the intervention to observe for the intended effect and any known side-effects, and if ongoing assessment in implementing this nursing activity reveals any of these, they will be recorded on the patient's nursing notes, and side-effects would be reported to the doctor.

It is possible that there will be nursing activities related to defaecation written on the patient's plan (not related to a patient's problem which is amenable to nursing — the nurse-initiated part of nursing) resulting from medical prescription, for example:

- preparation of the bowel for:
  barium enema
  proctoscopy
  sigmoidoscopy
  operation on the bowel
- rectal lavage
- total colonic lavage
- preparation of the bowel to ensure a clearer X-ray of the kidneys
- preparation of the bowel prior to surgery other than on the bowel.

There may well be instructions in the nursing plan only indirectly related to the patient's problems. For example, 'inspect the product of each defaecation' requires details of the place and the vessel into which the product will be evacuated so that it can be inspected (as a means of ongoing assessment). It is not an acceptable standard of nursing just to tell an ambulant patient to use a bedpan in the lavatory because a stainless steel slipper bedpan tends to 'rock' on some lavatory seats, and a person with short legs may find the increased height unmanageable. To facilitate inspection of faeces (or a specimen for the laboratory) from an ambulant patient, there is a strip metal frame with four hooked supports (Fig. 14.7); it has a circular hole to accept a standard 20 cm stainless steel bowl. The apparatus is placed across the lavatory pan; the support does not interfere with the normal lowering of the seat. If it is not available on the ward, the nurse could send in a written requisition for one.

If a specimen of faeces for the laboratory is to detect the presence of microorganisms, then it has to be kept at as near human body temperature as possible, and delivered to the laboratory as soon as possible. A specimen of

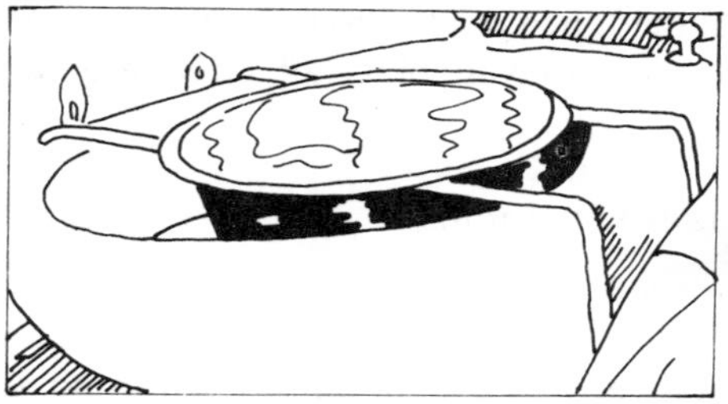

Fig. 14.7 Frame for collection of a specimen of faeces

faeces which is to be examined for its contents, for example the amount of fat present, does not have the same urgency — but the varying members of staff thoughout the 24 hours may not know these details unless they are summarised on the nursing plan.

It may be that the medical microbiologist and the Control of Infection Committee recommend the disinfection of faeces from patients with particular medical diagnoses. These recommendations should be clearly stated in the nursing plan so that each nurse involved in the nursing of such a patient can accept responsibility and accountability for carrying out the recommendations.

Ward planning

Ward planning in a more general context has to be considered in relation to a patient's defaecating habits. 'Ward rounds' of giving out bedpans should be a thing of the past in relation to 'individualised nursing'. The individualised planner's first choice of nursing intervention might be two nurses to help a patient walk to the lavatory. The rationale for this might be:

- helps to fulfil the nursing intervention at 'mobilising'
- helps to prevent pressure sores
- helps to prevent deep venous thrombosis
- helps to prevent pulmonary embolism and so on.

But ward planning has to include the reality of whether or not sufficient nursing staff are available to help the patient to walk to the lavatory. A second best decision of a commode at the bedside should be recorded as such. It is factual evidence related to the quality of nursing because of unavailability of adequate nursing staff.

Generalised planning

It is not too early for students of nursing in a 3-year programme to begin to appreciate the importance of the generalised planning which has to be carried out to provide an adequate number of nurses so that first choice nursing interventions can be planned as mentioned in the previous paragraph. Registered nurses have a responsibility to feed this factual information to the appropriate level of management. After all, how is 'management' to know if it is not given the facts? If human resources are not available to offer bedfast patients post-bedpan handwashing facilities, then the alternative of moist wipes can be provided.

Generalised planning is also necessary to provide the material resources at clinical level which can enhance or constrain the standard of nursing that can be planned. The following list suggests the sort of resources which are relevant to nurses helping patients to eliminate.

- number of lavatories available
- provision of type of toilet paper; servicing of its presence throughout 24 hours
- provision for cleanliness of lavatories throughout 24 hours
- provision of clean and efficient post-toilet handwashing facilities, recommended by relevant health education programmes
- number of commodes available
- provision for patients' privacy when using a commode
- minimal noise when wheeling commode — helped by regular removal of fibre, dust and hairs which inevitably collect around wheels, and prevent easy forward wheeling. Some older commodes are very noisy in transit; this is especially distressing to patients who require to use them during the night; the newer ones are almost noiseless in transit.
- the type and number of bedpans and urinals available
- provision for stainless steel ones to be clean and warm when wanted
- provision for efficient disposal of bedpan contents and subsequent washing of bedpan
- provision for regular servicing of this equipment to avoid breakdown.

Implementing

Glancing back at the discussion about individualised planning (p. 186), the goals and nursing interventions were stated in more detail than in some of the other chapters. The implementation resulting from a medication prescription was mentioned on page 186. Possible nursing activities as a consequence of other medical prescriptions were suggested on page 187. And those related to inspection of faeces and taking a specimen of faeces for the laboratory were outlined on page 187. When any of these prescribed nursing actions are carried out, the fact is recorded on the patient's nursing notes together with any other relevant information, some of which will provide summative evidence on the day set for whether or not the goal is being/has been achieved.

When writing nursing plans it is imperative that the place and the vessel to be used are stated, and that implementation of the instruction is recorded. The plan may change fairly rapidly as for instance, on admission of a patient exhausted from a severe attack of diarrhoea, it may state 'use commode at bedside'; in 2 or 3 days there may be marked improvement and the patient may ask to go to the lavatory which he has observed is not far from his bed. So it is important that the instruction on the plan is changed to 'use lavatory independently', otherwise the patient will be embarrassed by a nurse continuing the implementation of offering a commode at the bedside. It is equally important that each nurse reads the nursing plans at the beginning of each shift to note changes. If she fails to do so another embarrassment could occur; she might reprimand the patient for being at the lavatory — he is implementing the changed plan! Either way the patient could be forgiven for thinking that the nurses do not know what they should be doing.

Concentration on learning to think in a process of nursing context, should not blind us to the fact that the conciseness which is essential when writing nursing interventions on the nursing plan, cannot convey the artistic dimension of nursing — the cognitive and psychomotor skills required to carry out these interventions safely and effectively. In this final section of implementing, helping a patient to use a commode and a bedpan will be used as examples.

Helping a patient to use a commode

The more natural position on a commode prevents a patient suffering the discomfort of retention of urine (Fig. 11.2 p. 128), flatulent abdominal distension and constipation. He is spared the further discomfort and embarrassment of relief of such conditions by catheterisation, flatus tube, suppository or enemata. Less frequent performance of these techniques is also timesaving for the staff and a hospital economy. Fewer aperients are necessary. Use of the commode affords an easy means of inspection of excreta before disposal and allows for collection of a specimen of urine and/or faeces. Page 180 gives some of the details of lifting a patient from bed to commode and vice versa, and Figures 14.1 and 14.2 illustrate these procedures. Safe and effective lifting helps to prevent low back pain to which nurses are prone (p. 159). To prevent nosocomial infection (p. 257) both nurse and patient should wash their hands after use of a commode.

Helping a patient to use a bedpan

We now come to the minority of bed patients for whom there seems to be no other solution but using a bedpan. It is good practice to convey to the patient that you are aware of the increased anxiety associated with needing help for such an intimate procedure.

Where an ordinary bed is in use, the standard method of giving a bedpan to a *recumbent* patient is illustrated in Figure 14.8. In the absence of a mechanical lifting aid, a lifting pole

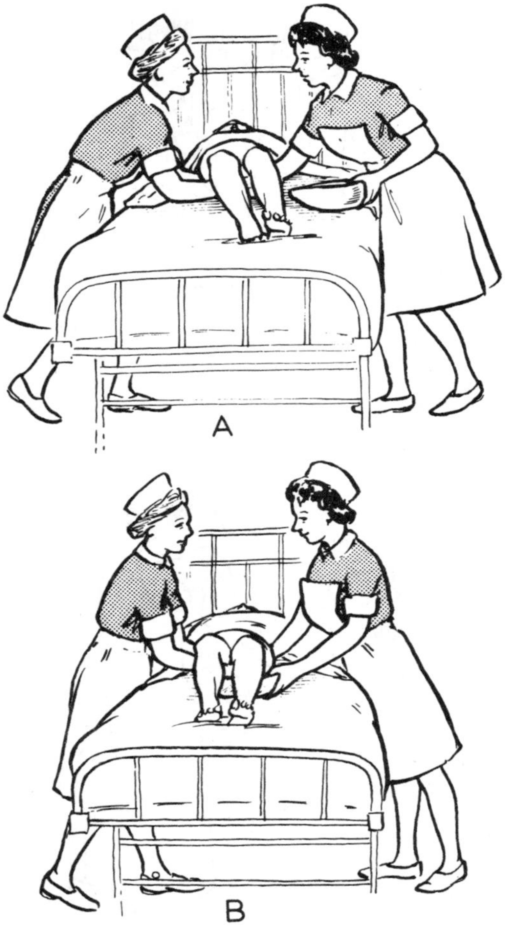

Fig. 14.8 Giving a bedpan to a recumbent patient (A) Ready to lift (B) Insertion of bedpan

should be attached to the bed so that where possible the patient can help, even if this is minimal. At the start of the lift the nurses have one foot in front of the other, the anterior thigh against the bed rail and the forearms on the mattress supporting the patient's pelvic girdle. As the nurses' legs are straightened the patient's lower trunk is lifted on three forearms, the fourth arm inserts the bedpan (Fig. 14.8B).

One method for giving a bedpan to a patient who is sitting up in bed is illustrated in Figure 14.9A. In the presence of a lifting pole many nurses prefer this method to the shoulder lift, as at the end, the patient is more easily turned on to his side for post-bedpan toilet. Where there is no

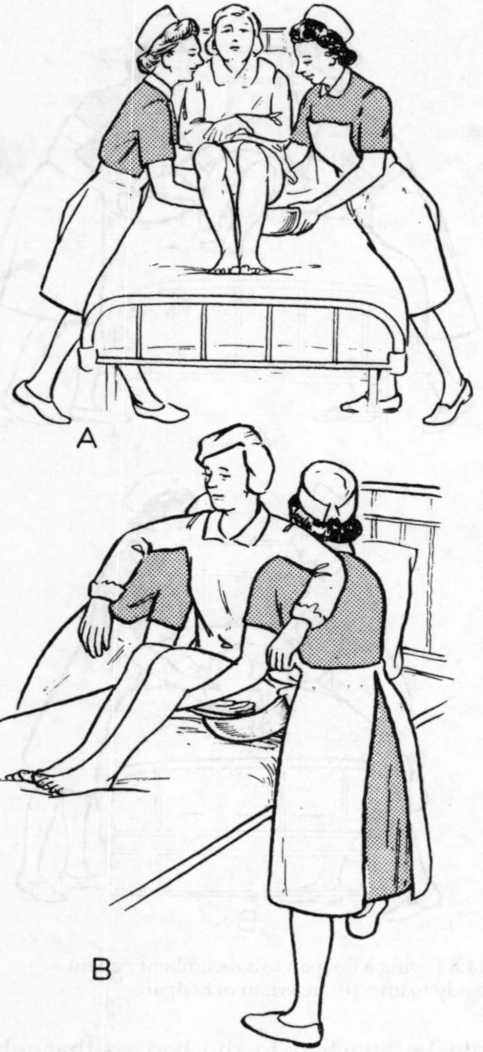

Fig. 14.9 Giving a bedpan to a patient who is in the sitting position in bed (A) Using the three arms lift (B) Using the shoulder lift

lifting pole, when using the shoulder lift each nurse has one hand free for placing the bedpan under the patient (Fig. 14.9B). After removal of the bedpan, post-bedpan toilet can be performed by one nurse before lowering the patient onto the bed. If necessary the patient can be turned to one side to complete the toilet in a position in which the nurse can see what she is doing.

It will be seen that this is another nursing activity which has other dimensions, preventing nosocomial infection, and low back pain.

And now back to 'process thinking'.

Evaluating

The fourth phase of the process of nursing is interpreted by the majority of nurses as an activity which is carried out on a set date to discover whether or not the set goal has been achieved. However, as we are gaining more experience of using the process, we are realising that it is a concept which has much wider implications.

For example in the context of defaecation and the giving of an enema or suppository, the assessment information would confirm the reason for administration — constipation, or any one of those mentioned on page 187 — and the state of the patient. The goal would be emptying the lower bowel of faeces. Planning would include preparation of the patient, the environment and the equipment for the procedure. Implementing would be the actual carrying out of the procedure. Evaluating would compare the state of the patient before and after the procedure: evaluating the faecal result would be immediate. It would seem that we rely on the nurse's notion of a 'normal stool'. It may be that rather than write 'good result' or 'poor result', the stainless steel bowl (p. 187) or the bedpan could be weighed before and after defaecation to give a factual recording of weight of faeces.

For rectal lavage approximately the same mode of thinking could be carried out, but in this procedure a large bore catheter is passed into the rectum; a funnel is attached to the fluted end of the catheter into which warm water is poured and allowed to flow into the rectum, after which the funnel is held at a low level in a bucket to receive the returned fluid. There has to be immediate assessment of the returned fluid — are there bits of broken up faeces in it? Flaky bits of faeces? How faecal-stained is the returned fluid? Another funnelful is allowed to flow into the rectum and the procedure repeated until evaluation is achieved of the return of clear, unstained liquid. The amount of fluid required to achieve this is recorded.

To return to the accepted interpretation of the

evaluating phase of the process of nursing — evaluating on a set date whether or not the set goal has been achieved. This confronts us with the circularity of the process. Evaluating depends on the quality of the implementing of nursing interventions and activities; implementing depends on the quality of the nursing plan and the clarity with which the goals are stated in observable and, where possible, measurable terms; goal statements are dependent on the quality of the statement of problems as the patient is experiencing them, and this in turn depends on the quality of the assessment data.

Glancing back at the assessing section, factual information can be used when evaluating in relation to constipation and diarrhoea. When evaluation reveals that the problem of constipation has been solved to the patient's satisfaction, it will continue to be a potential problem if the patient fails to comply with the life-style advocated by the nurses, to prevent constipation. Discomfort is a subjective experience and when evaluating one can only accept the patient's feeling that he is more, the same as, less — bloated, blown up, distended or whatever words he used to describe it, and we have to rely on the nurse's written record of the patient's description of the pain being experienced. This would alert nurses on subsequent shifts to explore with the patient whether current pain experience is more than, the same as, less than the previously recorded description. Some operations such as haemorrhoidectomy are particularly painful in the early postoperative days and it would be a good standard of nursing to use a painometer (p. 52) as an evaluative tool. Investigation of patient satisfaction could be used for evaluation of the continuance of defaecation habits of paraplegic, tetraplegic and stoma patients who are admitted for another reason. In the individualised planning section (p. 186) several examples are given of goals and nursing interventions with subsequent evaluations. With regard to anxiety (p. 186), nurses of the future will probably become more involved in using well-tried anxiety scales such as those used by Wilson-Barnett (1978) in relation to barium enema investigations.

After this somewhat detailed consideration of patients' defaecating habits, discussion of their micturating habits follows. It will necessarily be shorter because the vessels used for both activities are the same. The skill of giving a bedpan to a recumbent patient (Fig. 14.8), and to a patient who is in the sitting position in bed (Fig. 14.9) is the same for eliminating faeces and urine.

MICTURATING IN A PROCESS OF NURSING CONTEXT

The objective in using the accepted four phases of the process of nursing is to 'individualise nursing'. This means that the nursing plan must take into account the person's previous well-established habits of passing urine. Even though an older person may need to void during the night, it need not be a 'problem' for him. The fact would be recorded on the assessment form and it would be ascertained that the patient knows the way to the lavatory and agrees to be independent for this night time activity. In the interest of economy of paperwork, all nurses should realise that what is written on the assessment form (patient profile, nursing history) is necessary information throughout the patient's stay in hospital, and does not need to be re-written on the nursing plan. Night nurses on subsequent shifts will not be surprised to find the patient visiting the lavatory during the night.

However, if the patient takes a 'sleeping pill' in hospital because of the changed circumstances, for example a single as opposed to a double bed; sleeping alone in bed rather than with another person; being in a four or six bed area, or a Nightingale type of ward, a clinical nursing judgement may be that it will be safer to void into a commode at the bedside. This change in nursing prescription will only be made after considering that there are sufficient commodes to permit one at the bedside throughout the night, and it will be written on the nursing plan. It is not good nursing practice to leave the responsibility with the patient to 'ask' for a commode; he may lie awake with the desire to pass urine because he is not sufficiently assertive 'to ask'.

Assessing a patient's micturating habits

Some relevant information can be found in Chapter 11 which is about helping incontinent patients. The items concerned with assessing incontinence are recognisable by the title or annotation (p. 123). The nurse will collect as much of the information as possible, requested by the assessment form, from other sources before the initial interview with the patient. Some of this information might alert the nurse to the fact that a detailed investigation about the habits of passing urine will be necessary. A general question such as 'Would you like to tell me about your daily pattern of passing water?' will probably bring most of the required information. But the nurse needs to have a scheme in mind, which she can use as prompts to fill in possible omissions in response to the general question. The scheme might include such questions as:

- how many times is urine passed during the day?
- how many times is urine passed during the night?
- how much urine is passed each time?

  passage of a small amount of concentrated urine (oliguria). There are many causes of this condition, which include:

  any febrile state
  dehydration
  lack of fluid intake
  excessive loss of fluid — sweating
  — vomiting
  — diarrhoea
  — bleeding
  an acutely inflamed kidney

  no urine is passed (anuria)

  can occur in the first 24h postoperatively. It can be caused by obstruction in a ureter. The anuria from pressure of an enlarged prostate gland results in retention of urine in the bladder.

  urine is not secreted (suppression)

  this will obviously result in anuria. It can occur in emergency, for example when a patient collapses and the blood pressure is insufficient to produce filtration in the kidney.

  a large amount of urine is passed (polyuria)

  the most frequent cause is diabetes mellitus, which may or may not be insulin dependent

  a rare cause is deficiency of the antidiuretic hormone secreted by the pituitary gland (diabetes insipidus)

  an increased amount of urine is passed

  results from taking diuretics which are frequently prescribed as treatment for high blood pressure

- when did you last pass urine? This would be appropriate when retention of urine is suspected.
- how much fluid is taken daily? (cups of, mugs of, can only be interpreted approximately because of the varying size of cups and mugs)
- has there been any recent change/s in voiding habits?
- has there been any problem with passing water in the past?
- when?
- how long did it last?
- what treatment was given?
- is there any leakage between visits to lavatory?
- is there any perineal soreness in women?
- is there a steady flow?
- is the flow interrupted?
- is there any pain on passing urine?
- can it be described?
- are any medications which influence the amount of urine being taken?

It cannot be stressed too strongly that it will never be necessary to ask all these questions of one patient. They are to be borne in mind so that they can be used as prompts to elicit relevant information and they, together with experience, become part of professional judgement. But putting them together does show the complexity of nursing knowledge required to appreciate the rationale behind any prompting questions.

The purpose of collecting assessment information is to identify any problems which the patient is experiencing in relation to passing urine, stated in the words which the patient uses to describe them. On page 7 an example is given of problems written from a woman's perspective when the medical diagnosis is cystitis. On page 128 another example of problems as the patient might experience them is given when the medical diagnosis is the cause of incontinence.

Planning, implementing, evaluating

The result of planning, the accepted second phase of the process, is the written individualised nursing plan. It starts with consideration of the patient's problem/s. If the medical diagnosis is 'enlarged prostate gland', the patient's problems which are amenable to nursing intervention might be:

- sweating profusely (body's attempt to get rid of some fluid)
- restlessness (due to discomfort and physiological imbalance)
- a feeling of 'being ill' or whatever words the patient uses — he will certainly feel far from 'well' (due to electrolyte imbalance)
- a bloated, stretched feeling across the lower abdomen (from a grossly distended bladder).

Taking the last problem first because its relief would have the highest priority, there will be a medical prescription to catheterise the bladder, but the procedure will be carried out by a nurse. Roper, Logan & Tierney (1985) recommend two parts of the nursing plan to cope with this, so that nurse-initiated interventions are recorded separately from delegated nursing interventions. However, this particular delegated nursing intervention will be the first priority and it may well lessen the patient's other problems. It will now be considered, and then the other three patient's problems in the context of planning, implementing and evaluating.

- the goal would be relief of abdominal discomfort. The delegated nursing intervention would be catheterisation, followed by establishment of a closed drainage system, and the technique of emptying the bag. The technique will have been advocated by the Control of Infection Committee to prevent nosocomial infection (Ch. 20). Urinary infection causes approximately 30% of the approximately 9% of nosocomial infections in hospital patients (Meers 1981). A corresponding planned, delegated nursing intervention would be an intake and output chart. Implementation of these interventions would be recorded on the patient's nursing notes. Regarding the intake and output chart, it will probably only be necessary to record a daily summary in the notes. Evaluation would be subjective information from the patient, unless abdominal girth had been assessed with a tape measure. The amount of urine drained will be indirect evidence of less distension. Whenever catheterisation is carried out, the standard of nursing practice is evaluated by the presence or absence of urinary infection.
- the goal might be refreshment of patient by removal of stale perspiration.
  The planned nursing intervention would be bedbath with water at body temperature. The plan would be implemented. Evaluation would be almost immediate and might consist of asking the patient how he felt — not, 'do you feel refreshed?' There may be visible evidence of decreased sweating. This cannot be only attributed to the bedbath, since draining the bladder will have contributed.
- the goal might be reduced/absence of restlessness.
  The planned nursing intervention would include those comforting measures deemed to be appropriate. There are likely to be medical prescriptions for investigation of blood electrolytes and subsequent intravenous infusion to correct any imbalance. They will result in delegated interventions on the nursing plan. As planned nurse-initiated and delegated nursing interventions are implemented, the fact is recorded on the patient's nursing notes, together with any relevant information. Evaluation will

compare current state of restlessness with the description on the assessment form. An open-ended question such as 'How are you feeling now?' will give the patient's subjective information. There may be visual evidence of lessened restlessness.

- the goal might be feels less (whichever word the patient used).

The planned nursing intervention would include any activities to help the patient to understand what was happening to him. Most men are aware of the fact that in middle age some of them have trouble with their 'waterworks'. But what does the patient mean by this? It is important that nurses 'listen' to what patients think is wrong with them; only in this way can we learn to help them when they feel ill, poorly, unwell, badly, out of kilter or whatever word the patient used. Implementing the nurse-initiated and delegated nursing interventions for the other problems which were identified, with this patient, will most probably have helped to make him feel 'a bit better'.

What was written earlier in this chapter about commodes, sanichairs, Clos-o-mats, bidets, bedpans and urinals is equally applicable to helping a patient to pass urine. The same is true of ward planning and generalised planning. Readers must be aware of the complexity of helping patients to eliminate and the tremendous sensitivity required to do this in such a way that patients retain their dignity.

Finally, a discussion of micturating would not be complete without offering some background information about catheterisation and bladder infection. The questions in the assessing section, if they elicited an increased frequency of passing urine would alert the nurse to the possibility of cystitis. But a common cause of bladder infection is catheterisation.

CATHETERISATION AND BLADDER INFECTION

Urethral catheterisation is an invasive procedure and is therefore carried out using an aseptic technique. The article by Gibbs (1986) gives the principles of aseptic technique in tabular form. Between 5 and 10% of patients admitted to hospital develop a nosocomial infection; of these, urinary tract infections head the list at 30%, the majority being associated with indwelling catheters. Many factors enter into estimating the annual cost to the NHS such as increased patient stay, use of antibiotics, apparatus, swabs, lotions and nursing time. The current estimate for the UK is £60 million (O'Neil 1986) each year. This does not take account of the pain and discomfort experienced by the patient, nor the inconvenience to his life style of spending extra days in hospital. The items in the Reading Assignment contain research-based knowledge which will permit a registered nurse to practise safely, and thereby minimise nosocomial urinary tract infection.

In this chapter the equipment which can be used to facilitate patients' elimination was described. In the section on assessing, possible problems were discussed; in the planning section the notion of individualised ward, and generalised planning was introduced. The principle — helping patients to eliminate — was considered in a process of nursing context.

APPLYING THE PRINCIPLE

A registered nurse must be capable of:

- using bedpan washers, sterilisers, special beds and lifting apparatus, and getting maintenance staff to check efficiency of same at intervals
- teaching staff to use these properly
- disinfecting and sterilising bedpans, commode pans, urinals, etc. without special apparatus, and teaching these methods
- transmitting to authority the patients' needs to gain improvement of their facilities
- transmitting to authority the staff's needs regarding non-noisy equipment, lifting devices, etc., to enable the patients' basic

functions to be carried out in the most humane way possible
- providing psychological support for the patients
- lifting and positioning a patient on a bedpan, commode or sanichair comfortably and with safety to all concerned
- giving a bedpan without contaminating its external surface on any ward surface before insertion into the bed
- removing a bedpan without injuring the patient's skin (sweaty skin tends to 'stick' to the bedpan)
- attending to patient's post-bedpan toilet
- safe placing of the used bedpan during this attention
- giving sanitary utensils with as little germ-dissemination as possible and without contaminating uniform
- observing contents of pan before disposal
- recognising abnormalities of excreta and the act of excretion; communicating these to the rest of the staff; recognising their significance — taking any immediate steps necessary, for example the patient may need to be barrier nursed. Communicating all these skills to others
- treating the subject of excretion and elimination in such a way that no member of staff looks upon it as 'junior' nursing
- instilling the attitude that it is worthy of high regard
- disinfecting excreta before disposal and teaching other members of staff safe methods
- accurate reporting, verbal and written, of excreta and the act of excretion; teaching staff to do the same
- collecting faeces for macroscopic examination on the ward and for microscopic examination and chemical analysis in the laboratory
- administering antidiarrhoeal drugs, laxatives, aperients and purgatives with discretion and safety
- administering suppositories, flatus tubes, and enemata to be returned or retained
- recognising the need for, and performing manual evacuation of the rectum
- collecting a specimen of urine; (a) for ward testing and testing it; (b) for chemical analysis in the laboratory; (c) by the midstream method (from male and female patients) for culture and sensitivity tests in the laboratory
- collecting a 24-hour specimen of urine
- organising as foolproof a method as possible for intake and output charts
- administering urinary antiseptics and diuretics, performing catheterisation, bladder drainage and lavage
- organising a safe routine for barrier nursing
- applying the principle — helping patients to eliminate — in a process of nursing context.

WORKING ASSIGNMENT

Topics for discussion

- *Nurse A*: We have 12 bed patients. If we give them bedpans before a meal what about the smell? Of course it would mean that they had had their hands washed *before* the meal. You just can't win every time, can you?
  Nurse B: I've heard of something you can spray into the bedpan for one second, before use. It will remain air suspended long enough to cope with all noxious effluvia and render it entirely innocuous.
- *Nurse A*: What's the use of doing research about bedpans? They'll be obsolete in another 10 years.
  Nurse B: Obsolete? Not on your life. There'll always be patients tied to their beds. What about traction and plaster casts?
  Nurse A: Go on, any more to add to your interesting list?
- there is a great need for an efficient, pleasant smelling 'hospital disinfectant'
- it is quicker to give round bedpans than to lift patients on to commodes
- *Patient*: I've had a disturbed night. I was

up at the lavatory at 4 o'clock this morning and I've been twice since. I still have a griping pain as if I want to go again. Nurse came in last night with two Senakot tablets. I told her that I didn't need them, but she said it was routine and I would have to take them.

- you visit an elderly lady in hospital. You lift her used nightdress from the locker to take it home to wash. You notice brown stains on the nightdress. With a look of shame the old lady says, 'I'm sorry it is marked. I cannot attend to myself when I have used a bedpan. I always ask nurse if I'm clean and she assures me that I am. I hate this happening, but what can I do?'
- accountability
- responsibility
- the patient's right to privacy when passing urine and faeces.

Writing assignment

- how much urine does the average adult pass in 24 hours?
- name some conditions in which there is an increased urinary output
- name some conditions in which there is a decreased urinary output
- what are the dangers of retention of urine?
- state the weight of faeces to be passed daily
- describe how you would collect a specimen of urine for ward examination
- describe how you would collect a 24-hour specimen of urine
- name the vitamins manufactured by the intestinal flora
- give the causes of constipation
- give the means of overcoming constipation
- name the materials of which bedpans can be made. Give the advantages and disadvantages of each.
- define the following:

acetone
accountability
aerosol
amenorrhoea
analeptic
anal fissure
anti-emetic
anuria
anus
aperient
atomiser
barium enema
bidet
catheterisation
chronic
clinical thermometer
constipation
coryza
costive
cyanosis
cystitis
debilitation
defaecation
dehydration
diabetes insipidus
diabetes mellitus
diarrhoea
discomfort
douche
dyspnoea
effluvia
electrolyte
embolism
emesis
enemata
epidemiology
faeces
febrile
fistula
food poisoning
gastrocolic reflex
haemorrhoids
halitosis
hypothermia
imperforate anus
innocuous
irritable bowel syndrome
ketones
laryngitis
latent heat
laxative
leucorrhoea
linctus
macroscopic

meconium
melaena
microorganisms
microscopic
micturition
mucoid
mucolytic
mucopurulent
mucopus
mucus
nebuliser
oliguria
ostomy
pain
paraplegia
parenteral
perianal
peristalsis
pharyngitis
piles
pneumonia
polyuria
postural drainage
proctocolectomy
proctoscopy
protein
purgative
pyloric stenosis
rectal lavage
rectum
responsibility
retention of urine
retention with overflow
rhinitis
rhinorrhoea
seropurulent
serous
sigmoidoscopy
sinusitis
sphincter
sputum
stool
stoma
stress incontinence
suppository
suppression of urine
thrombosis
tetraplegia
total colonic lavage
toxins
turgor of skin
urine

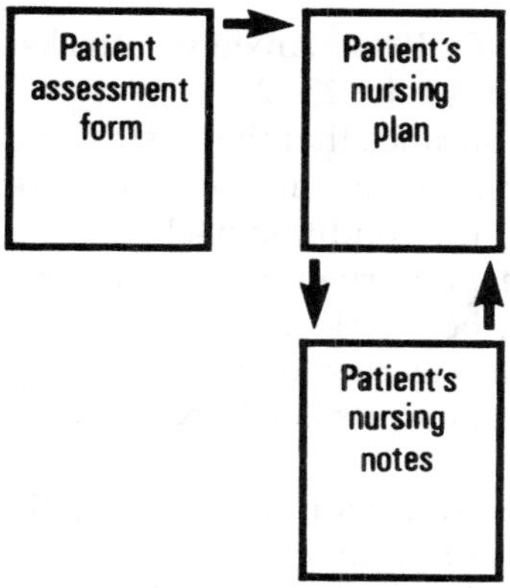

15

Helping patients to breathe

READING ASSIGNMENT

Agius L, Gregg I 1984 The role of the practice nurse in the management of asthma. Nursing: The Add-On Journal of Clinical Nursing 2 (28) August: 815–819
What is asthma and what causes it? Drug Therapy. Nurses' role in assessment, treatment and managing severe attacks.

Ashworth P 1979 Psychological and social aspects of respiratory care. Nursing 7 (November): 295–299
Illustration of a 'Nursing care plan'.

Bakshi Mrs 1984 Asthma — a personal account. Nursing: The Add-On Journal of Clinical Nursing 2 (28) August: 819–821

Boyd G 1984 Drugs and the respiratory system. Nursing: The Add-On Journal of Clinical Nursing 2 (27) July: 805–806
Describes the various bronchodilators and aerosol inhalers among other drugs.

Boylan A, Brown P 1985 Respiration. Nursing Times 81 (11) March 13: 35–38
Gives a detailed account of what to observe about respiration supported by biological rationale.

Brown S E 1979 Respiratory physiotherapy and the nurse. Nursing 6 (September): 257–259
Illustrated.

Campbell D 1984 An inspired tale of the old iron lung. Nursing Mirror 159 (15) October 24: 32–36
Describes the nursing care of a patient in

an iron lung.

Chilver W L C 1978 On being a patient in an intensive therapy unit. Nursing Mirror 146 (14) April 6: 33–35
Noisy ventilator; warm humid atmosphere.

Cochrane G M 1978 Saving a life after cardiac arrest. Nursing Mirror 147 (2) July 13: 17–20
Description of resuscitation.

Corrigan A 1984 Home ventilation. Nursing: The Add-On Journal of Clinical Nursing 2 (28) August: 840
Rarely patients who are unable to breathe without a ventilator can be at home if there is adequate family and health service support.

De Carle 1985 Tracheostomy care. Occasional Paper 81 6 Nursing Times 81 (40) October 2: 50–54
Gives an 'ideal' model of care pre-operatively, postoperatively and in the long-term.

Dickins B F 1979 David: a case for ventilation. Nursing 7 (November): 310–314
Explains intermittent positive pressure ventilation (IPPV) and a tracheostomy.

Douglas A 1978 A disease of hospitals: venous thrombosis and pulmonary embolism. Nursing Mirror 147 (17) October 26: 44–46
Nurses should be on their guard to identify patients most at risk.

Durie M 1984 Respiratory problems and nursing intervention. Nursing: The Add-On Journal of Clinical Nursing 2 (29) August: 826–828
Cough; sputum; dyspnoea, bronchospasm, haemoptysis.

Evans P M, Massey R M 1979 Helping the patient with respiration. Nursing Times 75 (25) June 28: 1106–1107
It is vital to inspire confidence in patients distressed with respiratory embarrassment.

Felstein I 1970 Snoring: the sufferer who doesn't suffer. Nursing Mirror 148 (15) April 12: 42–43

Glover A 1986 Hyperventilation. Nursing Times 82 (49) December 3: 54–55
Describes how nurses can assist patients to correct their faulty breathing.

Hek F A 1987 Living with asthma. The Professional Nurse 2 (6) March: 168–169
Research shows that sufferers are often given little information or education about their condition.

Hek G, Carswell F 1986 Anxiety attacks. Community Outlook July: 23– 24
Parents need reassurance that their asthmatic child is not going to die, and much more information about the condition itself.

Howe P 1979 The respiratory effects of surgery. Nursing 7 (November): 324–327

Jackson H 1979 Nursing care of patients with chest injuries. Nursing (Issue 7) November: 303–309
Illustration of a central venous pressure (CVP) line and under water drainage.

Johnson S 1984 Ventilators. Nursing: The Add-On Journal of Clinical Nursing 2 (28) August: 836, 838–839
Describes the principles on which modern ventilators work and illustrates four of them: Pneu-Pac; Oxford Mk1; Servo and Accutronic model Mk800.

Kirkman P A S 1979 The Heimlich manoeuvre. Ambulance Journal September: 238, 241
Technique to be used for choking because of food obstructing airway.

McMillan E Oxygen therapy. Nursing: The Add-On Journal of Clinical Nursing 2 (29) August: 822-825
Indications for; acid-base balance and blood gases; equipment; humidification; nursing responsibilities; long-term therapy.

Mortimer B, Froud A 1984 Respiratory infections. Nursing: The Add-On Journal of Clinical Nursing 2 (28) August: 831–835
General nursing care of a patient with respiratory infection; common cold; influenza, bronchitis; pneumonia; Legionnaire's disease; tuberculosis; principles of infection control; patients receiving immunosuppressant drugs.

Ng A 1984 Chronic bronchitis. Nursing: The Add-On Journal of Clinical Nursing 2 (28) August: 829–830
Clinical features; management; nursing care study — Mr T. a 66-year-old bachelor was admitted as an emergency patient to a medical ward on 30th March 1983. His condition was very poor. Since November 1982 he had been admitted to hospital five times with cor pulmonale and chronic bronchitis.

Nursing Mirror 1980 Allergy: when the body

takes a stand. Nursing Mirror Supplement 150 (10) March 6
Describes the immune response; mechanism of the allergic reaction; allergens; clinical allergies and symptoms.

Rifas E M 1980 How you and your patient can manage dyspnoea. Nursing 80 10(6) June: 34–41
Illustrations of how to help a dyspnoeic patient get his breath; assessment form for dyspnoea.

Roper N, Logan W, Tierney A 1983 Using a model for nursing. Churchill Livingstone Edinburgh p 11

Roper N, Logan W, Tierney A 1985 The elements of nursing, 2nd edn. Churchill Livingstone, Edinburgh

Siegler D 1977 Pneumonia. Nursing Mirror 146 (2) January 12: 27–28

Siegler D 1977 Chronic bronchitis and emphysema. Nursing Mirror 145 (25) December 22: 17–18
Defined on the basis of symptoms; largest cause of absence from work in this country and is therefore of major economic importance.

Stephens D S B, Boaler J 1977 The nurse's role in immediate postoperative care. Nursing Mirror 145 (13)September 29: 20–23
Results of a survey of nurses' knowledge.

Thompson M C 1984 Physiotherapy — essentials of chest care. Nursing: The Add-On Journal of Clinical Nursing 2 (27) July: 796, 798– 800
Describes initial and continuous patient assessment with regard to respiratory function: preoperative and postoperative chest physiotherapy.

Twohig R G 1984 Respiratory function tests. Nursing: The Add-On Journal of Clinical Nursing 2 (27) July: 807–810
Describes how the nurse plays a very important role in the care of patients undergoing respiratory function tests.

Weatherstone R M 1978 The pattern of pneumonia today. Nursing Mirror 146 (16) April 20: 22–24

Williams R F 1980 Infection of the respiratory tract and lungs in cystic fibrosis. Nursing Times 76 (12) March 20: 517–520

Hospitals and smoking

Beales A 1984 The lure of the weed. Nursing Mirror 149 (8) September 5: xii, xiv–xvi
Asks why one-third of Britain's population still smokes cigarettes even though their harmful effects on health have been undeniably proved.

Belcher M, Hajek P, Stapleton J 1986 Nursing Times 82 (32) August 6: 48–49, 51
Why do some people find it difficult to stop smoking? Some answers are provided and the methods used at one smokers' clinic are described.

Black P 1984 Who stops smoking in pregnancy? Nursing Times 80 (19) May: 59–61
Report of a small study which concluded that individual support was essential if the message was to have any impact.

Darbyshire P 1986 Hiding behind the smoke-screen. Nursing Times 82 (29) July 16: 48–50
The tobacco lobby has manipulated the feminist spirit of independence for its own monetary gain. Nurses, since nursing is a predominantly female profession, have enormous potential to lead a mass revolt against smoking.

Garvey J P 1984 An anti-smoking clinic. Nursing Times 80 (33) August 15: 38–39
The clinic was set up by an occupational health nurse and employees were informed, and the results given concerned a group of 10 people.

Gaze H 1986 Making it the last one. Nursing Times 82 (11) March 12: 16–17
Discusses the work carried out by Chelsea College 'Helping people to stop smoking — the nurse's role.'

Holmes P 1985 How health hit the headlines. Nursing Times 81 (15) April 10: 18–19
Discussing health education and the media, the question is asked, How successful was the National No Smoking Day?

Hutton I 1985 Kicking the habit. Nursing Mirror 160 (24) June 12: 29–30
A survey revealed that 44% of the Glasgow population smoke. The study discovered some interesting regional and socio-economic variations in smoking habits.

Loysen E, Silmen 1986 Dangerous smoke signals. Nursing Times 82 (3) January 15: 42–43
Contains a Table of the effects of smoking on health.

Mulcahy R 1985 Passive smoking. Irish Nursing Forum 3 (4) Winter: 18–19
Examines the effects of chronic exposure to cigarette smoke on the exposed non-smoking individual.

New Scientist 1984 Low tar cigarettes. New Scientist September 20: 7
May be more dangerous than medium tar brands.

Nursing Standard 1986 Stub out smoking trends. Nursing Standard 429 January 9: 2
Announces that the government is launching a major drive to counter teenage smoking. Gives numerical indices of the size of the problem.

Nursing Times 1985 Tutors use stress therapy to prevent smoking. Nursing Times 81 (12) March 20: 7
The best thing to do about smoking is prevent it, so there will be health education at the beginning of the programme.

Nursing Times 1986 Women still ignore smoke signals. Nursing Times 82 (44) October 29: 5
DHSS chief medical officer says that studies are under way to find the reasons for the increased number of young girls smoking, and why women are less susceptible to anti-smoking propaganda than men.

Sanders D 1985 Weeding out the weed. Nursing Mirror 161 (12) September 18: 20–22
Routine health checks, which include advice for those who want to give up smoking, are being offered by practice nurses. Clearly outlines that nurses need to find out the smoker's viewpoint.

Watson L 1984 Helping people to stop smoking. Nursing Times 80 (33) August 15: 34–37

BACKGROUND INFORMATION

All people admitted to hospital have at some time been able to manipulate their environment, whenever they wanted a breath of fresh air. Each person has blown his nose and cleared his throat at intervals to keep his air passages patent. Most people have had a cold and know how to deal with it. Some have a greater or lesser degree of 'catarrh' (sinusitis) evident from their 'catarrhal voice'. These people may be in the habit of inhaling steam (p. 290) during an attack. Some people have asthma. They may or may not know what starts an attack. Similarly some people have attacks of 'hay fever' (rhinitis) and again, they may or may not know what starts an attack. They may be in the habit of inhaling drugs from a nebuliser or atomiser. Some people may have come from a warmer clime and may not have had time to adapt to the colder air, or to build an immunity to the microorganisms in the ward atmosphere. The minority will be in the habit of doing some breathing exercises.

We attempt to interfere as little as possible with our patients' previous breathing habits by keeping the ward atmosphere as fresh as possible, free from unpleasant odour and at an acceptable temperature and humidity. We turn the top corners of blankets down and see that there are no heavy bedclothes over the chest.

Much attention has been given in recent years to the provision of a dust-free ward atmosphere, but still the dreaded 'hospital' Staphylococci, some of which have become resistant to the antibiotic methicillin, have ample opportunity to be wafted here and wafted there. Since 50 to 60% of normal people carry Staphylococci in the nose there is considerable pollution of the ward atmosphere from this source. Cubicle curtains are within the 180 cm respiratory range of the patient and frequently within closer range of the staff. Gentle drawing of curtains, as opposed to swishing, will cause less atmospheric pollution (and in addition produce a more bearable noise!). Curtains are best made of dust-repellent, bacteriostatic or bactericidal material to lessen pollution of the ward atmosphere. There is a great deal of research to be done to render the ward atmosphere as safe as possible.

Deep breathing

Even in wards with different clinical labels, there are patients whose nursing plans have an intervention 'remind to take six deep breaths

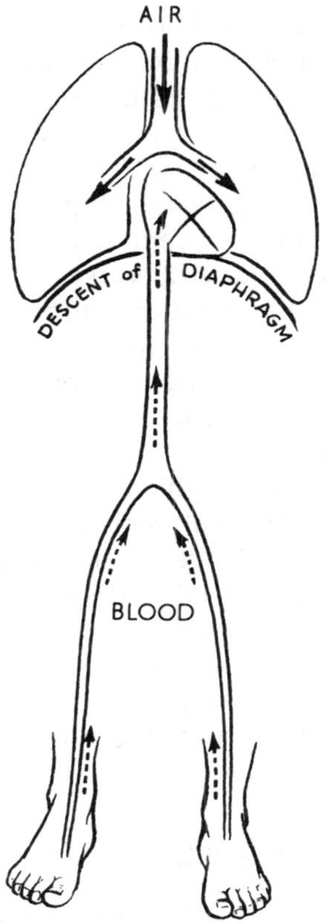
AIR
DESCENT of DIAPHRAGM
BLOOD

Fig. 15.1 The effect of deep breathing

hourly'. So a discussion of deep breathing follows, before considering it in a process context

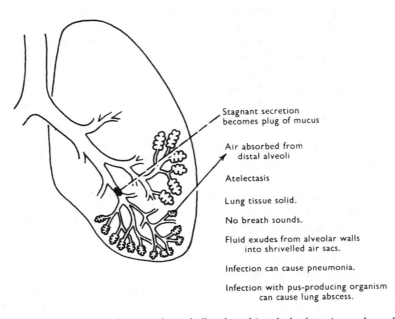

Most schools teach children deep breathing exercises but few people continue this excellent health habit. Most patients are now encouraged to take six deep breaths (Fig. 15.1) hourly. In this way they can increase tissue oxygen supply which facilitates the increased metabolism following injury and operation (p. 147); they can aerate their lung bases and prevent stagnation of secretion therein. Stagnant secretion can solidify and act as a plug in a bronchiole. There are no breath sounds in the lung tissue distal to the plug of mucus. The air already in this distal tissue is absorbed (atelectasis). Fluid exudes from alveolar walls into the shrivelled air sacs; infection can cause pneumonia; infection with pus-producing organisms can cause lung abscess (Fig. 15.2). The negative thoracic pressure that draws air into the lungs at the same time sucks blood up the inferior vena cava, thus preventing blood stagnation in the calf veins, with consequent danger of thrombosis and possible pulmonary embolism (Fig. 15.8). The physiotherapists often teach the exercises which will be written on the nursing plan but the nurse

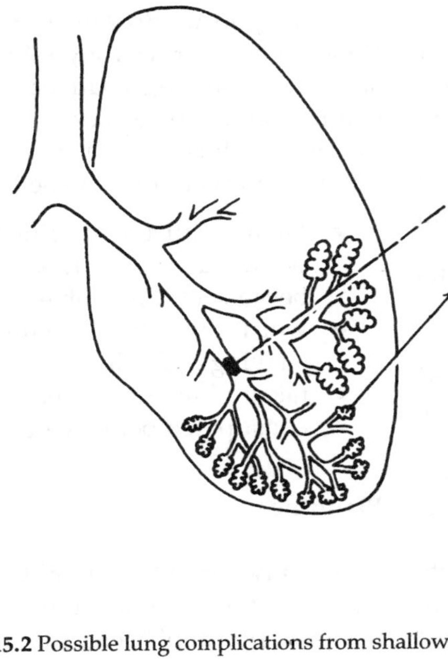
Stagnant secretion becomes plug of mucus
Air absorbed from distal alveoli
Atelectasis
Lung tissue solid.
No breath sounds.
Fluid exudes from alveolar walls into shrivelled air sacs.
Infection can cause pneumonia.
Infection with pus-producing organism can cause lung abscess.

Fig. 15.2 Possible lung complications from shallow breathing, lack of turning and coughing

needs to help the patients to carry them out throughout the day and record the fact in the patient's nursing notes. Evaluation of the efficacy of the exercises will be that the previously mentioned potential problems have not become actual ones.

BREATHING IN A PROCESS OF NURSING CONTEXT

One objective in using the process of nursing is to identify the nursing contribution to total health care. The essential nature of this everyday living activity is taken for granted until something goes wrong, and so many things can go wrong. When a person collapses and appears to have stopped breathing, first-aiders can carry out cardio-pulmonary resuscitation (p. 213) and many members of the public realise that this has to be effective within 4 minutes as there can be permanent brain damage when that organ is deprived of oxygen for any longer.

The respiratory tract is usually considered in two parts — upper and lower — because the shape and size of the component parts of each are so different. The upper respiratory tract comprises the nose, pharynx and larynx which can be rendered less effective by trauma, infection, and tumour which can be innocent for example nasal polyps, or cancerous. There may be minimal, medial, maximal effect on breathing. The 'emergency' which can arise in the upper respiratory tract is 'choking'. Kirkman (1979) describes a technique to be used because of food obstructing the airway.

The lower respiratory tract comprises the trachea, bronchi and lungs. The trachea can become infected (tracheitis), but rarely suffers other afflictions. The bronchi can be infected (bronchitis); any tumour formation is likely to be malignant (cancer). Some patients will have pneumonia and you will discover that many different microorganisms can inflame the lung. Figure 15.2 suggests other medical conditions which can affect breathing — and there are lots more, some of which are included in the Reading Assignment (Durie 1984, Mortimer & Froud 1984, Ng 1984). You may encounter a patient with broken ribs complicated by pneumothorax; and road traffic accidents can result in a stove-in-chest. Head injuries and some neurological conditions can paralyse the muscles of respiration, in which instance the highly skilled intervention of nursing a patient on a respirator (ventilator) will be required. Nurses have no control over the type of ward to which patients with these medical diagnoses will be admitted. Hence the rationale of describing a principle of nursing as 'helping patients to breathe'.

With such a wide spectrum of traumatic and pathological conditions which can disturb breathing it is obvious that registered nurses require adequate knowledge of the biological sciences to understand the rationale of the delegated nursing interventions which they will have to implement. But introducing this knowledge within a nursing context does help understanding of how nursing differs from doctoring.

Assessing a patient's breathing

The patient with a respiratory medical diagnosis may well be admitted as an emergency via the Accident and Emergency department. Rifas (1980) illustrates an assessment form for patients with dyspnoea. Boylan & Brown (1985) and Roper, Logan & Tierney (1983) also tackle the subject of assessing a patient's breathing. Here, a continuously breathless patient's possible problems which would be amenable to nurse-initated intervention, will be identified:

- talking difficult; gasping between each few words; agrees he has become withdrawn because of this problem
- worn out after washing and dressing; shaving difficult
- takes a long time to eat so loses appetite
- constipated because he cannot 'push'.

Planning

The first two problems might be alleviated by an entry on the patient's nursing plan 'nurse in upright position' (Fig. 15.3) to give more

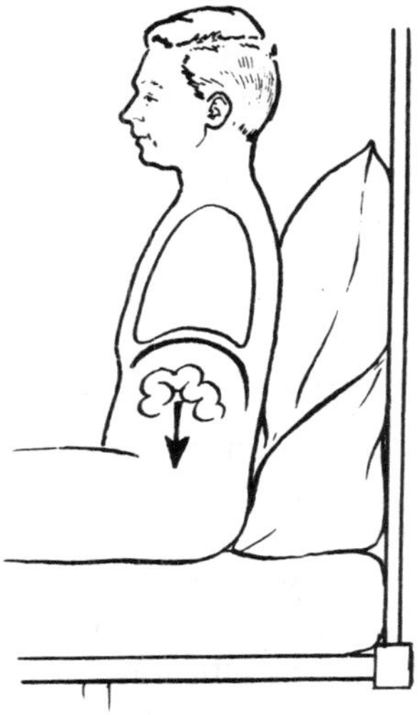

Fig. 15.3 Upright position – more diaphragmatic freedom

diaphragmatic freedom; 'spare muscular activity'; 'observe for cyanosis' (each body movement uses oxygen and produces carbon dioxide). The interventions are stated sufficiently broadly to facilitate the nurse's creative response, for example 'nurse in upright position' means that on a fine day the patient could be lifted into a wheelchair and wheeled to a window or even outside. 'Spare muscular activity' would permit the nurse to collect current ongoing assessment information, and decide with the patient, who would do what, in relation to washing, dressing and shaving on that particular morning or evening. An entry in the patient's nursing notes will permit the level of dependence/independence to be traced. Conversation with the patient should be so worded that it requires minimal contribution from him.

The last two problems will also have some nursing interventions in common. This is another example of there being no special order in which to collect assessment data. Here information about dietary habits would become appropriate. A continuously breathless patient is likely to be in the older age group and to have well established eating habits. The goal would be to achieve a sufficiently soft stool to be expelled with minimal muscular effort. However, the discomfort from constipation might provide the motivation to eat more fibre and drink more fluid. Discussion with the patient established that he wanted to continue to feed himself. The nurse-initiated interventions might read:

- will feed self with small portion (loses appetite)
- serve his meal first (he eats slowly)
- patient will provide and eat snack between meals (because of smaller meals)
- monitor that diet contains increased fibre and fluid intake
- monitor bowel movement and state of faeces.

Probably more than any other everyday living activity, helping a patient to breathe consists of a whole range of delegated nursing activities. There is likely to be medical prescription for blood investigations, respiratory function tests, X-rays, bronchoscopy, postural drainage, suctioning of the tract, giving oxygen, giving intermittent positive pressure breathing therapy and so on. There will be instruction on the patient's plan about the delegated nursing contribution to these procedures, and there will be a record in the nursing notes when it has been implemented. And of course there is likely to be a prescription for medication on the Kardex which is signed as each dose is given. The appropriate nursing intervention on the nursing plan is to observe for positive signs that the drug is having the desired effect, and the appearance of any known side-effects.

Implementing

Implementing, the accepted third phase of the process of nursing has already been mentioned and this is yet more evidence of the 'circularity' of the process and the ongoing nature of each of the phases. To practise process thinking, it was suggested that 'nurse in upright position' could be implemented as lifting the patient into a wheelchair. It is feasible that it could be implemented as making the patient comfortable in bed in the sitting position (Fig. 15.3). The availability of equipment could influence these implementations and registered nurses have a responsibility to inform management of equipment which would raise the standard of nursing in the ward. Implementing has already been mentioned in relation to the nurse-initiated intervention 'spare muscular activity' by deciding with the patient, who would do what, related to morning and evening toilet each day and adjusting conversation so that it requires minimal patient input. If it is possible for the patient to shower in the sitting position, this may be the preferred implementation of 'spare muscular activity'. Although the patient prefers to feed himself, this does not relieve the nurse of the responsibility to implement monitoring how much food the patient actually eats; to monitor that the patient does receive his meal first to accommodate his slow eating; that he is in fact taking a snack between the smaller meals; that his diet does contain increased fibre and fluid, and that he passes soft faeces without difficulty. The patient's nursing notes should reflect these implementations.

Evaluating

For the evaluating phase of the process of nursing one has to refer to the statement of the patient's problems which are amenable to nursing intervention (p. 204). The goals may have been stated as:

- less gasping when talking
- less withdrawn
- less tired after morning and evening toilet
- no cyanosis.

The evaluation will only be as good as the recorded descriptions on the patient's nursing notes. One of the essential skills required in nursing is to be as factual as possible when recording subjective information. For this continuously breathless older patient, as well as improvement from implementing the nursing interventions with the goal of 'resting' to reduce oxygen need, there is likely to be some improvement from the medications prescribed by the doctor and given by the nurse — or indeed the delegated nursing activity might be supervising while the patient takes his own medicine, and it could possibly include teaching the correct use of a nebuliser.

A continuously breathless patient's possible problems which would be amenable to nursing intervention have been used to illustrate the four phases of the process. However the illustration does not capture all the points about a breathless patient so before leaving this subject, further discussion follows.

The breathless patient

Breathlessness is evidence that a compensatory mechanism is at work to try to get more oxygen for the person's tissues. The breathlessness can be normal, due to exercise; it can be brought on by a less than normal amount of exercise because of anaemia. It can be continuous and distressing due to lung or heart disease. Every movement of the body uses up oxygen and produces carbon dioxide; breathless patients are therefore spared muscular activity. A patient who is continually breathless exhibits signs of oxygen-lack (hypoxia), more frequently, but less accurately referred to as anoxia. Cyanosis appears first under the finger nails, then in the lips, ear lobes and cheeks; the inner cheek mucous membrane is the most sensitive index in a dark-skinned person. The nurse may need to help a cyanosed patient with the administration of warm, moistened oxygen (p. 292). This may have to be continued after the patient goes home (Fig. 15.4). The staff instruct the patient and his relatives about this procedure; feedback from them will help the nurse to assess their understanding, and give opportunity for further explanation if there is misunderstanding.

When looked after at home a breathless patient is often nursed continuously in a chair. Special beds make the sitting position more comfortable for the patient and less hazardous for the staff in hospital. Failing a special bed, the nurse needs to be skilful at placing the patient in the upright position, using pads and pillows to give support and relieve pressure where required (Fig. 15.3). A bedtable with a pillow, on which the patient can rest his arms, may give relief.

The breathless patient's mouth gets very dry. Milky drinks need to be followed with a little clear fluid to prevent a 'dirty' mouth. Breathless patients appreciate a covered drink within reach

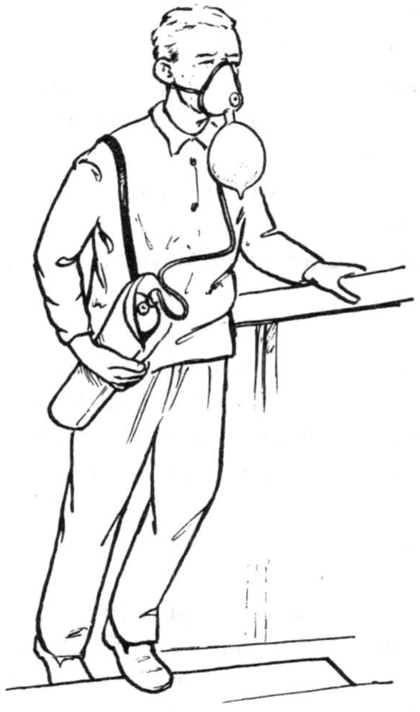

Fig. 15.4 Portable oxygen cylinder and face mask

so that they can have frequent sips. If they are on restricted fluids a covered, pleasant tasting mouthwash is acceptable. They need help to prevent cracked lips; a film of grease will prevent evaporation from same. Lip salve is the best; failing that white petroleum jelly can be offered.

The dyspnoeic patient experiences further embarrassment to his breathing if he lies down (Fig. 15.5). The abdominal organs slide against the under surface of the diaphragm and make movement of that powerful respiratory muscle more difficult.

If the breathless patient cannot be lifted out for bedmaking, then the nurse is faced with solving the problem of changing the bottom sheet and drawsheet with the patient remaining in the upright position. There are several methods of doing this, but in all, the basic principles of bedmaking need to be complied with (p. 171).

PEOPLE WITH POTENTIAL BREATHING PROBLEMS

It would seem that smokers should head the list

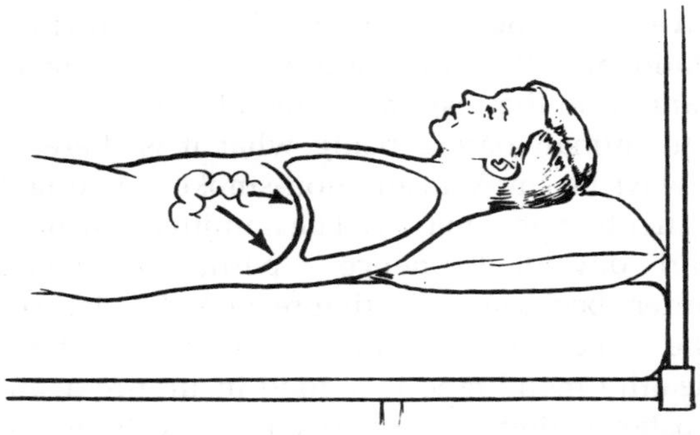

Fig. 15.5 Recumbent position – less diaphragmatic freedom

of people with potential breathing problems. Hiccoughs can be problematic if they last more than 10 minutes, even if only for the social embarrassment! Some people with asthma are free from breathing problems between attacks; others have a consistent problem with low grade chest infection. Inhalation of a general anaesthetic can sometimes cause irritation of the respiratory membrane, and absence of the cough reflex puts the patient at risk, as will be explained later. A person who is unconscious from any other cause will naturally be at risk. These potential problems will be discussed in this order.

Smokers

Whereas at one time, cancer of the lung was the dreaded disease from smoking, it is now customary to speak of the smoking related diseases. The Health Education Council published a leaflet in 1983 entitled 'The facts about smoking: what every nurse should know' and it lists the three main physical diseases as:

- coronary heart disease
- cancer of the lungs or bronchus
- chronic bronchitis and emphysema.

Roper, Logan & Tierney (1985) on pages 143–144 discuss composition of tobacco smoke and the effects of compounds based on information from the leaflet. On pages 146–147 they discuss the politicoeconomic factors related to tobacco. There is adequate discussion in the items in the Reading Assignment and it is obvious from them that nurses are expected to encourage patients to give up smoking and to offer help to do so. Rationally, the inhalation of hot tobacco smoke cannot do the respiratory membrane any good. But human nature being what it is there will always be smokers and non-smokers among the patients. Some may well be admitted during the early days of abstinence — perhaps on doctor's orders because of existing respiratory disease or the need to have an anaesthetic — when a healthy membrane is a good insurance against postanaesthetic respiratory complications. Is it right to put such patients into a ward where the other patients are allowed to smoke? Is it right to have a no-smoking rule in the ward? Is there a place for smoking and no-smoking day-rooms? Is this the right time and place to encourage patients to break with the habit?

There is one situation in which the patient has to be protected from smoking and denied its pleasure, that is during administration of oxygen, as oxygen supports combustion (p. 292).

People with hiccoughs

Hiccoughing is a respiratory interference caused by spasm of the diaphragm, so that it fails to synchronize with the intercostal muscles and results in an uncontrollable expiratory grunt. The patient needs to be in the upright position, be it standing, sitting in a chair, or in bed. Should the patient be in a hip spica raising the head of the bed may help. The everyday remedies aim at holding the breath in the hope that at the next breath the muscles will work in unison. Taking several sips of water without a breath in between sometimes works, as does blowing up a paper bag or balloon, or sniffing smelling salts or ammonia. Occasionally hiccoughs are persistent and distressing; one sometimes hears in the news of a person who has hiccoughed for days. Prolonged hiccoughing in a patient is considered a serious sign and occurs in the late stages of uraemia.

There may be a medical prescription for:

- inhalation of carbon dioxide and oxygen
- inhalation from a crushed amyl nitrite ampoule
- instillation of one drop of ammonia in each nostril, followed by a few minutes inhalation of oxygen
- application of ½% cocaine (local anaesthetic) to the nasal mucous membrane
- subcutaneous injection of 0.3 to 0.6 mg atropine
- intramuscular injection of 50 mg chlorpromazine.

These prescriptions would of course result in delegated nursing activities which would be written on the patient's plan; implementation would be recorded on his nursing notes.

People with asthma

Continuing to breathe adequately is difficult for the patient in an asthmatic attack. Asthma is a reaction to an allergen, for example dust from a feather pillow or a cat. The non-cartilaginous muscular tubes entering the alveoli go into spasm, so that the alveolar air cannot get out. Oxygen is absorbed from this static air, then the patient experiences oxygen-lack and carbon dioxide retention. He is naturally frightened and in a severe attack becomes livid. The alveolar walls continue to secrete mucus increasing the 'tightness' of the chest.

Unlike most forms of dyspnoea this is of expiratory origin. A man in an attack is reputed to have said, 'If I get rid of this breath, I'll never take another.'

An afflicted person may or may not know what acts as the allergen to set off an attack. At the initial assessment the nurse needs to enquire so that she can make the hospital environment as safe as possible for such a sensitive patient. The atmosphere in a single room will contain less allergens than that in a large open ward. Foam or Dunlopillo pillows and mattress may be needed. The nurse can tactfully tell relatives and visitors if any flower, perfume or pollen affects the patient adversely.

The patient may well be used to coping with an attack. Treatment usually consists of a bronchial dilator in an inhalant spray. Until the drug becomes effective the patient can be encouraged to do breathing exercises. He may find benefit

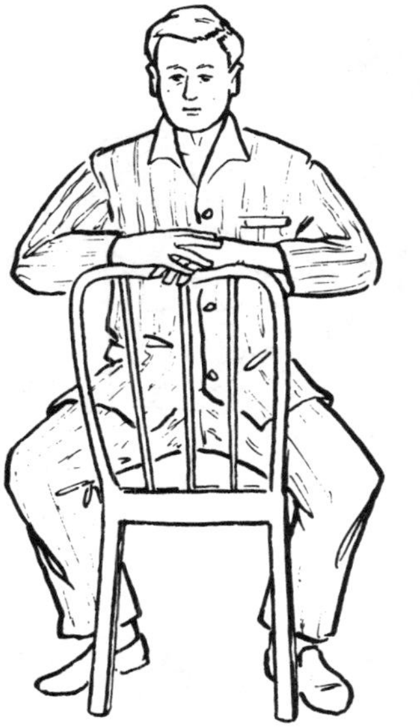

Fig. 15.6 Sitting position which helps in dyspnoea

from sitting backwards on a chair (Fig. 15.6), arms and hands supported on the back of the chair to steady the shoulder girdle and bring the accessory muscles of respiration into play. The mere presence of a nurse may help him to feel less frightened. When rested after the attack he needs encouragement to cough and get rid of the sputum.

People with a cough

There is a normal mucoid secretion from the moist membrane lining the respiratory tract. Since the nasal cilia normally waft towards the pharynx, it is more physiological to hawk nasal secretions into the back of the throat and then expectorate them. It is acceptable behaviour in less sophisticated cultures, but spitting on the ground is to be discouraged as it is a health hazard. Disposable tissues should be used. In sophisticated society secretion from the upper tract is blown into a handkerchief. Paper ones are most hygienic. Patients should be supplied with these and discouraged from keeping used linen handkerchiefs in the locker drawer together with sweets and chocolates. A paper bag should be supplied for disposal of paper hankies and other rubbish.

Secretion from the nose is increased (rhinorrhoea) during the common cold (coryza), when there is inflammation of the nasal mucous membrane (rhinitis), the pharynx (pharyngitis), and the nasal sinuses (sinusitis). Early symptoms must be reported to the doctor immediately if there is any question of the patient needing an anaesthetic. Such a patient, admitted for elective surgery, may well be advised to go home to bed and arrange admission when he has fully recovered. The common cold can easily occur in a long-stay patient and the common sense treatment that a nurse gives to herself should be offered.

The normal mucoid secretion from the lower respiratory tract is dealt with by 'clearing the throat'. This in fact means that it is coughed up into the throat and swallowed. People deal with anything more than this 'normal' amount by spitting it into a paper handkerchief and putting it into a disposable bag.

When there is inflammation of the lower tract membrane and/or lung tissue it causes coughing. The product coughed up is called sputum. Patients with such inflammation may well have difficulty in breathing and insufficient gas exchange in the lungs leading to cyanosis. They experience tiredness, apathy and weakness and they need help with the evacuation of tenacious sputum which affords some measure of relief. Expectorant medicines contain respiratory stimulants, analeptics and liquefying agents. For the patient to get the best benefit from them they are given half an hour after a meal. It is best if the patient can take them undiluted, but if this is not possible a little hot water is added. An hour later the patient is encouraged, preferably by a physiotherapist, to breathe deeply, to cough and to expectorate. Postural drainage may also be instituted. Direct liquefaction of sputum can be obtained by spraying the back of the throat with a mucolytic agent, delivered as an aerosol from the nebulizer or atomizer. Some patients can do this themselves; others need assistance. They should all understand that in an hour's time the mucus will be loosened and will need to be coughed up.

A debilitated patient requires help and encouragement with coughing. Provided the patient understands what is expected of him he can apply firm pressure on the anterior abdominal wall, gradually increasing it until the explosive action, then releasing it. Should there be a wound one hand must cover it. The patient may or may not be able to hold his sputum mug. Sometimes it is beneficial to encourage the patient to rest his forehead in the nurse's outstretched palm (Fig. 15.7A). Nurse can give further assistance by wiping the lips free of the last 'threads' of viscous sputum (Fig. 15.7B). Many patients are exhausted after a coughing bout; a posture conducive to rest should be adopted and a soothing drink may be acceptable.

'Coughs and sneezes spread diseases, trap them in your handkerchief,' should be observed by all. A patient with a tuberculous lung infection learns to lift the lid of his sputum carton to allow nurse to observe the contents. He replaces the lid, puts the used sputum carton on one side of a tray and removes a clean sputum carton from the other side. A person with pulmonary tuberculosis is taught not to breathe directly on any person.

Some patients will have a dry, irritating cough which serves no useful purpose because there is no sputum. A drink of water, sucking a sweet or lozenge, sucking honey from a spoon or inhaling steam or vapour, for example from such things as camphorated oil or Vick applied to the chest, are all worthy of trial. Should these fail the doctor will probably prescribe a linctus. These syrups have a direct soothing effect on the pharyngeal mucous membrane. They are taken undiluted, sipped slowly and are not followed by a drink of water.

The anaesthetised patient

There are parts of nursing knowledge, for example about the anaesthetised patient, which do not lend themselves to description in process format, yet it is knowledge which has to be borne in mind while nursing a patient in the pre- and postoperative phases, using the patient's nursing plan, nursing notes, medication Kardex and whichever 'charts' are appropriate — in other words the nursing documentation system which is used in the hospitals in which you work.

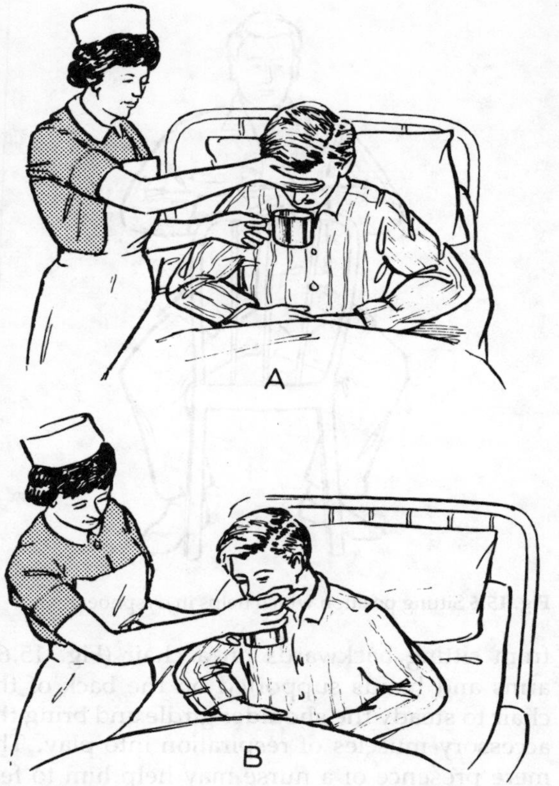

Fig. 15.7 Nurse offering assistance to patient who is coughing

The nurse accepts the responsibility for making arrangements for removal of dentures prior to anaesthesia as, if they become dislodged, they will cause respiratory obstruction.

The anaesthetist accepts the responsibility for the patient continuing to breathe adequately while he is in the operating theatre. The anaesthetist visits the patient in the ward and orders pre-anaesthetic drugs. The nurse accepts the responsibility of giving and recording these drugs accurately and at the appointed time. The practice of giving pre-anaesthetic drugs intramuscularly to achieve quicker and more complete absorption — as opposed to subcutaneously (hypodermically) — is spreading. In some hospitals all premedications are given intravenously in the anaesthetic room. These drugs directly affect the patient's safety while inhaling the anaesthetic. Atropine and hyoscine (scopolamine) inhibit secretion from the salivary glands and respiratory membrane. A dry membrane is less likely to become irritated or inflamed by the anaesthetic, and there is less likelihood of a plug of mucus causing obstruction. At the same time these drugs inhibit gastric and intestinal secretion and movement (peristalsis), thus reducing the possibility of postanaesthetic vomiting, with its attendant danger of inhalation or aspiration pneumonia. By inhibiting the slowing action of the vagus nerve on the heart, they help to prevent cardiac arrest. (Some physiologists say that the popular dose is too low to accomplish this.) Cardiac arrest is a possible early complication of a general anaesthetic. It can lead to venous stasis, with the possibility of thrombosis which can result in pulmonary embolism, thus interfering with breathing (Fig. 15.8).

Atropine reduces the laryngospasm associated with intravenous barbiturates; it inhibits the secretion of sweat, making the skin warm and flushed, so overheating should be avoided.

Most patients having an abdominal operation are given a muscle relaxant drug (curare derivative) intravenously, the action of which can last for 24 hours. It can be reversed by giving neostigmine intravenously, but neostigmine slows the heart beat (bradycardia) and this can lead to venous stasis, thrombosis and embolism (Fig. 15.8). To offset this, neostigmine can be given with atropine to inhibit the vagus nerve and so quicken the heart beat.

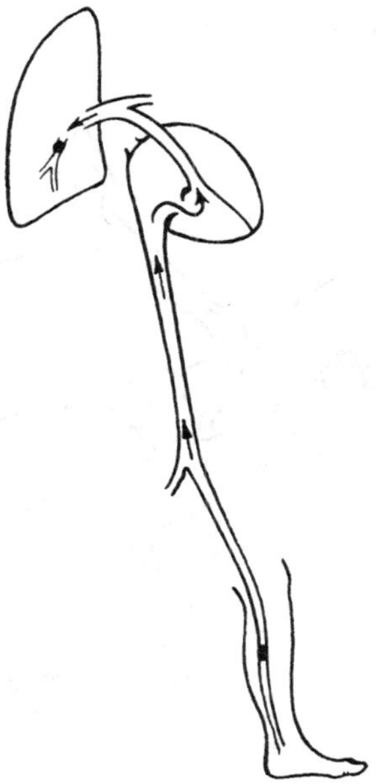

Fig. 15.8 The route of a pulmonary embolus

The safest position for the continuance of breathing in an anaesthetised patient is currently called the semi- or three-quarter prone position (Fig. 15.9) — sometimes with the feet raised. The terms 'lateral' or 'tonsil' position were once popular and are still used.

In this position the tongue is less likely to fall back against the posterior pharyngeal wall and occlude the passage of air from the nose and mouth. Lack of tone in the jaw muscles and tongue predispose to this happening (Fig. 15.10) but it can be prevented and treated by supporting the jaw as illustrated in Figure 15.11. It is less likely to happen if an airway is in situ (Fig. 15.12). As the cough reflex returns the patient attempts to spit the airway out. The nurse can remove it into a bowl of sodium bicarbonate solution 1 in 160 (later to be cleaned and returned to the operating theatre). The cough reflex may not be 100% effective at this stage, and there may still be danger from gullet regurgitation. Other methods of drawing the tongue forward are illustrated in Figures 15.13 and 15.14. They pull the epiglottis away from the glottis. A wedge to part the teeth, and a gag to hold the mouth open may be required.

In the three-quarter prone position, any regurgitated material from the gullet has a free descending pathway into the mouth, from where it is easily removed. It discourages 'pooling' at the back of the throat. Besides secretions being more difficult to remove from the back of the throat, they can be sucked down the larynx and trachea to cause 'inhalation' or 'aspiration' pneumonia.

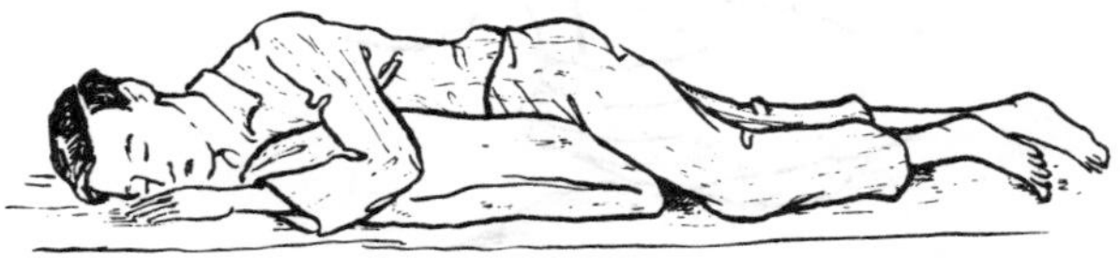

Fig. 15.9 Safest position for the anaesthetised patient

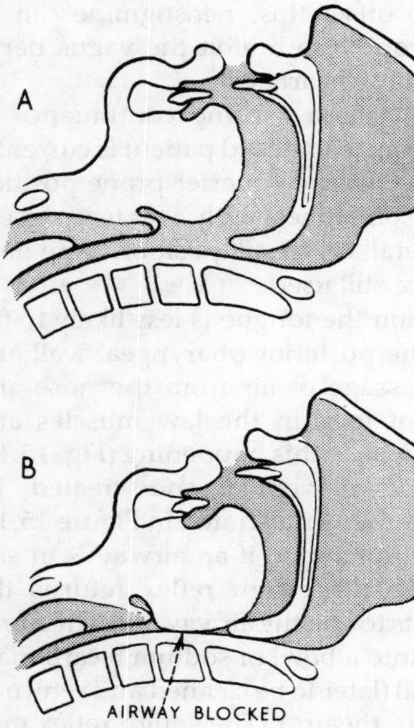

Fig. 15.10 Flaccid tongue and jaw muscles interfering with breathing

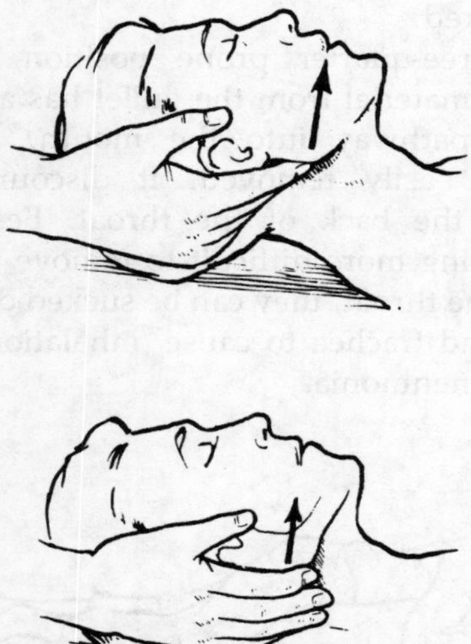

Fig. 15.11 Two methods of holding the jaw forward to prevent the tongue falling back

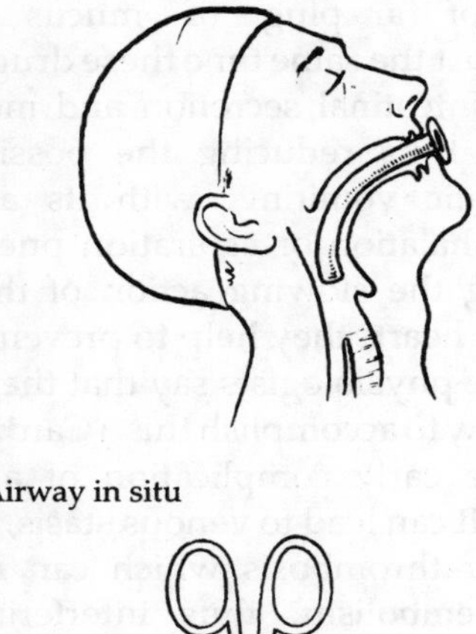

Fig. 15.12 Airway in situ

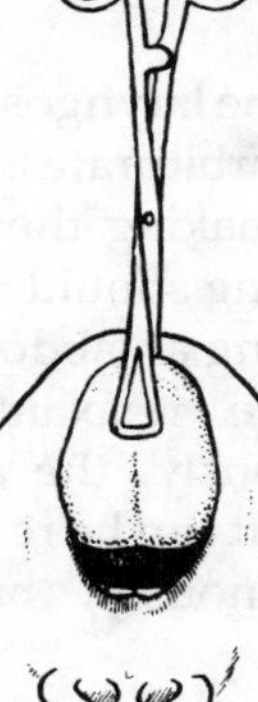

Fig. 15.13 Application of tongue forceps

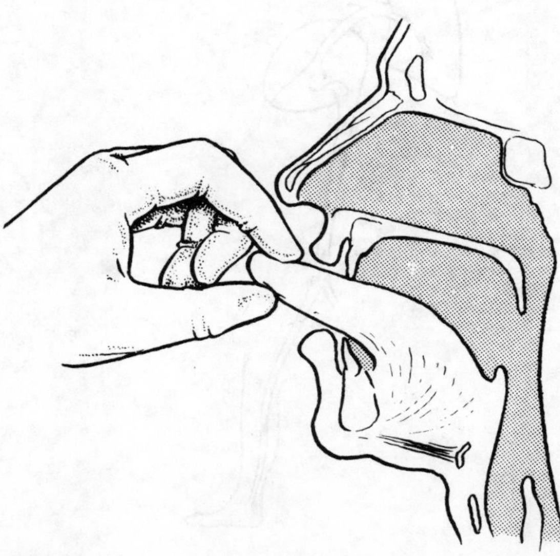

Fig. 15.14 Finger and thumb traction on tongue

The presence of an airway after anaesthetic can create a false sense of security. The nurse must make sure that there is adequate chest movement, as well as in- and out-flowing air. She can assess the latter by placing the back of her hand near the airway (or nose and mouth). Chest movement is assessed by placing an outstretched palm on each side of the rib cage.

A patient who has had a muscle relaxant may be drawing in some air with minimal chest expansion. There may be drawing in of the soft tissues around the neck and between the ribs in an attempt to get a better air intake (paradoxical breathing). These efforts may be accompanied by stertorous breathing (snoring). The heart may show signs of labouring with insufficient oxygen and changed pressures within its chambers; this can produce back-pressure, visible as distended neck veins. The pulse may well be bounding and more rapid in an early compensatory effort. The patient will have insufficient oxygen for the rest of his body needs, manifested by blueness of the finger nails, lips and ear lobes. He should be given warmed, moistened oxygen (p. 252) for at least the first hour.

If the respirations are very shallow or the patient stops breathing, he requires expired air resuscitation. Mouth to nose (Fig. 15.15) or mouth to mouth breathing can be started immediately as no apparatus is required.

Expired air resuscitation is easier (and more aesthetic) if performed with a Brook, Safar, Resuscitube or similar tube (Fig. 15.16). Some people find it difficult to achieve an effective airtight seal and at the same time support the jaw and compress the nostrils. In order to overcome these difficulties the mouth guard of the Brook airway has been replaced by that of the German oral mask 42010. The nose clip, which is attached by a chain to the mouth guard, effectively seals the nostrils, and the loops which are attached to the sides of the mouth guard, enable the thumbs of the resuscitator to achieve a perfect seal. In this way the fingers of each hand are left free to support the jaw effectively and maintain a clear airway (Fig. 15.17). Other apparatus achieving the same objective are the Ambu bag illustrated in Figure 15.18, the Oxford bellows (Fig. 15.19) and Waeco pulmonator (Fig. 15.20) and there are several others, Smith Clark, Barnett, Blease, Cape and Bird.

Suction apparatus can be used to remove excessive secretion from the respiratory tract, so that emergency inflationary methods have the best chance of being effective. There are many types of suction apparatus (Figs 15.21 and 15.22). Each member of staff must know where such apparatus is kept and how to use it.

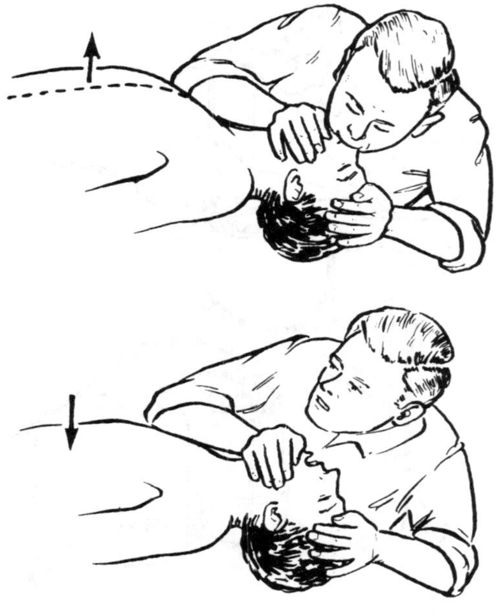

Fig. 15.15 Mouth to nose expired air resucitation

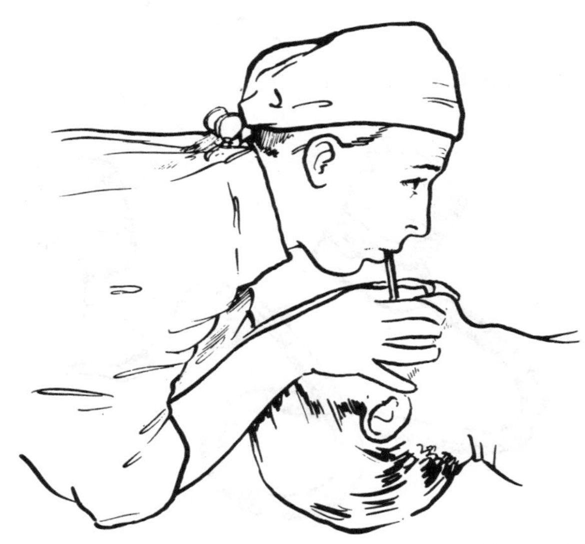

Fig. 15.16 Expired air resuscitation with Safar tube

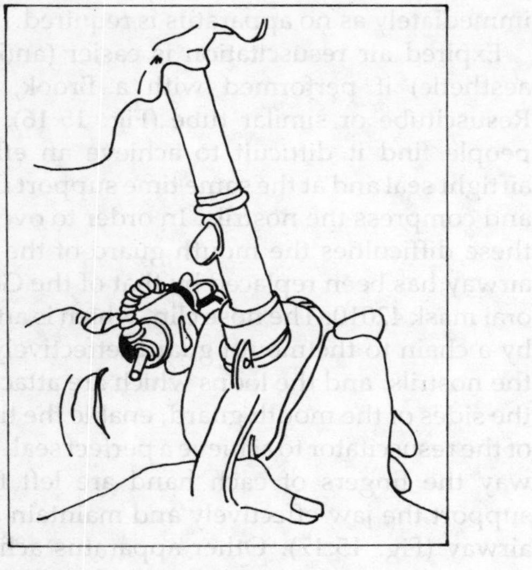

Fig. 15.17 Modified resuscitation tube

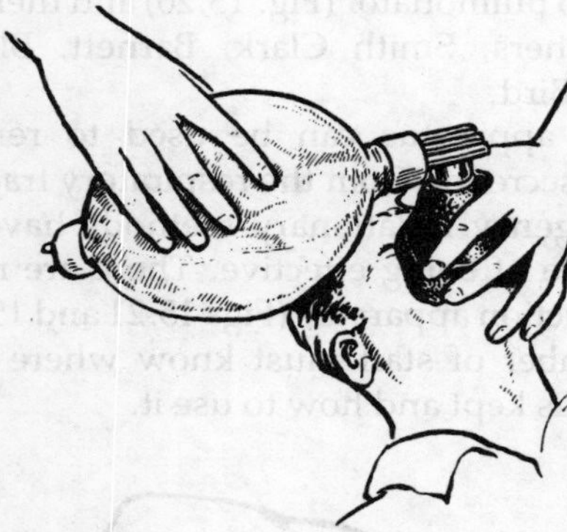

Fig. 15.18 Ambu bag in situ

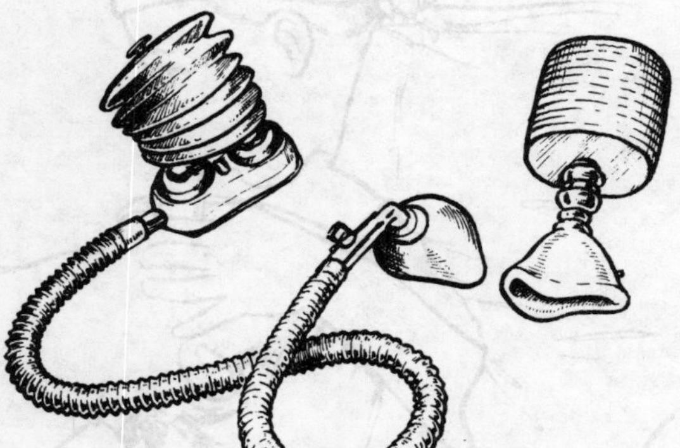

Fig. 15.19 Oxford inflating bellows

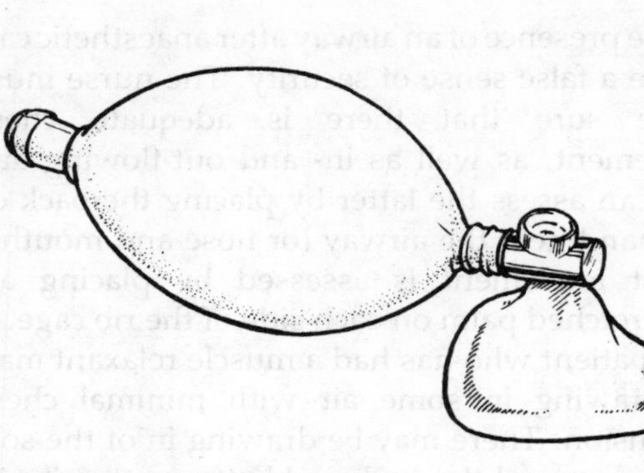

Fig. 15.20 Waeco pulmonator

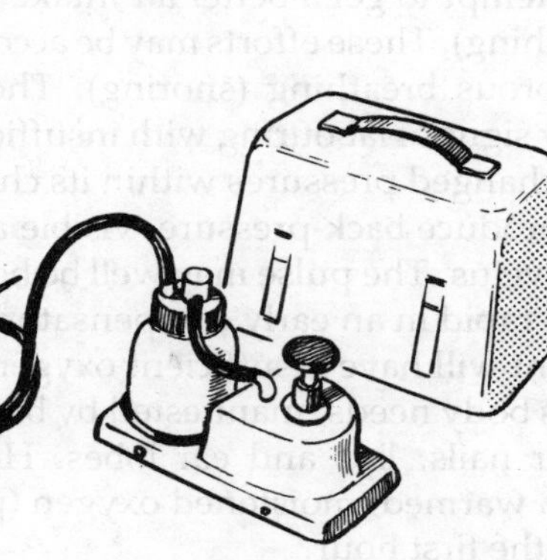

Fig. 15.21 Lightweight foot-operated suction pump

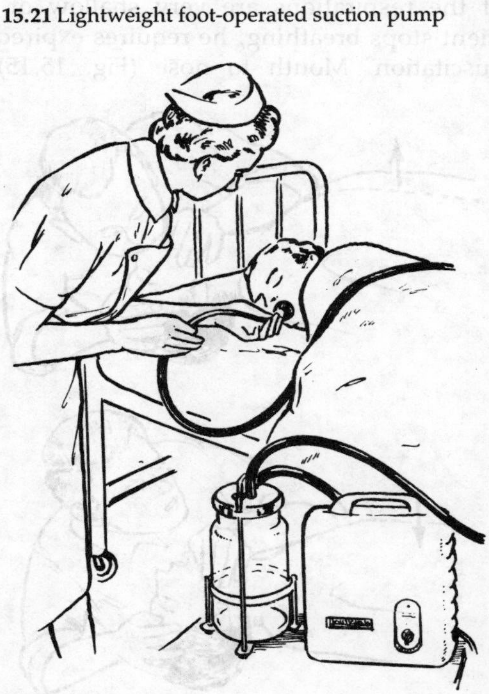

Fig. 15.22 Mechanical suction through an airway

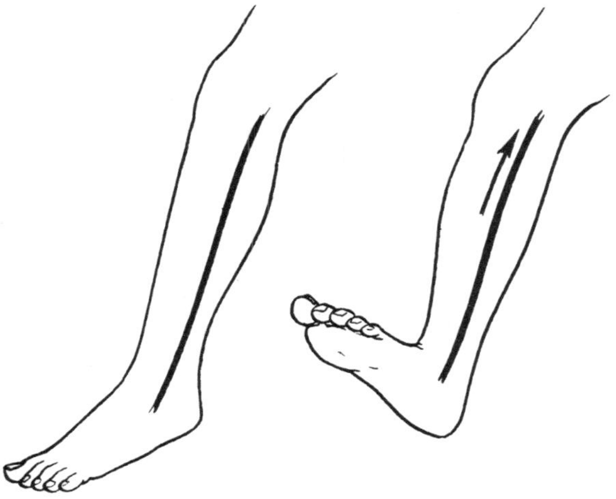

Fig. 15.23 Toe and foot movements 'milking' blood along veins

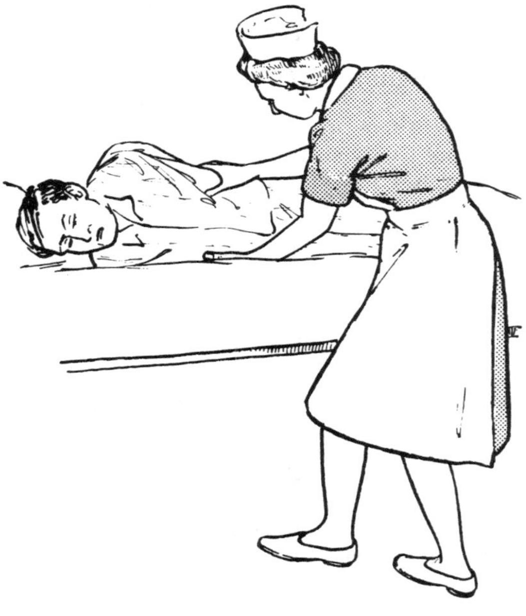

Fig. 15.24 A type of 'artificial respiration' to help the unconscious patient

With adequate respiratory movement, cough reflex, absence of vomiting and return of continuous consciousness, there is less hazard to the patient. He can be helped into the position in which he has to be nursed. He still needs to do deep breathing, coughing and foot movements hourly (Fig. 15.23).

The unconscious patient

All that has been said about helping the anaesthetised patient to continue to breathe safely applies to the unconscious patient. In such patients arrangements have to be made for more prolonged aids to breathing. In some instances tracheostomy is performed, a cuffed tracheostomy tube preventing inhalation of secretions and vomit. The cuff is deflated for 1 minute in each hour, or as prescribed by the doctor, to prevent necrosis, which on healing will shrink and can lead to tracheal narrowing (stenosis). Suction is applied through the tracheostomy tube to keep the bronchial tree free from secretions in which infection can arise. To help to prevent a plug of mucus causing atelectasis (Fig. 15.2), an Alevaire or other mucolytic spray can be administered via the tracheostomy. The patient needs to be turned from side to side hourly, or 2-hourly, and the uppermost chest wall percussed after each turning to help to move stagnant secretions. At each 'turning' the nurse can place her outstretched hands on the lower rib cage on either side. In time with the patient's breathing she can press sufficiently to deflate the lung bases — similar to artificial respiration (Fig. 15.24). The negative thoracic pressure thus produced will reinflate the lungs.

Intermittent positive pressure breathing apparatus (iron lung/artificial ventilator) has sometimes to be used for an unconscious patient, who may have an endotracheal tube inserted, or a tracheostomy performed. In this way the lungs are mechanically inflated with air at a predetermined pressure and rhythm.

In this chapter the merits of deep breathing were mentioned, before discussing the principle — helping patients to breathe — in a process of nursing context. The opportunity was taken to discuss several specific potential problems, as they are so important when considering the essential nature of breathing.

APPLYING THE PRINCIPLE

A registered nurse must be capable of:

- making the best use of ventilation and heating devices so that the air is of an acceptable freshness, temperature and humidity; free from pronounced odour and as dust-free as possible

- estimating respiratory rate, recognising abnormality in rate or type of breathing. Giving a factual report, oral and written, and teaching these skills
- teaching the value of deep breathing and coughing and giving assistance to some patients
- giving drugs and treatment that affect the respiratory system directly, for example expectorants, linctus, mucolytic aerosols, ephedrine sprays, oxygen and steam, with safety and maximum benefit to the patient
- knowing the drugs which depress the respiratory system and thereby put the patient in danger of stagnation of secretions at the lung bases; taking steps to prevent this
- positioning an unconscious patient to prevent respiratory obstruction and 'inhalation' pneumonia
- applying suction to the respiratory tract
- conducting postural drainage
- nursing a patient
  - (a) with a tracheostomy
  - (b) having positive pressure breathing
  - (c) in a respirator
- applying the principles of bedmaking and adapting them for each patient
- recognising the signs and symptoms of respiratory obstruction and failure; taking first-aid measures to deal with these, for example using the postoperative tray for care of an unconscious patient, giving artificial respiration
- organising emergency equipment in the ward so that it is easily available and readily usable. Instructing staff about these measures
- organising procedure in her ward for detection of early venous thrombosis and reporting it immediately to the doctor.
- applying the principle — helping patients to breathe — in a process of nursing context

WORKING ASSIGNMENT

Topics for discussion

- smoking
- turning off the ventilator when the required two doctors have diagnosed brain death
- it is more important in hospital than anywhere else 'to have a place for everything and everything in its place'. Failure to achieve this resulted in the following questions being asked in Parliament about the death of an asthma patient, aged 32:

> Is it true that at 10 pm as this patient was dying on his deathbed his parents witnessed a frantic search by members of the staff for the necessary apparatus to drain the mucus from his chest, and heard one state, *There is never anything ready in this place?'* When some apparatus was finally found, is it a fact that the electric plug was a different size from the socket over the patient's bed?

Writing assignment

- why does a dyspnoeic patient breathe more easily sitting up?
- at what temperature should the average ward be kept?
- what help can be offered to a hiccoughing patient?
- what are the possible consequences of shallow breathing, lack of turning and coughing in a bedfast patient?
- how would you help a breathless patient to keep his mouth clean?
- what help would you offer a patient at the beginning of an asthmatic attack?
- what does the vagus nerve do to the heart?
- name a drug which inhibits the vagus nerve
- name a drug which reverses the action of muscle-relaxant drugs
- state the nurse's responsibility for the anaesthetised patient's respiratory safety
- state the nurse's responsibility for the unconscious patient's respiratory safety
- state the potential problems of stagnant secretions in the lung bases.

define the following:

acidosis
adenoidectomy
air hunger
Alevaire
allergen
alveoli
anoxia
anticoagulant
apnoea
arteriosclerosis
asphyxia
aspiration pneumonia
atropine
bactericidal
bacteriostatic
barbiturates
bradycardia
bronchi
bronchial asthma
bronchiectasis
bronchitis
bronchography
bronchoscopy
bronchospasm
carcinoma
cardiac asthma
cerebral
Cheyne-Stokes breathing
cholecystectomy
chronic obstructive airways disease
coma
common cold
concussion
congestive heart failure
cor pulmonale
cough
craniotomy
curare
cyanosis
deep vein thrombosis
diaphragm
dyspnoea
embolism
ephedrine
expectorants
fibrinolysin
gastrectomy
haemoglobin
haemoptysis
haemorrhage
haemothorax
hiccough
humidity
hyoscine
hyperpnoea
hypodermic
hypoxia
immunosuppressant drugs
influenza
inhalation
pneumonia
intercostal
intracranial
intramuscular
intravenous
ketosis
laryngectomy
larynx
Legionnaire's disease
linctus
meningitis
methicillin
mucolytic
muscle relaxants
neostigmine
nephritis
opium
orthopnoea
oxygen therapy
paradoxical breathing
passive smoking
peristalsis
peritonitis
pharynx
pneumonia
pneumothorax
positive pressure breathing
postural drainage
pulmonary embolism
respirator
respiratory distress syndrome
scopolamine
sedative
sinusitis
sputum
staphylococcus
stertorous
stridor
stove-in chest
subcutaneous
thoracocentesis
thoracic
thoracotomy
thrombosis
tonsillectomy
trachea
tracheostomy
uraemia
venous stasis
venous thrombosis
ventilators

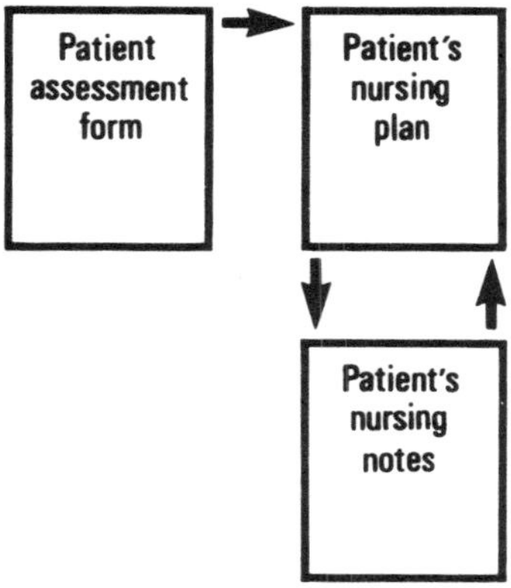

16

Helping patients to maintain body temperature within normal range

READING ASSIGNMENT

Aikens R M 1977 Hats and lamps in the prevention of neonatal hypothermia. Nursing Mirror 144 (16) April 21: 65–66
Report of a small study; illustrated.

Boyland A, Brown P 1985 Temperature. Nursing Times 81 (16) April 17: 36–40
Contains an illustration of core and body shell temperature and a detailed account of thermoregulation. No references.

Bramwell S 1977 Thermometer versus moodstone. Nursing Mirror 145 (11) September 15: 14–15
Laboratory investigation for simple method of detecting the 0.5°C increase in women's body temperature in the second half of the menstrual cycle.

Brislen W, Collins A M, Smart G I 1976 Assessment of single-use clinical thermometer. Nursing Times 72 (6) February 12: 235–237

Campbell K 1983 Taking temperatures. Nursing Times 79 (32) August 10: 63–65
One hundred measurements of body temperature using a clinical mercury thermometer, followed immediately by using a digital thermometer, are compared. One of the nurses' comments was that temperature taking would continue to be a 'task allocation' even if digital thermometers were provided!

Close J 1987 Oral temperature measurement. Nursing Times 83 (1) January 7: 36–39
Discusses the problems inherent in using the

oral cavity as the site of choice for measuring body temperature.

Davies S P, Kassab J Y, Thrush A J, Smith P H S 1986 A comparison of mercury and digital clinical thermometers. Journal of Advanced Nursing 11 (5) September: 535–543.
This report contains statistical methods which are more advanced than student nurses need to know. It is included here as the reference supporting a 3 minute placement time for a clinical mercury thermometer.

Drummond G 1979 Hypothermia. Nursing Times 75 (49) December 6: 2115–2116
Its causes, effects and treatment in the very young and the very old.

Feinmann J 1986 Some don't like it hot. Nursing Times 82 (29) July 16: 21, 24.
Describes heatstroke.

Gooch J 1986 Taking temperatures. The Professional Nurse 1 (10) July: 273–274

Goodall C 1986 Heat trials. Nursing Times 82 (8) February 19: 46–47
To facilitate learning about research, students of nursing carried out a temperature-taking project.

Hillman H 1987 The cold that kills. Nursing Times 83 (4) January 28: 19–20
Describes the stages of hypothermia and its treatment.

Hughes K I T, Patterson G et al 1985 Detection of fever with infrared thermometry: a feasibility study. Journal of Infectious Diseases 2: 301–306

Kearns A 1985 Keeping cool when taking temperatures. Nursing Mirror 160 (5) January 30: 12 (Letter to editor)

Moorat D S 1976 The cost of taking temperatures. Nursing Times 72 (20) May 20: 767–770

Nichols G A, Kucha D H 1972 Oral measurements. American Journal of Nursing 72 (6): 1091–1093

Nursing Times 1978 A digital sphygmomanometer. Nursing Times 74 (48) November 30: 1974
Illustrated; description of its use.

Quattrucci J 1977 The hygiene of stethoscopes. Nursing Times 73 (6) February 10: 193–195

Sims-Williams A J 1976 Temperature taking with glass thermometers: a review. Journal of Advanced Nursing 1 (6) November: 481–493

Skidmore E, Marshall A 1976 Towards a more accurate measurement of blood pressure. Nursing Times 72 (10) March 11: 376–378

Stevens J 1986 Catching the cold ones. Community Outlook November: 19, 21
Describes a multidisciplinary project which included doctors, nurses, social workers, housing officers, home helps, clergy, care assistants and voluntary agents.

The Professional Nurse 1986 Hypothermia: one of winter's threats to the elderly. The Professional Nurse 1 (5) February: 136–137
Describes three scenarios to illustrate some of the risk factors and appropriate nursing interventions.

Tam G 1979 A comparison of two electronic sphygmomanometers with the traditional mercury type. Nursing Times 75 (21) May 24: 880–885

Walker M 1986 When the going gets hot. Nursing Times 82 (32) August 6: 44–47
Gives an account of heat regulation in the human and describes exertion-induced heat illness.

The body's defence against infection

Stronge J L, Meers P D 1980 Combating infection. Nursing Times 76 (25) June 19: Hospitals … should do the sick no harm

Watson K 1979 Immunology
Part 1 The immune system: cells involved in immune response. Nursing Mirror 148 (9) March 1: 26–28
Part 2 All about antigens and antibodies. Nursing Mirror 148 (10) March 10: 35–37
Part 3 Reactions to antigens can produce clinical states of disease. Nursing Mirror 148 (11) March 15: 40–41
Part 4 Malfunction of immune response: major laboratory investigations for suspected immunodeficiency. Nursing Mirror 148 (12) March 22: 44–45
Part 5 Protection against infection. Nursing Mirror 148 (13) March 29: 40–42
Part 6 Autoimmunity and disease. Nursing Mirror 148 (14) April 5: 42–44
Part 7 Why many transplants fail. Nursing

Mirror 148 (15) April 12: 38–40
Part 8 Investigations in the laboratory. Nursing Mirror 148 (16) April 19: 30–32

An occasional item from the Reading Assignment of the third edition has been retained, even though a more recent one about the same subject has been added, on the grounds that the two articles take a different stance. Otherwise items have been deleted when an updated item discusses the same area of knowledge required by a registered nurse. The 'Medical microbiology' section has been deleted as it is now so highly specialised. The background information is broad and wide-ranging to encourage readers to remember that patients entering the health service, whether at a health clinic, an outpatients' department or a hospital ward, have a well-established experience of what for them is a comfortable body temperature.

BACKGROUND INFORMATION

Many factors enter into consideration of a 'comfortable' (normal) body temperature, taking this to mean that a person is not aware that any part of his body is hot or cold. For healthy adults the range of this lack of awareness is a body temperature between 36 to 37.5°C. From the crying which ensues, it would seem that even small babies are aware of being uncomfortable when they are too hot or too cold.

Among the population are the open air types who can usually withstand cold and there are the 'hot-house plant' types who can withstand heat. Some people quickly feel sickly when subjected to a warmer atmosphere than that to which they are accustomed. Some people quickly feel miserable when subjected to a colder atmosphere than that to which they are used. In their homes and in some places of work people are able to control factors, and achieve that temperature of the atmosphere in which they feel comfortable.

Some people wear a lot of clothing; others wear scanty attire, but all are in the habit of choosing clothing according to the atmospheric temperature.

After admission to hospital an ambulant patient in a single room can continue to cater for his own needs if shown how to manipulate the windows and the heating apparatus, provided the latter is controllable in each unit and both are in working order. The nurse has to adjust the heating and ventilating devices in accordance with the wishes of a bedfast patient. In the event of a patient who is unable to speak, the nurse must use some other means of communication before she can manipulate the environment, for example, after tracheostomy a patient requires pencil and paper to make his needs known; many people with a right hemiplegia are dysphasic and the nurse learns to interpret wishes from signs.

Patients in a two-, four-, six or eight-bedded ward/room, provided that communication is good between them, usually come to an amicable arrangement about heating and ventilation. If a patient complains of draught, the nurse may need to provide a screen between the bed and window, and offer or advise extra clothing for shoulder warmth.

The problem is much more complex in an open (Nightingale) ward. Some hospitals have a régime whereby the atmospheric temperature is charted twice daily in each ward and department. At the end of the week, the charts are sent to the chief engineer; from them he assesses the adequacy of heating and ventilating plant throughout the hospital. In a permissive atmosphere patients feel free to say they are too hot, too cold, or in a draught and the staff feel free to suggest a remedy. Dysphasic patients in an open ward need an observant nurse who can act as interpreter.

Female patients may find that their fashionable, flimsy nightdresses, dressing-gowns and mule slippers provide inadequate warmth when visiting the lavatory, bathroom, dayroom and other hospital departments. When they discover this, capable patients who are well visited will be able to get warmer garments. Sometimes it is necessary for the nurse to ask the visitors to bring warmer clothing. In some instances the nurse needs to offer warmer garments from hospital stock. Elderly patients feel the cold more readily and the nurse should remember that two thin layers of clothing, for example, vest and nightdress, are usually warmer because of the layer of air (which is a bad conductor of heat) entrapped between them, than one thick layer. Patients sitting up in bed or in a chair usually appreciate extra warmth on the shoulders. Many patients bring their own bed-jackets or capes and many hospitals provide shoulder capes. Capes provide the warmth where it is needed without increasing warmth in the axillae.

The amount of bedclothes needed to maintain a comfortable body temperature varies. Nurses need to avoid becoming rigid in their thinking and comfortable in encouraging patients to express their preference in this direction.

Thermometers and measuring body temperature

The conventional instrument for measuring body temperature is the clinical thermometer. British Standard Specification 691 demands a 'maximum error' and reputable British manufacturers guarantee that their thermometers are accurate to within 0.1°C (0.2°F) and they are engraved with BSI Kite mark. However, some hospitals use imported thermometers and they are unlikely to comply with British Standards. The General Conference on Weights and Measures in 1948 favoured the Celsius thermometric scale, which is in use in several continental countries; like the Centigrade scale, boiling point is 100°, freezing point 0°.

A Continental-type, enclosed scale clinical thermometer is now available in this country (Fig. 16.1). The outer glass case is oval which reduces the risk of dropping it. With the refined construction, shaking down the mercury after use is a simple matter of two flicks with the wrist. The firm 'Chester-care' has produced a precision mercury thermometer which will be a boon to those with poor sight: the blue mercury becomes even easier to see when the thermometer is

Fig. 16.1 Continental-type thermometer

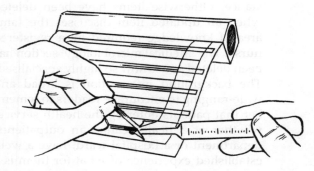

Fig. 16.2 Steri-temp thermometer sheath of disposable plastic

replaced in its case which has a built-in magnifying lens.

A thermometer for each patient is a fairly recent innovation; an error in a thermometer may give an inaccurate reading, but if used for only one patient it will measure change in that patient. Another objective achieved by individual thermometers is that temperature taking is no longer a possible cause of cross infection. When the fashion first swept through the wards a stout test-tube was attached to the head of each bed with a spring clip. Some hospitals put a little shelf above each bed for the thermometer in its container; some attached the container to the wall at each bedside. Now that so many patients are ambulant this can create problems so some hospitals have devised a portable test-tube rack for the thermometers.

The Steri-temp thermometer sheath made of disposable plastic may also help when ambulant patients who are sitting away from their bed need to have their temperatures taken. Figure 16.2 shows the thermometer being inserted into one sheath on a roll of sheaths. It not only protects the thermometer from actual contact with oral or rectal contents, but because of a

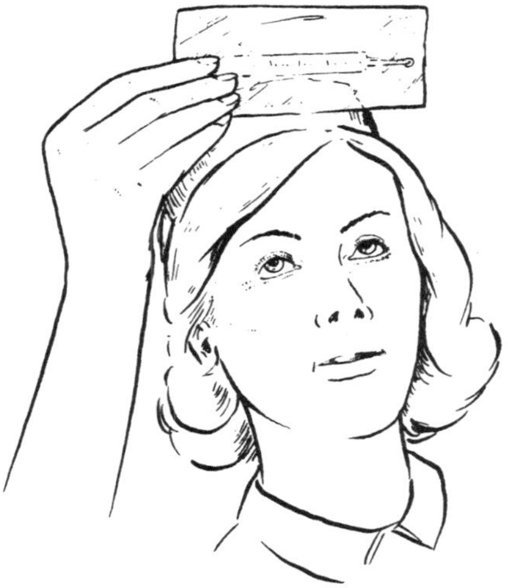

Fig. 16.3 Nurse reading thermometer through a transparent bag.

device which turns the sheath inside out on removal, these contents are enclosed in the removed sheath and the level of mercury is read with maximum safety and hygiene. It seems an ideal method for general practitioners and district nurses.

In Canada, the Ottawa Civic Hospital has a thermometer service in its central sterile supply department. Used thermometers are cleaned with an alcohol and soap solution, rinsed in cool water, dried, placed in selfseal envelopes and gas-sterilized.

Denmark found that 6.5% of rectal and 8.3% of oral thermometers were contaminated with *Staphylococcus aureus* so the used thermometers are immersed in a 1 in 1000 solution of benzalkonium chloride for 2 hours. They are then washed and dried and put in a plastic bag. The thermometer is removed by the patient, who takes his temperature, replaces the thermometer in the bag, through which nurse reads it (Fig. 16.3), then sends it to be disinfected.

Remembering that the mercury bulb of a thermometer needs to be in contact with the tissue of which it is recording the temperature, it is one of those accepted misnomers to speak of a 'rectal' temperature. Strictly speaking it is the temperature of the anal tissues which is measured (Fig. 16.4).

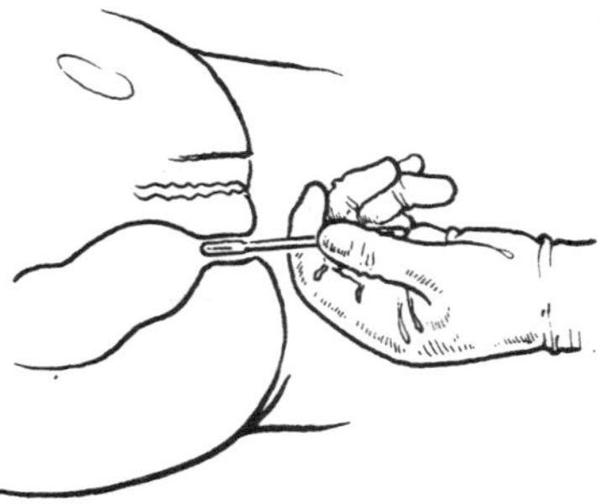

Fig. 16.4 Thermometer in situ in anal canal.

Sims-Williams (1976) reviews the research literature on temperature taking with glass and mercury thermometers and this should be considered essential reading for members of the Nursing Procedure Committee. She quotes the work of Nichols & Kucha (1972) in which six oral recordings were taken of 480 subjects; only in 13% of the subjects was the maximum recording reached after 3 minutes. These researchers recommended the following thermometer placement times:

8 minutes for men in room temperatures of 65–75°F;
9 minutes for women in room temperatures of 65–75°F;
7 minutes for all adults in room temperatures of 76–86°F;
7 minutes for febrile children in room temperatures of 70–82°F;
10 minutes for afebrile children in room temperatures of 70– 82°F.

These are exacting placement times and conditions both for the nurse and the patient. In the early 1980s, as nursing practice was beginning to pay attention to these research results from 1972, many Nursing Procedures Committees took a rational decision of 3 minutes and currently this is the most commonly used placement time. This decision has now been upheld; in a sophisticated piece of research reported in 1986, Davies et al found that when making clinical measurements with mercury thermometers there is no clinical advantage in using a measurement time longer than 3

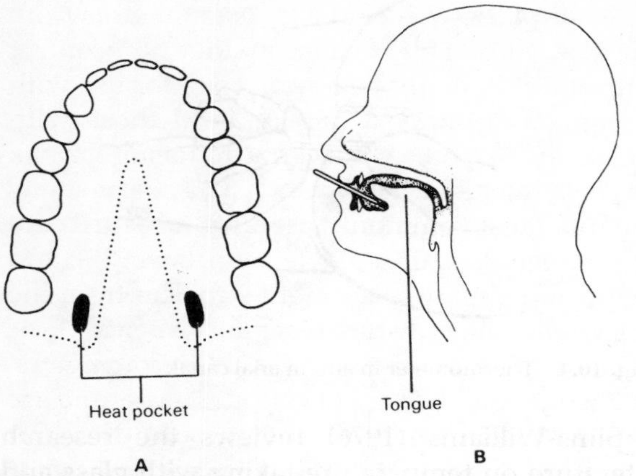

Fig. 16.5 Sublingual heat pockets.

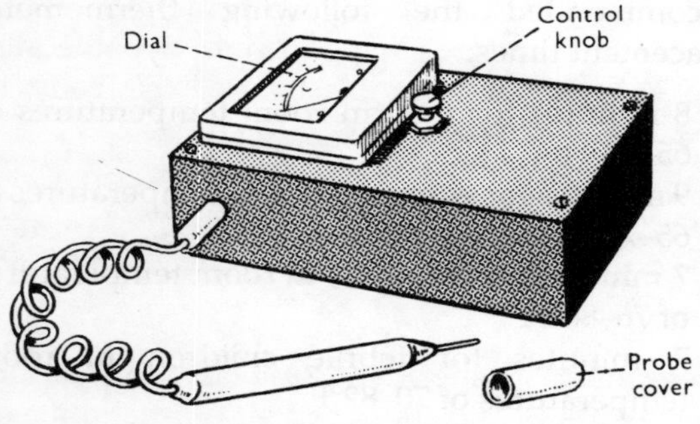

Fig. 16.6 Dependatherm electronic thermometer.

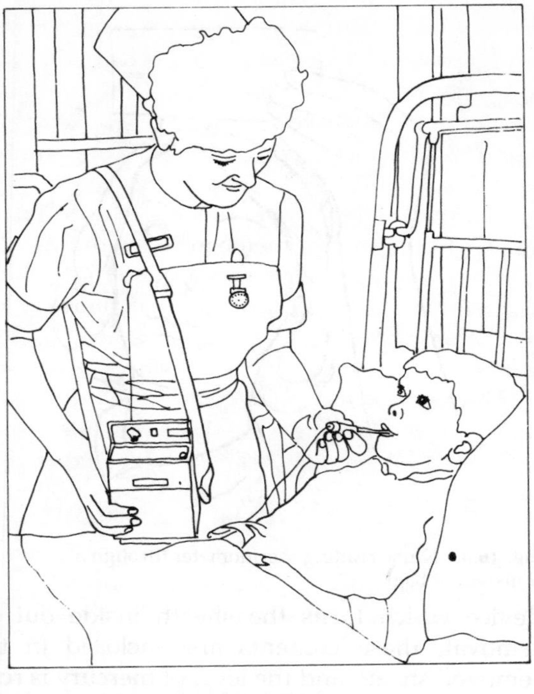

Fig. 16.7 Ivac electronic thermometer

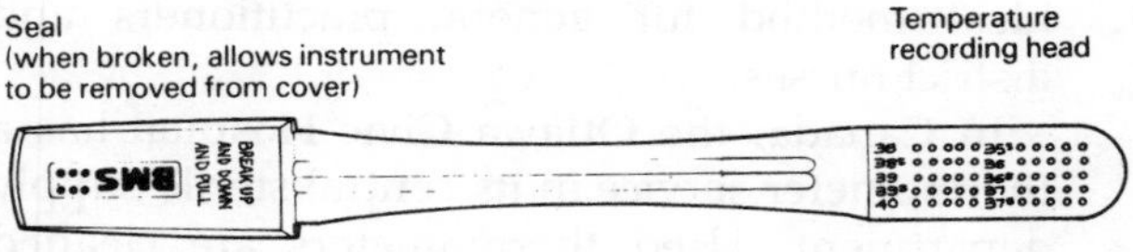

Fig. 16.8 The 'Temtake' single-use thermometer

minutes. Another point which was established was that the right or left sublingual heat pocket must be used for placement of the thermometer (Fig. 16.5). This is an example for students to realise that when they become registered nurses they still need to read nursing journals to update their knowledge according to the most recent research reports.

The dependatherm electronic thermometer uses a probe (Fig. 16.6) in the same way as a clinical thermometer. After depression of the control knob the temperature registers in 3 seconds. The dial is marked in both Fahrenheit and Centigrade. Manual recording is necessary even with the dependatherm electronic thermometer.

The Ivac electronic thermometer (Fig. 16.7) is a probe which, covered by a plastic sheath, rests along and under a patient's tongue to reach the right or left sublingual heat pocket (Fig. 16.5). It takes only seconds to register the temperature in large numbers which remain until the instrument is switched off. It is powered by a rechargeable battery. The carrying strap leaves nurse's hands free.

As might be expected there have been several studies comparing mercury and digital clinical thermometers. The previously mentioned study by Davies et al (1986) had that as its main objective, and they found that in both laboratory and clinical studies there was no significant difference in the accuracy of the two types of thermometer. Campbell (1983) carried out a project in which there were 100 participants. The temperature was taken using a mercury thermometer, followed immediately by using an electronic thermometer. Of the 100 comparative readings, only 18% registered the same temperature. Higher readings were recorded on the electronic thermometer in 58%, and 24% of readings were lower. She concluded that 'taking temperatures by the conventional mercury-in-glass thermometer does not accurately reflect body temperature'.

The main constraint on both these measuring tools (glass and mercury thermometer, electronic probe) is their rigidity. This fact was taken up by industry in 1970 (USA), which developed a plastic 'Temtake' thermometer (Fig. 16.8). It uses colour changes along a scale of calibrated holes to tell the temperature. It is sometimes referred to as 'the chemical dot' thermometer; it still needs to be placed in the right or left sublingual heat pocket. Brislen et al (1976) undertook an evaluation and found it to be convenient. It measured the oral temperature accurately in 60 seconds and being disposable, its single-use eliminated any risk of cross infection. Moorat (1976) carried out a comparative study, costing the nurses' time in using the glass and mercury thermometers and Temtakes, and the cost of both tools used in the study and found that using Temtake was more economical.

The Temtake seemed to fall into oblivion in the late 1970s/early 1980s, but a new version called TempaDot is currently being marketed in the UK. It certainly overcomes the rigidity problem; it is accurate to 1/10th degree (according to the firm's research); it takes only 6 seconds to record; being disposable it cannot contribute to nosocomial infection, but its efficacy depends on correct placement in the right or left sublingual heat pocket. The fact that some people wear dentures, whether upper only, lower only, or both, does not seem to have been investigated, yet it seems reasonable to presume that the presence of nearby plastic as opposed to nearby human tissue may have some effect on measurement of oral temperature.

Industrial technologists are trying to overcome the problem of efficient placement by using infrared thermometry (Hughes et al 1985). The detector probe was held 6 to 8 centimetres from the site. Close (1987) suggests that non-contact with the skin might be appropriate for use with sleeping or confused patients and those with facial injury or burns, as well as reducing the risk of cross-infection. However, the axillary site is the one most commonly used for measurement of shell temperature, (Boyle & Brown 1985), and one wonders how placement 7 to 8cm from the site would fail to disturb sleeping patients.

There are a few liquid crystal 'thermometers' on the market; they are of various shapes and are applied to the forehead; the amount of colour change is calibrated on a numerical scale corresponding with other clinical thermometers. It is thought that they will be especially useful for babies, children and the elderly.

After this brief consideration of thermometry in relation to measuring body temperature and before discussing 'Maintaining body temperature in process context' it is pertinent to pay attention to patients with changed body temperature — fever, pyrexia, hyperpyrexia, hyperthermia, hypothermia, and the inflammatory reaction of the body to infection, in that order.

Patients with abnormal change in body temperature

Everyone has some change in body temperature each 24 hours and the accepted normal range is 36 to 37.5°C. Above or below this range is abnormal. In the case of a slight abnormality most people are capable of acting to return to a comfortable body temperature. When feeling hot, people act in a commonsense way by, for example, removing an article of clothing, taking a cool drink, opening a window, moving into the shade, fanning the face, showering with cool water as appropriate in the circumstances. Readers can probably add to this list of suggestions and can apply the line of thinking to people who feel cold. Although the person may be comforted by these commonsense activities, the abnormality may be such that it requires help from the nurse to implement planned nurse-initiated interventions and delegated interventions from medical prescription.

Fever

Fever is mentioned here because many lay people use the word, particularly when parents say that a child is feverish. When prompted to describe the child, a parent might use all or some of the following words — hot, sweaty, crying, irritable, restless. Most medical dictionaries give fever and pyrexia as synonyms with febrile and pyrexial as their adjectives.

The word 'fever' is also of interest to nurses because it is used in several medical diagnoses, typhoid and paratyphoid fever, scarlet and yellow fever are examples. In all of them an increased body temperature is part of the syndrome and the patient's nursing plan will contain nurse-initiated and medically delegated interventions to reduce it.

What follows is merely an illustration of encouraging readers to diversify their knowledge: much more will be learned about these fevers in a 3-year nursing programme. It is included as practice in the complexity of 'process thinking'.

It is appropriate to point out that the first two fevers are spread by the faecal-oral route; the nursing plan would therefore contain instruction about nurses' and patients' diligent handwashing after elimination from the bowel and before eating food; and the method (usually prescribed by the Control of Infection Committee) for disinfection of faeces. Scarlet fever still occurs in some countries and the nursing plan will contain a prescription for bedrest until the medically delegated nursing intervention of giving penicillin takes effect and the danger of rheumatic fever and glomerulonephritis has passed. Yellow fever is endemic in the tropical regions of South America and Africa. As there is no specific therapy, a patient's recovery is dependent mainly on 'good nursing' — as was the case with pneumonia before the advent of chemotherapy and antibiotics and currently with AIDS.

Initial assessment will necessarily be detailed because the patient is likely to be experiencing problems with several everyday living activities other than helping to control body temperature. And similarly the patient's plan will need to be detailed if the nursing interventions are to be the main contribution to achieving the overall goal of regaining health. The patient is likely to be very ill for as long as 10 to 14 days, so several weeks convalescence will be desirable. This will entail setting short-, medium- and long-term goals. Nurses travelling to endemic areas can take preventive action by being immunised.

Pyrexia

Even though fever and pyrexia are synonyms, considering them separately can be useful and there is an accepted medical diagnosis 'pyrexia of unknown origin'. The main tool which provides objective information at the initial and subsequent occasions of ongoing assessment is one of the clinical thermometers. At the same time, the pulse is counted; it rises four points to each degree rise in temperature: and counting the respirations which increase with the emotional response to the physiological changes.

Subjective information can be collected from the patient at initial and ongoing assessment. Many people have been chilled and had a febrile reaction so that they recognise the feeling. While the core temperature is rising, the patient may 'feel' cold. To offset this there will be a physiological response of goose-flesh and shivering, both of which most patients can recognise and describe and the nurse can observe. The cessation of shivering and absence of goose-flesh can be observed by the nurse. The patient begins to feel warmer and as the core temperature rises he feels hot. The nurse can confirm this by using touch, and it can be verified by using a clinical thermometer. It is likely that at this stage sweat will be visible on the skin.

Information gained at the initial assessment is recorded on the patient assessment form (patient profile or nursing history), and that from ongoing assessment on the patient's TPR chart and nursing notes. Information from all these sources will be analysed, with the patient whenever he is able to co-operate, in order to identify any problems as the patient is experiencing them. Identification will influence the goals set, and the selection of nurse-initiated interventions to achieve them and these will be written on the patient's nursing plan. That which is considered problematic by one patient may not be so for another patient, hence individualised planning. The rationale behind selected nurse-initiated interventions is that visible sweat needs to evaporate to cool the underlying tissues. Movement of air over the body will hasten evaporation and the nurse might prescribe 'electric fan near patient: lower room temperature to 25°C'. The last will depend on whether this is possible, which serves to show that individualised planning has to take account of the resources available. Implementing the planned nurse-initiated interventions will be recorded on the patient's TPR chart and nursing notes. Evaluating will be immediate on the TPR chart, and summative evidence of achieving goals will be written on the nursing notes. When goals have been achieved, or partially achieved, instruction on the nursing plan may need to be changed so that nurses on succeeding shifts will know exactly what nursing interventions they are required to implement, and can record them on the appropriate document.

Hyperpyrexia

The prefix 'hyper' means that this condition is greater than the suffix 'pyrexia'. There may be a medically delegated nursing intervention with the goal of increasing evaporation.

When implementing this, the nurses' goal is to maintain the patient's dignity while removing night clothes, applying a loin cloth and inserting two bedcradles underneath a sheet which is arranged around the patient's neck as a modesty drape (Fig. 16.9). The bottom is left open and a fan placed nearby. The convection currents evaporate sweat as it appears on the skin. Discomfort from soaking wet clothing and bedclothes is avoided, and the patient is spared the muscular activity associated with changing these frequently. Another 'planned', but currently medically delegated, nursing intervention might be 'suspend three icebags from

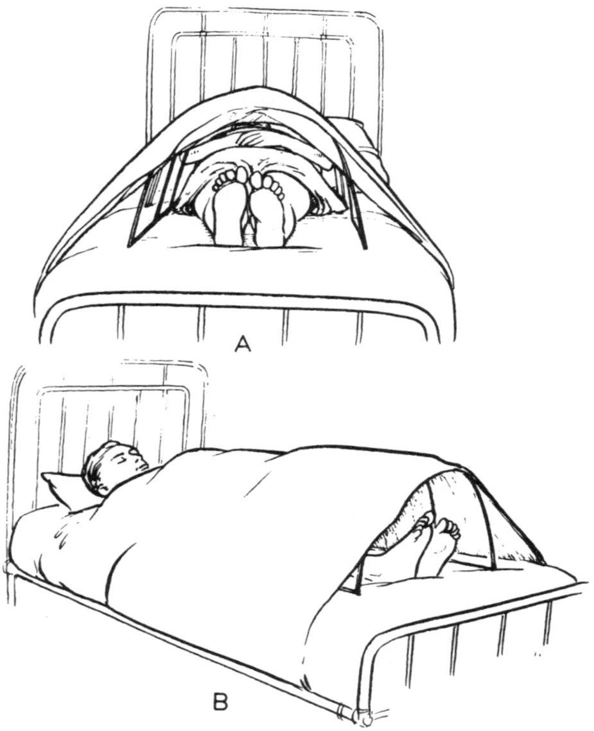

Fig. 16.9 Increasing evaporation, radiation and convection

the cradles' the rationale being to lower the temperature of circulating air without increasing its humidity. Cooling to the point of the patient feeling chilled has to be judiciously avoided. And, of course, there is likely to be a medication prescription in the Kardex and at each 'implementation' the nurse signs that the drug has been given. The nursing plan will carry an instruction to observe for signs of whether or not the drug is having the desired effect, and the appearance of any known side-effects. Should a side-effect occur, it will be reported to the doctor, and written in the nursing notes. The patient outcome will be 'return to previous range of core body temperature'. It will be evaluated by using a clinical thermometer, and subjectively — by the patient feeling better, and by the nurse observing that there is general improvement.

It is appropriate to include here some other planned nurse-initiated interventions which might be necessary to nurse the hyperpyrexic patient safely and effectively. He is likely to have a headache and in 'process thinking' could be written like this:

assessing: patient's description of headache: it may be necessary to use a painometer, for example if the headache is due to meningitis
patient's problem: headache
patient outcome: no headache
nurse-initiated intervention: cold compress to forehead each hour
evaluation: patient's current description against description at initial assessment, or, comparison from use of measurement tool — painometer

The fluid lost through perspiration has to be replaced as well as maintenance of the usual daily intake. The patient may or may not have a problem — thirst; if not, he has a potential problem of electrolyte imbalance if the fluid balance is not maintained. Consequent planned nursing interventions might be:

- maintain accurate intake and output chart
- offer iced glucose drinks hourly (iced drinks will help to cool the patient; glucose will supply ready-to-be-absorbed extra kilojoules (calories) required because of the increased rate of metabolism).

Sweat contains sodium chloride; with normal blood chlorides there is excretion of 5.7 g chloride in 1000 ml urine; less than this is indicative of chloride shortage. The kidneys are involved in filtering the toxic products from for instance inflammation, and being overworked they can excrete urine containing albumen. To identify early stages of these abnormalities, a planned nursing intervention might be:

- test urine daily for albumen and chlorides

When the patient's temperature has returned to normal, the bed is arranged to suit the circumstances, for example, the cradles may be removed, the patient may be able to have a gown placed round him; he may have only the sheet covering him or he may desire a second article of bed clothing. After he has rested, that is within the next 24 hours, he needs to be bathed to prevent odour from decomposing perspiration.

The patient with a **high temperature** and a **dry skin** needs help in the form of tepid sponging (p. 94). The reduction of temperature achieved by this process may be maintained without further disturbance of the patient by the exposure method described previously. It allows the body to continue to lose heat by radiation, conduction, convection and evaporation (this process is continuous even when there is no visible sweat). Any rise in the patient's temperature must be dealt with, by repeating tepid sponging. There is not the danger of salt depletion as in a sweating patient. There is no 'extra' perspiration on the skin, so that the patient can be bathed at his customary time.

Hyperthermia

Hyperthermia (as opposed to hyperpyrexia) is the word used when the increased temperature is induced for therapeutic purposes. In the main local and general heat treatment is less popular than formerly. However, there are fashions in therapy. What is considered by some people to be old fashioned today may well come back into fashion in the near future. The student can be expected to become skilful only in those procedures in use in the wards to which she is allocated. In many hospitals heat is applied locally in the form of a protected hot water bottle, electric pad, kaolin poultice or foot or hand immersion bath. Prevention of burning and scalding is the nurse's main responsibility. These treatments rarely increase the general body temperature. If they do, simple measures, such as opening a window, removing an article of personal or bed clothing usually suffice.

Application of dry heat to the total body surface with the main therapeutic objective of raising the body temperature is coming back into fashion and is being used to treat certain malignant diseases. The application of moist heat in the form of a hot wet pack is useful for relieving muscle spasm, for example, in poliomyelitis. The procedure has been greatly simplified by a washing tub with an attached wringer or a spin drier. Such packs are bound to increase the body temperature temporarily and the nurse will be able to deal with this situation from what has already been written. Hot baths are given for many purposes; the temporary increase of body temperature is easily dealt with.

Hypothermia

Hypothermia is a condition in which the core body temperature falls below normal measured by using a low reading thermometer. Hypothermia can occur in the newborn due to failure to adjust to external cold. Aikens (1977) describes a small study in which hats and lamps were used to prevent neonatal hypothermia. The condition can also occur insidiously in the elderly due to impaired circulation and lessened ability to react to external cold. Lack of intake of sufficient kilojoules may play a part in its production. The articles in the Reading Assignment by Hillman (1987), Drummond (1979), Stevens (1986) and The Professional Nurse (1986) provide adequate knowledge of hypothermia in the young and old. Lowered body temperature due to over-exposure to the elements can occur by accident or due to lack of proper precautions. Prevention of tissue damage (frost-bite), attention to adequate diet and clothing, provision of general warmth in the form of an immersion bath (temperature carefully graded and prescribed by the doctor) and provision of an above average atmospheric temperature throughout the 24 hours all play a part in bringing the core body temperature up to normal.

Hypothermia can be artificially induced to as low as 26 to 32.5°C to permit major cardiac, cardiovascular and neurological surgery to be carried out.

Sometimes the temperature does not need to be as low as 32°C and is achieved with tepid to cold sponging (p. 94), and arranging the patient under cradles as described for hyperpyrexia.

Hypothermic patients are prone to chest infection and preventive measures are carried out in the same way as for an unconscious patient (p. 215). One of the scoring scales for risk of developing pressure sores will be used, and the result will guide the selection of planned nursing interventions to achieve the patient outcome 'absence of pressure sores'. Diet will be prescribed by the doctor according to the degree of hypothermia induced. It will be of lower kilojoule value than that needed by tissues at normal body temperature. The nursing intervention is monitoring food intake and gradually increasing it as the core body temperature rises to normal.

Cooling of one limb (local hypothermia) can be used for a patient with an ischaemic lower limb which threatens gangrene. He is helped into a comfortable, recumbent position. The head of the bed may be raised to increase bloodflow to the feet. Under a cradle the limb is exposed to cool air from a fan, and the rest of the body is kept warm. By a complicated reflex the opposing temperatures increase blood supply to the cool tissues. Convection currents also keep the limb dry which helps to prevent infection in these tissues which have poor resistance to micro-organisms. (Warmth and moisture encourage bacteria to multiply at their maximum rate.) Metabolism is decreased in cool tissues, so that they are helped to survive on the lessened oxygen which they are receiving.

Gangrene is excruciatingly painful; a painometer may be used as a tool to evaluate whether or not the goal of 'no pain' has been achieved by implementing the delegated planned nursing intervention of giving analgesics. The patient should be encouraged to take extra protein and vitamins A and C for repair of tissue and prevention of infection.

Inflammation

Many of the patients needing the treatments discussed in this section have an inflammatory lesion. Considerable economy of learning can be achieved by understanding this basic process.

Inflammation is a protective phenomenon and is the reaction of living tissue to infection, injury or an irritant. Some examples are given in Table 16.1 on page 231. However, Gooch (1986) states 'It is a popular misconception that a fever must indicate the presence of infection.' The commonest cause of a raised body temperature is tissue injury and this includes surgical operations. The injured cells release pyrogens which are fever-producing substances. The increased temperature speeds up all chemical reactions and this facilitates healing (Boylan &

Brown 1985). Lack of increased temperature indicates a poorly functioning healing process. But an increased body temperature is also a characteristic of infection.

Infection can be acute or chronic. One of the body's inflammatory reactions is to produce more white blood cells to fight the infection and clear up the debris. This physiological increase is called leucocytosis, as opposed to a pathological increase which is known as leukaemia.

In acute inflammation leucocytes predominate; in chronic inflammation lymphocytes predominate so that a differential white cell count may aid diagnosis.

At the site of inflammation there will be some or all of the following signs and symptoms; swelling, heat, redness, pain and loss of function. The nearby lymphatic vessels may become involved in the inflammatory process. Lymphangitis in the limbs is evidenced by a red streak rising from the focus of infection. The draining lymphatic nodes (glands) may enlarge in an attempt to perform their filtering function more effectively (Fig. 16.10). They may become palpable, especially those in the neck, axilla and groin. They may be inflamed (lymphadenitis), and an abscess may form. They may fail in their filtering, and germs and their toxins may flood into the blood stream. Toxaemia, pyaemia, bacteraemia, bacillaemia, septicaemia and viraemia are terms used in these conditions.

The patient with an inflammatory process experiences general malaise (Fig. 16.11). The body temperature rises and the pulse becomes rapid. A rise of 10 in the pulse for each degree rise in the temperature is considered average. The respiratory rate is increased in an attempt to get more oxygen for the increased rate of metabolism. The skin is hot and dry at first and, later, sweating occurs; it is usually a prelude to a fall in temperature. The patient complains of thirst, dry mouth, sordes, furred tongue, anorexia, nausea, vomiting and constipation. He passes only a small amount of concentrated urine. He often complains of headache, restlessness and insomnia and he may become delirious.

In the sweating stage the patient requires the care given on page 227. The temperature,

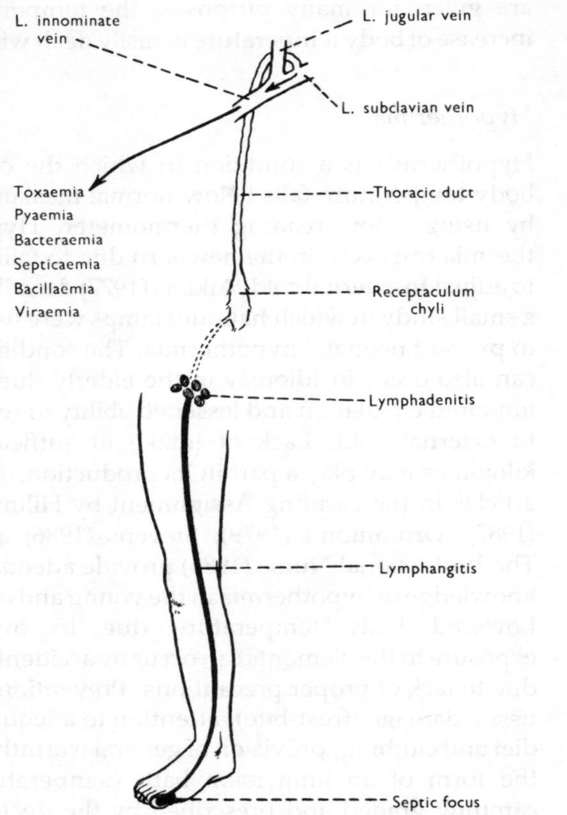

Fig. 16.10 Results of inflammation

1. General malaise
2. ↑T.P.R.
3. Hot dry skin

Digestive system:

4. Thirst
5. Dry mouth
6. Sordes
7. Furred tongue
8. Anorexia
9. Nausea
10. Vomiting

Bowel:

11. Constipation

Urinary system:

12. Small amount of concentrated urine

Nervous system:

13. Headache
14. Restlessness
15. Insomnia
16. Delirium

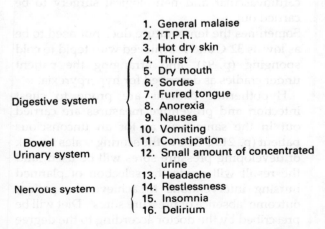

Fig. 16.11 General signs and symptoms of inflammation

Table 16.1 Inflammation

Inflammation of	Technical name	Agent causing infection
Tonsil	Tonsillitis	Streptococcus
Mouth	Stomatitis	*Candida albicans* (fungus)
Nose	Rhinitis	Virus
Hair follicle	Furuncle (boil)	Staphylococcus
Eye lash	Hordeolum (stye)	Staphylococcus
Lung	Pneumonia (pneumonitis)	Pneumococcus
		Staphylococcus
		Mycobacterium tuberculosis
		Various viruses
Appendix	Appendicitis	Bacteria
Gall bladder	Cholecystitis	Bacteria
Digestive tract	Gastritis	Streptococcus
	Colitis	Staphylococcal toxin
	Enteritis	*Salmonella typhi*
	Gastro-enteritis	*Salmonella paratyphi*
	Proctitis	*Bacillus flexner*
	Food poisoning	*Bacillus shiga*
		Bacillus sonne
		Entamoeba hystolytica
		Vibrio cholerae
		Clostridium botulinum
Kidney	Nephritis	Streptococcus
Brain coverings	Meningitis	Meningococcus
		Pneumococcus
		Influenzal virus
		Mumps virus
		Streptococcus
		Staphylococcus
		Mycobacterium tuberculosis
Skin		Staphylococci
		Streptococci
Injury	Irritant	
Insect bite	Corrosive chemical	
	Dust, Feathers, Pollen	
	Chlorine gas	
	Phosgene gas	
	Silica	
	Faecal impaction	
	Thread worms	
	Stones which form from precipitated bile	
	Chemicals	
	Poisonous berries and fungi	
	Toxins from other bacteria	
	Chemicals	
Flame, Radium, Friction, Boiling Liquids, Electricity, 'Flash' burns from radioactive explosion, Frost-bite, X-rays, Pressure, Heat	Pollen	
	Metal	
	Corrosive chemicals	
	Wound	

pulse and respiration is taken at least 4-hourly as part of ongoing assessment and is evaluated against the previous recording. Careful observation of the pulse is necessary for several days after the temperature returns to normal. Continuance of a rapid pulse after fall of temperature may mean that the toxins have had an adverse effect on the heart muscle. This is reported to the doctor.

Some or all of the following nursing activities will be written on the nursing plan:

- encourage extra glucose fluid
- offer fresh fruit drinks
- oral toilet 2 hourly
- test urine daily for protein, chlorides
- progress to light, then full diet with extra protein, vitamins A and C.

Glucose is ready to be absorbed; it spares digestive activity and provides kilojoules (calories). Fresh fruit drinks help to cleanse the mouth. The fluid intake should be sufficient to replace that lost by sweating, and to help in the elimination of toxic substances by the kidneys. If the cells in the glomerular capsules of the kidney become inflamed by toxic substances, they may allow passage of the large molecule of protein. The urine must be tested daily for protein, so that this complication can be detected early. As soon as possible the patient progresses to light, and then to full diet. Extra protein is necessary to repair tissue, vitamin C to help with protein synthesis and vitamin A for its anti-infective property.

Rest is necessary for the inflamed tissues. An arm can be put in a sling or splint; a leg can be put in a splint or on traction if the inflammation is in a joint. Tonsils can be rested by spitting out some of the saliva, thus reducing swallowing. With an inflamed lung the patient is inclined to lie on the affected side; the external pressure minimises movement of the chest wall. But this patient does need to cough up sputum. He can be helped by giving an analgesic (which is not a respiratory depressant) before coughing exercises, during which manual support is applied to the chest wall. The digestive tract is rested by attention to the diet; soothing, low residue foods are given. The kidney is rested by withholding protein in the early stages and increasing it gradually as the inflammation subsides. As a rule fluids are restricted in the early stages of nephritis. The patient is spared muscular effort so that he does not use body protein, the end-product of which the kidneys have to excrete. A patient with meningitis or encephalitis is often more restful in a quiet, darkened room. There should be a minimum number of people with whom he needs to establish a relationship. Passive entertainment will need to be instituted according to the patient's likes and dislikes.

The doctor is likely to order chemotherapy or antibiotics for those patients with body temperature above or below normal.

Having discussed in this section fever, pyrexia and hyperpyrexia in process context; followed by discussion of hyperthermia, hypothermia and inflammation in a general context, it is time to use the four phases sequentially as further practice in process thinking related to the principle 'helping patients to maintain body temperature within normal range'.

MAINTAINING BODY TEMPERATURE IN PROCESS CONTEXT

After collection of as much information as possible from other sources, the nurse will have some idea of whether or not the patient might require help in maintaining body temperature within normal range. Those admitted from the waiting list are unlikely to have a problem per se, but they might require the commonsense sort of help because the atmospheric temperature at which hospitals are maintained is often higher than the temperature which they can afford to maintain in their own home. For patients admitted as 'emergencies' via the Accident and Emergency department the initial assessment of TPR is likely to have been carried out in that department and be recorded on the case notes brought to the ward. This may not be the case for patients admitted as an 'emergency' from an Outpatients' Clinic. Even patients who are seriously ill may not have a problem related to maintaining body temperature. Only the initial assessment of using a clinical thermometer to provide objective evidence will confirm this.

Assessing maintenance of body temperature

From what has been written so far about patients with abnormal change in core body temperature, readers will have some idea of observations to be made at the initial assessment. If day clothes are being worn are they appropriate for the atmospheric temperature? People whose thyroid gland is over-secreting can feel very hot on the coldest winter day and be outside in shirt and pants. Whereas when the gland is under-secreting the opposite can happen. Does the skin feel hot or cold to the touch? Does it feel dry or moist? Is there any visible perspiration? Does the hair seem moist with perspiration? Is there any restless irritability? Have convulsions occurred? This is more likely to be so in babies. And in some instances, gross change in core body temperature, for example severe hypothermia, is accompanied by change in the level of consciousness. It may therefore be pertinent at this point to use a tool such as the Glasgow Coma Scale (p. 66) to assess level of consciousness.

The objective in collecting assessment data is to discover whether or not the patient has any actual or potential problems which are amenable to nursing intervention. A clear statement of these problems as the patient is experiencing them is a nursing diagnosis.

Exploring the assessment data with the patient, he agrees on the problems he is experiencing; so for a patient with a medical diagnosis, 'pyrexia of unknown origin', a comparison of the diagnosis might be:

Medical diagnosis:
 pyrexia of unknown origin
Nursing diagnosis:
 headache
 tiredness
 feeling hot and sweaty
 obnoxious body odour

Planning

Writing the patient's nursing plan is the identifiable activity associated with the second phase of the process — planning individualised nursing. For each identified problem, an outcome (goal) would be discussed and agreed with the patient. These might be:

- no headache
- less tiredness
- decreased body temperature and perspiration
- absence of smell of stale perspiration.

This would lead to discussion of possible nurse-initiated nursing interventions to achieve the patient outcomes (written on the nursing plan) and these could be:

- cold compresses to forehead hourly
- kilojoules (calories) are needed to produce energy. Discussion with the patient about what flavoured fluids would be most acceptable. Glucose is useful because it is not sweet to taste and can therefore be added to most drinks.
- wash patient all over (bedbath), gradually lowering temperature of water: dab skin dry, no friction (this will also solve patient's fourth problem).

Implementing

Implementing, the accepted third phase of the process, is probably the best understood by nurses — the active phase — which other people can observe.

- each time the cold compress is applied to the forehead there will be ongoing assessment of the patient's headache and both will be written on the nursing notes. The last point will provide cumulative evidence towards the goal 'no headache'
- each fluid intake (quantity and quality) will be recorded on the patient's nursing notes, together with perceived progress (agreed with patient) towards the goal of 'less tiredness'
- each bedbath with cool water will be recorded on the nursing notes with observation on the state of perspiration. This together with recordings on the TPR chart will provide summative evidence towards the goal, 'decreased body temperature and perspiration'

- the previous implementation will help to achieve the fourth goal 'absence of smell of stale perspiration' and the agreed patient's and nurse's subjective information from using their sense of smell after each bedbath will be used in recording summative evidence on the nursing notes.

But nurses will have to learn to convince others that diversity and synthesis of knowledge are necessary in the current cognition (thinking) which precedes the 'doing'. From the foregoing text readers will begin to realise that these precedents are essential in facilitating the safe and effective nursing of patients, in this instance one of pyrexia of unknown origin. The precedents include a considerable knowledge of:

- thermometry
- research work which has been carried out about placement of a thermometer in the oral cavity (it is not just 'under the tongue' as many lay people believe, and some nurses continue 'to do')
- abnormal core temperatures, their association with medical diagnoses, and their implications for nurse-initiated as well as medically delegated nursing interventions.

Evaluating

To evaluate, which is the accepted fourth phase of the process, nurses need to consult:

- the assessment data
- the statement of the patient's problems which are amenable to nurse-initiated interventions
- the statement of goals (patient outcomes)
- the selected nurse-initiated interventions to achieve the goals (nursing plan)
- the record of implementation of the nurse-initiated interventions (TPR chart, and patient's nursing notes).

This surely is evidence of the complexity of nursing!

It was stated previously that the patient outcome (goal) would be discussed and agreed with the patient and this might be:

- no headache
- less tiredness
- decreased body temperature and perspiration
- no smell of stale perspiration.

Without further repetition in the text, can you suggest how these goals, might be evaluated?

In this chapter, thermometers and other measuring equipment have been discussed. Various changes in body temperature were mentioned in relation to the nursing required by the patient and finally the principle — helping patients to maintain body temperature within normal range — was discussed in process of nursing context.

APPLYING THE PRINCIPLE

A registered nurse must be capable of:

- introducing a patient to his environment so that he feels free to manipulate any heating and ventilating devices
- reporting inadequacies of heating and ventilation to the appropriate authority (Perseverance may be necessary to report these daily until they are attended to!)
- estimating and recording temperature, pulse and respiration, and blood pressure, recognising abnormality, reporting these verbally and in writing. Teaching staff these skills
- facilitating the first year student's acquisition of these skills by seeing that she does a little of it daily, rather than a lot weekly, for example, making six estimations daily results in more efficient learning than making 30 estimations once weekly
- recognising a patient with an increased body temperature and taking the necessary steps to deal with it. Nursing a hyperpyrexic patient
- recognising a patient with a decreased body temperature, and taking the necessary steps to deal with it. Nursing a hypothermic patient

- carrying out any cold or hot applications or immersions prescribed by the doctor with safety and maximum benefit to the patient
- organising and teaching a safe method for chemotherapy and antibiotic administration
- applying the principle — helping patients to maintain body temperature within normal range — in a process of nursing context

WORKING ASSIGNMENT

Topics for discussion

- how is cross-infection from thermometers prevented in your ward?
- I've worked in a hospital where the students didn't shake the thermometer down after use before returning it to its container, so that, if necessary, an experienced nurse could check the reading
- grease is a bad conductor of heat. Discuss this in relation to the taking of a 'rectal' temperature
- at 02.00 hours Mr Jones is sleeping soundly; his intramuscular injection of antibiotic is due. What will you do?
- you are working in a ward where the patients' temperatures are not taken routinely. What personal observations and/or comments from a patient would lead you to take his temperature?
- did you read in the *Medical News* that in a 500-bed hospital, temperature taking was cut from twice to once daily, at 19.00 hours; from 4-hourly to thrice daily at 07.00, 14.00 and 19.00 hours, thereby saving 3500 nursing hours in a year?
- if TempaDot has the advantages of being made of flexible plastic, registers core body temperature accurately to 1/10th degree in 6 seconds and is disposable so that it cannot contribute to nosocomial infection, why don't we use it in this hospital?

Writing assignment

- give an example of a bacterial infection
- give an example of a viral infection
- give an example of a protozoal infection
- state the normal body temperature on the Fahrenheit scale
- state the normal body temperature on the Centigrade scale
- define the following:

  antibiotic
  antipyretic
  antitoxin
  bacteria
  diphtheria
  dysphasia
  dyspnoea
  endemic
  faecal-oral route
  glomerulonephritis
  hemiplegia
  hyperpyrexia
  hypothermia
  immunisation
  inflammation
  influenza
  leucocytes
  leucocytosis
  leukaemia
  malaria
  osteomyelitis
  paratyphoid fever
  pathogen
  penicillin
  pneumonia
  protozoa
  pulse
  pyrexia
  rheumatic fever
  rigor
  scarlet fever
  specific
  Staphylococcus
  Streptococcus
  syndrome
  toxaemia
  toxin
  tracheostomy
  virus
  yellow fever
- at what temperature should a ward be kept?

- give the normal pulse range in an adult
- give the normal pulse range in a baby
- name some conditions in which there is an increase in body temperature
- name some conditions in which there is a decrease in body temperature
- define the following:

albuminuria
aneurysm
apnoea
apyretic
atrial fibrillation
bradycardia
bronchiectasis
bronchitis
chemotherapy
Cheyne-Stokes breathing
constant pyrexia
convulsion
crisis
cyanosis
delirium
emphysema
empyema
febrile
fever
feverish
heat stroke
intermittent pyrexia
inverse pyrexia
lysis
mediastinal
orthopnoea
palpitation
pyaemia
remittent pyrexia
sinus arrhythmia
stertorous
stridor
tachycardia
thyroidectomy
tuberculosis
typhoid fever
vasoconstriction
vasodilation

- name some conditions in which there is a rapid pulse
- name some conditions in which there is a slow pulse
- give the technical word for fever
- give the technical word for difficulty in breathing
- define the following:

acidosis
air hunger
amyl nitrite
anaemia
arteriosclerosis
asphyxia
atropine
blood pressure
cholecystectomy
coma
concussion
core temperature
coronary artery disease
dicrotic pulse
digitalis
extra systole
gastrectomy
haemorrhage
heart block
hyperpnoea
infection
intracranial
mitral stenosis
moribund
morphia
myxoedema
narcotic
opium
Pel-Ebstein fever
pleurisy
polyuria
pulsus paradoxicus
pyelitis
pyrogens
sedative
shell temperature
shock
side-effects
stethoscope
thyrotoxicosis
uraemia

- how much chloride is normally excreted in urine?
- at what level of urinary chlorides is extra salt in drinks needed?
- in what way is a clinical different from any other type of thermometer?
- define the following:

  anorexia
  arrhythmia
  ascites
  bacillaemia
  bacteraemia
  bronchial asthma
  carcinoma
  cardiac asthma
  conduction
  convection
  craniotomy
  dysphasia
  encephalitis
  evaporation
  hemiplegia
  jaundice
  ketosis
  latent heat
  lymphadenitis
  lymphangitis
  lymphocyte
  meningitis
  nausea
  nephritis
  paroxysmal tachycardia
  pathological
  peritonitis
  pyaemia
  radiation
  septicaemia
  sulphonamide
  therapeutic
  tracheostomy
  viraemia
- where does one feel the pulse in the radial artery?
- where does one feel the pulse in the temporal artery?
- where does one feel the pulse in the facial artery?
- where does one feel the pulse in the carotid artery?
- what factors are observed when taking the pulse?
- define the following:
  agranulocytosis
  analgesic
  diastolic blood pressure
  frostbite
  gangrene
  hyperthermia
  hypothermia
  streptomycin
  subclinical
  systolic blood pressure
  thrush.

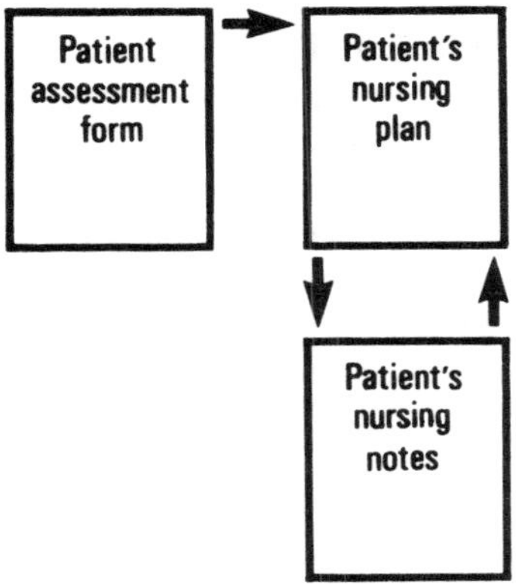

17 Helping patients to avoid environmental dangers

READING ASSIGNMENT

Boardman K P 1977 Fractures in an elderly population in a psychiatric hospital. Nursing Mirror 144 (9) March 3: 52–57
Collection of data over 1 year.

Chase R 1978 Blindness averted. Nursing Mirror 146 (13) March 30: 17-18
Easy for toddlers to become victims of accidental poisoning: nursing care study.

Colver A, Pearson P 1985 Safety in the home: how well are we doing? Health Visitor 58 (1) February: 41–42
A study in which health visitors gave accurate, detailed and realistic information about hazards which they observed at the time of the visit. Over half the families made changes in their home to make them permanently safer.

Community Outlook 1984 Baby buggies and car seats. Nursing Times 80 (27) July 11: 252–253
A safety checklist in the form of a poster.

Devlin R 1984 Which should you choose? Community Outlook Nursing Times 80 (27) July 11: 284, 250
What are the pitfalls and safety points health visitors should advise parents on when they are choosing baby buggies, pushchairs and car safety seats.

Farmer E 1978 The impact of technology on nursing. Nursing Mirror 147 (13) September 28: 17–20

The nurse is the constant factor in patient care and therefore her awareness of the technology which supports her patients must be expanded.

Howie C 1984 Accidents will happen. Nursing Times 80 (13) March 28: 19

A report from a King's Fund conference about the reporting and recording of accidents.

Kendall S 1986 Home safety and accident prevention. Nursing: The Add-On Journal of Clinical Nursing 3 (12) December: 454–457

Commonly occurring accidents and their prevention are discussed for those in the age groups 0-3 months, 3-6 months and 6-12 months.

Kings J 1979 Playing with fire. Nursing Mirror 149 (7) August 16: 25–26

Account of student nurses' crash course in firefighting.

Nursing 1980 Poisoning. Nursing Issue 15 July: 668–671

Excellent overview compiled with help from staff in a Poisons Unit.

Roberts F 1985 Accidents in hospital. Learning from past mishaps. Nursing Times 81 (10) March 6: 24–26

An illustrated report of a research project in which a new data collection document was designed.

Ross T 1985 Why did it happen in my ward? Nursing Times 8 (10) March 6:27–28

Six accidents to patients were reported one winter's day in one hospital. They involved both sexes, all age groups, a variety of wards and on different nursing shifts.

Skeet M 1980 First aid in the street and home. Nursing Issue 14 June: 615–620

Turvey K 1984 Clinical standards in occupational health nursing. Occupational Health Nursing Supplement Nursing: The Add-On Journal of Clinical Nursing 1 (6) May: 5–7

Describes the various dimensions involved in carrying out preventive activities in the work area.

BACKGROUND INFORMATION

Some of the items in the Reading Assignment have been retained in this fourth edition because they are still useful. Eight new items have been selected to cover a wide area of knowledge which is required, not only by nurses working in hospitals, but also by those working in the community which includes midwives, health visitors, school nurses and occupational health nurses. It is hoped that readers will develop an awareness of possible dangers in the environment and what nurses can do to eliminate them or minimise their effects. The following account of background information is purposely wide ranging and then the text focuses to avoiding environmental danger in process context.

Increasing industrialisation and advancing technology have rendered the environment more hazardous, not only for people at work but also in the pursuit of their leisure activities. In an attempt to cope with this, governments pass legislation pertaining to health and safety at work and there are occupational health services to enact the legislation. Dangers at work are recognised and monitored by safety representatives appointed by the trade unions.

The government attempts to control safety in some leisure activities by having driving tests, compulsory wearing of crash helmets by motor cycle riders, fire regulations for public buildings and so on. Local authorities are encouraged to make the environment — street pavings, access to public conveniences and other buildings — safe for handicapped people.

The mass media, as well as being used by health educationists to encourage the public to make their domestic environment as safe as possible, also inform them of hazardous outdoor conditions by such items as weather forecasts and road conditions. As a consequence of all these factors, most people who are in need of nursing have some knowledge of the subject of avoiding hazards in the environment.

People develop various attitudes to the possibility of accident. At one extreme are the over-anxious and at the other extreme there are those who do not admit the possibility of an accident happening to them and they spurn precaution. The important thing is to be able to recognize danger and take preventive action before an accident occurs. Having taken all sensible precautions one's attitude should be free from anxiety.

AVOIDING ENVIRONMENTAL DANGER IN A PROCESS CONTEXT

Such environmental hazards as baths, bath mats and washing bowls were discussed in Chapter 8 under 'ward planning' (p. 92) and in the context of preventing patients acquiring a nosocomial infection. The immediate environment in contact with a person's pressure areas can be hazardous in those at risk of developing pressure sores and this was discussed in process context in Chapter 10. The hospital environment is a hazard because of its bacterial population and the ever-present risk of nosocomial infection which is discussed in Chapter 20. From these references readers will realise that an essential skill in nursing is the ability to synthesise knowledge from several sources in a given situation. In the following text a general approach to the wide-ranging subject of avoiding environmental dangers will be taken using the accepted four phases of the process.

Assessing a person's ability to avoid environmental dangers

Ability to avoid dangers is dictated by knowledge and awareness of them, as well as motivation to comply with sensible precautions. Health visitors have a special role in assessing three factors — the level of knowledge and awareness possessed by clients; their physical and mental ability to put these into practice; their physical environment for actual and potential dangers. The purpose in collecting this assessment data is to identify with the client any problems being experienced in relation to avoiding environmental danger — there may not be available money to buy a fireguard. There may be instances of health visitor perceived actual or potential problems which are not client perceived: there cannot be a formula for dealing with such an experience because of its individuality. Professional judgement will be necessary and this may well have an ethical component. For example a health visitor may observe a crying child who has different visible bruising on several successive visits. It is reasonably easy to discuss such a situation hypothetically; but in recent cases of child abuse, reality is much more complex. Occupational health nurses also have these three factors to consider in assessing employees and identifying with them any problems they are experiencing which are amenable to occupational health nurses' intervention. But the majority of nurses work in hospital where patients are usually suffering from an episode of acute illness, some of whom may also have a long-standing disability, and some who have been admitted for treatment of the disability.

Human beings can be afflicted with such a diversity of disabling conditions that any list of them can only be tentative: the following is offered to start readers thinking of the opportunity for an imaginative and creative initial assessment related to patients' ability to avoid environmental dangers.

• people who are blind or visually impaired	• explore how they usually avoid environmental dangers • discuss any problems which they anticipate because of admission to hospital • visual impairment was discussed in a communicating context (p. 23) but it is equally relevant when assessing a person's ability to avoid environmental dangers.
• people who are deaf or hearing impaired	• ambulant patients will be at risk of accident because they cannot hear approaching trolleys, commodes, wheelchairs and so on • cannot hear the alarm if that is the method of alerting a ward to fire • deaf and hearing impaired people were considered in a communicating context on page 24.
• people who do not have a sense of smell (anosmia)	• although many people's ambition is to see hospitals as no smoking areas, realistically in the foreseeable future there will be

	some smokers. People who do not have a sense of smell will not be warned of the charring smell from the fall of hot tobacco on to their clothing, bed or chair
• people who cannot appreciate the sensation of touch	• explore how they usually avoid environmental dangers, including pressure surfaces (Ch. 10) • discuss any problems which they anticipate because of admission to hospital
• people who are physically disabled	• the same applies as for those who cannot appreciate the sensation of touch
• people who are mentally handicapped	• assessment data may have to be collected from a secondary source, for example a parent.

When interviewing people from the aforementioned groups, the patient may have managed at home, for example to transfer safely and effectively from wheelchair to bed but will require nursing help in hospital because the beds may be higher than the wheelchair. Exactly how this is to be accomplished will probably be written as a nursing intervention on the patient's nursing plan.

The assessment data in all instances will be examined with the patient and any problems relating to avoidance of environmental dangers formulated as the patient is experiencing them, and/or any which he anticipates experiencing because of the changed circumstances. A clear statement of such problems is a nursing diagnosis. There will not be a comparable medical diagnosis for ability to avoid dangers in the environment.

Planning — individualised

Only a minimum of patients will have a problem requiring a written nursing intervention on the patient's plan, but it is important that it is stated in sufficient detail for it to be implemented by nurses on succeeding shifts, even relief nurses unfamiliar with the ward and patients. One example was given in the previous paragraph; others are to be found in the planning section of preventing pressure sores (p. 119), keeping the body clean and well groomed (p. 92), and preventing nosocomial infection (p. 260).

There obviously has to be ward policy and planning to minimise the environmental dangers to which patients can be exposed. Upcurled floor tiles, broken windows and frayed cords have to be reported and repaired before they cause accidents. Although floor washing is a domestic activity it is wise for nurses to discourage patients from walking during the danger period of slipping on a damp floor. There must be a policy with domestic superintendents as to who attends to spills on the floor which should be mopped up immediately. Fire exits must be clear and accessible at all times and more will be said about fire in hospital later.

There undoubtedly has to be generalised planning to keep patient areas as free from danger as possible. When one considers all the equipment which is in almost constant use in hospitals it is not surprising that the staff includes such personnel as specialist technicians, electricians, mechanical engineers and plumbers.

Implementing

Implementing, the third phase of the process of nursing, involves carrying out the planned nursing interventions and recording this on the patient's nursing notes, together with any relevant information about the particular implementation.

Using the word in a wider context, nurses implement ward and hospital policy with the objective of preventing accidents, about which more will be said later.

Evaluating

To carry out the fourth phase of the process of nursing, on the day appointed the nurse will consult the initial assessment information, the statement of the problem, the goal or patient outcome and the patient's nursing notes for any summative ongoing assessment information.

For example the patient outcome for the person whose sensation of touch was absent would be uninjured skin. Part of the planned nursing intervention would be to inspect skin every x h, so the patient's nursing notes would have a lot of summative evidence that the skin had remained uninjured. For those patients who did not have a problem with avoiding environmental dangers, one can presume that the principle 'helping patients to avoid environmental dangers' has been applied effectively to each of them who leaves the hospital without succumbing to the dangers.

ACCIDENT FORMS

An 'accident form' has to be filled in after any accident to any person on hospital premises. Roberts (1985) describes a research project in which a new data collection document was designed. There is an illustration of it. Howie (1984) reports a King's Fund conference about reporting and recording accidents. It is an acknowledged fact that immediately after an incident, the individual accounts of three witnesses vary in detail; the longer the time between the incident and giving an account of it, the greater the variance. After a long lapse of time, one's memory of an incident can be affected by subsequent events. In fairness to all concerned, it is therefore important that the 'accident form' in hospital is filled in as soon as possible after the event.

FIRE IN HOSPITAL

The hospital authorities in conjunction with the fire brigade work out a policy to be enacted in the event of fire in any part of the hospital. It is the responsibility of all staff to know the location of and how to use the fire extinguishers in their working vicinity. There will be a plan for evacuation of patients and staff should this become necessary. Fire drill should be practised regularly and members of staff admitted between the drills should be acquainted with the hospital's policy. In some hospitals each member of staff signs a book on receiving the fire drill notes.

It cannot be too strongly stressed that part of each new member of staff's *introduction* to a ward should *include showing* her the nearest *fire-alarm* and *extinguisher*. As each person is human, and in this instance capable of omitting this part of the introduction, we should *instruct* members of *staff* to *ask* about these things when they move to another ward or department. We could also consider writing the fire instructions for the area in the procedure book or displaying them in each ward and department.

In this chapter the background information covered a wide range of ideas about possible dangers in the environment and some ways of coping with them. The principle — helping patients to avoid environmental dangers — was then discussed in process of nursing context.

APPLYING THE PRINCIPLE

A registered nurse must be capable of:

- rendering the environment as safe as possible
- advising management on safety of ward structure and equipment
- checking that electrical equipment is tested quarterly by maintenance staff
- rendering and teaching first aid
- learning, teaching and carrying out hospital policy in the event of fire
- applying the principle — helping patients to avoid environmental hazards — in a process of nursing context.

WORKING ASSIGNMENT

Topics for discussion

- first-aid treatment for burns and scalds
- what does one do when the needle breaks while giving an intramuscular injection? Name two diseases which are transmitted by blood.
- how should the staff deal with a small accidental fire in the ward?

- what should be done if a thermometer breaks in a patient's mouth?
- what would you do if a known epileptic in your ward had a fit?
- what would you do if a patient fainted in the bath?

Writing assignment

- what is the first-aid treatment for a patient who has broken a bone?
- what is the first-aid treatment for a sprain?
- how would you treat a cut?
- how would you remove a splinter from a finger?
- how would you remove a foreign body from an eye?
- keep a list throughout your 3-year programme of situations with an 'accident' potential.

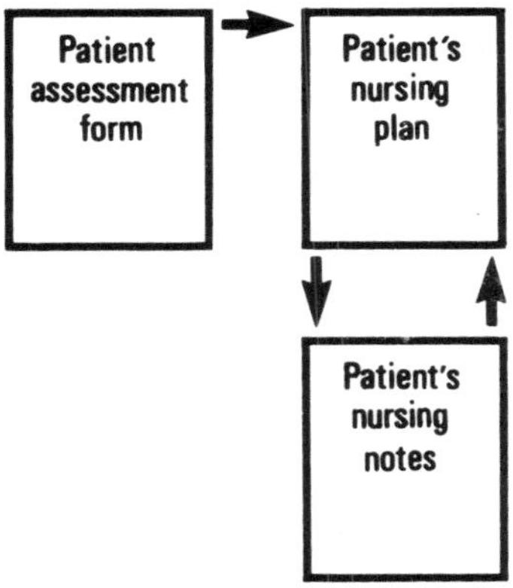

18

Helping patients to avoid misidentification

READING ASSIGNMENT

Nursing Times 1978 Personal identification aid. Nursing Times 74 (3) January 19: 104

RCN, The Association of Theatre Nurses, and the medical insurance organisations 1987 Theatre safeguards. Royal College of Nursing, London (Booklet)

BACKGROUND INFORMATION

Thirty years ago the patients' average length of stay in hospital was 14 days. They kept to their beds, at the bottom of which hung their temperature, pulse and respiration chart which displayed their name. The nurses worked longer hours, had shorter holidays and attended lectures in their off-duty. In this setting the patient had the security of knowing the ward staff; the ward staff had the security of being able to identify each patient.

Today the setting is very different; there is a rapid turnover of patients and only the minority of them are in their beds throughout the 24 hours. Some patients spend part or all of the day in a room away from their bed. The nurses work shorter hours, have longer holidays and attend college at the beginning and end of each module. To cover this there are 'part-time' staff who can experience insecurity because of the ever-changing ward population between spells of duty. The patient's security is lessened by the increased number of relationships they need to establish at a time when they may be less able to establish new relationships. After nights off or days off, the full-time staff can find the ward population considerably changed.

There is an increasing hazard of misinterpretation due to language difficulty. British staff meet inpatients and outpatients of many nationalities, especially in the areas with a large immigrant population. British patients meet staff of many nationalities. Proficiency in reading and writing a language other than one's mother tongue is quite different from understanding the spoken word, which can be of many dialects throughout any one country. It takes a long time to master the several thousand words used in a language. The problem is worldwide. The British Red Cross Society have prepared interpretation cards for many languages. Many Red Cross centres keep a list of people of other nationalities who are willing to help with interpretation for patients.

AVOIDING MISIDENTIFICATION IN PROCESS CONTEXT

Putting the principle of 'Helping patients to avoid misidentification' into process context does not result in use of a patient assessment form, a nursing plan or a patient's nursing notes. Yet the four phases of assessing, planning, implementing and evaluating are pertinent to the principle, but in a much broader context.

Assessing

Assessment (collection of data) is carried out because incidents of misidentification have to be reported. Analysis of the data reveals the problem — there has been misidentification of (fortunately relatively few) patients related to diets, investigations, medications, operations and treatments. The following examples are to help the beginning student to think about the subject:

- the misidentified patient has been operated on
- the misidentified (wrong) operation has been carried out on the correctly identified patient
- the misidentified side (left or right) has been operated on the correctly identified patient
- the misidentified digit has been operated on the correctly identified patient
- misidentified blood has been given to a correctly identified patient
- misidentified medication has been given to a correctly identified patient and
- a correctly identified medication has been given to a misidentified patient and so on.

Current planning and implementing

It is essential that the *right* patient is given the *right* medicine, diet, injection, treatment, transfusion, investigation or operation. The Royal College of Nursing (1987) advises that plans should be made so that patients in all acute areas including Accident and Emergency departments, 1 day and 5 day wards for surgical patients can be 'labelled' (Fig. 18.1), the minimum information being the patient's name and hospital number, as soon as possible after admission. This does not give a nurse the right to implement this precautionary (plan) policy

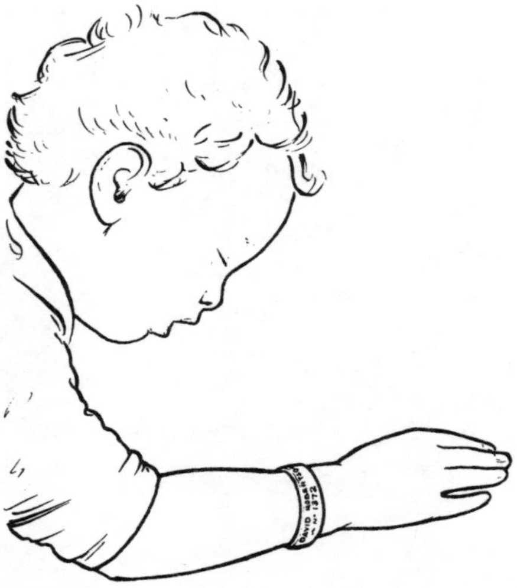

Fig. 18.1 Identaband

without explaining its purpose to the patient. What becomes routine to nurses can be degrading to patients unless an explanation is offered and compliance sought. Some patients may have unhappy memories of being 'labelled with a number' in prisoner of war camps.

Evaluating

Evaluating will not be carried out by nurses in the ward for individual patients, but by statisticians in whichever department customarily receives the reports of misidentification. As each incident is reported it will provide cumulative data which will probably be analysed annually to show increase or decrease in, for example, the whole hospital, or each clinical area in particular.

The number of incidents of misidentification may be an item in a quality evaluation system such as Performance Indicators, Qualpacs, Monitor or Quality Circles. The beginning nurse only needs to become familiar with these names and to realise that there is an increasing move towards trying to evaluate the standard of nursing — which is an extremely difficult task. As students progress towards registration they need to know more about these systems.

The problem of identification is complex and can only be solved in each hospital by discussion among all grades of staff, followed by formulation of a clear policy (plan) of action and by strict implementation of the policy (plan) by all members of staff in relation to medicines, diets, injections, treatments, transfusions, investigations and operations.

APPLYING THE PRINCIPLE

A registered nurse must be capable of:

- knowing, implementing and teaching the hospital's (plan) policy for identification of patients
- applying the principle — helping patients to avoid misidentification — in a process of nursing context

WORKING ASSIGNMENT

Topics for discussion

- two babies were mixed up in a maternity hospital and they were given to the wrong parents
- should a patient who is on medication, but is given a misidentified (wrong) medication be told?

Writing assignment

- write a short essay on the principle 'helping patients to avoid misidentification'.

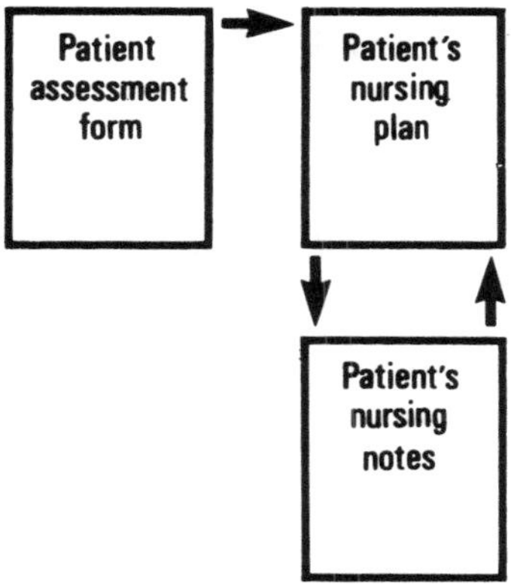

19

Helping patients to avoid loss of personal possessions

Background information

Loss of personal possessions in process context
Assessing
Planning
Implementing
Evaluating

Applying the principle
A registered nurse should be capable of:

Working assignment
Topics for discussion
Writing assignment

BACKGROUND INFORMATION

To help patients to avoid loss of personal possessions, the policy in some hospitals is to send a brochure to patients on the waiting list. It advises them not to bring jewellery and to bring only a small amount of money for current spending, for example a daily paper, letter cards or toothpaste. Where wardrobe and storage space are limited the patients are advised that someone should come with them so that outdoor clothes can be taken home.

Most women keep their money purse in their handbag, together with other personal items. They can rightly expect to be able to put them under lock and key while they go to the sanitary and washing area, and visit other departments. They will need them when visiting the day room where (as in any hotel), they will not expect the management to be responsible for loss. The Health Board must be covered by a notice to this effect.

Most men keep their loose change in their trouser pocket and notes in their inner breast pocket. Only a few men use a purse. If, in hospital, they solve their problem by putting their money in their dressing gown pocket, this can lead to coins rolling along the floor as the gown is rolled up to be put into its bedside locker space. In another department, such as X-ray or physiotherapy, they may be asked to hang their gowns in an adjacent room. Alternatively, if money is put into the locker drawer, it adds a questionable hygienic factor (for instance money in with sweets, chocolates and biscuits) to the safety factor.

People who suddenly become ill while on holiday or attending business or social functions and are admitted in emergency may be wearing expensive clothing and jewellery, and have large sums of money with them. A 24-hour hospital plan must be formulated to cope with these situations, and every member of staff must be conversant with the plan. Only visible facts are recorded about jewellery, for example a gold-coloured ring with a clear stone, *not* a gold ring with a diamond.

Patients' daytime and outdoor clothing is safest under lock and key in a wardrobe, at the bedside, or within the ward. Sometimes they are kept in a ward ancillary room or in a central clothes' store. In the last two instances each article needs to be clearly labelled with the owner's name.

Most people like to know the time of day and prefer to keep their wrist watch while in hospital; although a wall clock is provided in many wards, not all patients are capable of seeing it. Capable patients must understand that they are responsible for the safety of their own watches. When a patient is rendered unconscious for a short period by an anaesthetic, the staff accept the responsibility of locking up the watch and returning it when consciousness is regained. The watch belonging to an unconscious patient must be locked up until the time when the nurse can sensitively ascertain the patient's personal relationships, and this may have to await return of consciousness. To give an example of possible hazards, the legal next of kin, perhaps an ex-spouse, may not be in a meaningful relationship with the patient, whereas the 'significant other' may be a person of the same sex. Family quarrels can arise from the watch being given to a person whom the patient considers to be unsuitable.

Where personal night attire is worn it is usual to point out to the patient and his relative that the Health Board cannot accept the responsibility for such clothing. The patient and his relatives are responsible for it, though staff take every care to avoid loss of same (p. 105).

LOSS OF PERSONAL POSSESSIONS IN PROCESS CONTEXT

As nurses are gaining more confidence in using the accepted four phases of the process of nursing with the original objective of individualising nursing, they are beginning to realise that 'process thinking' can be used creatively in situations that do not result in using the customary documents which are associated with the four phases. The principle — helping patients to avoid loss of personal possessions — provides such an example.

Assessing

The document usually associated with this phase of the process is the patient assessment form. Very few of these forms request information about the patient's personal belongings, but considering the unpleasantness which can occur when patient's personal belongings go missing, perhaps too little attention has been paid to inclusion of such an item.

Even patients admitted from the waiting list who have had time to prepare for admission may not have given much thought to the fact that their handbag or wallet normally contains their cheque book, possibly a cash dispenser card, and various credit cards and they may not have thought of removing them. Patients who live alone may have felt that they did not want to leave these items in an empty house. The handbag or wallet of a newly admitted patient who had collapsed in the street or met with an accident while out shopping is likely to contain these articles.

The sort of questions which a nurse might bear in mind, but not necessarily ask, at an initial assessment could be — did the patient receive a brochure with information about personal possessions? Is the patient wearing jewellery unnecessarily, earrings for unpierced ears, ring with apparently precious stones and so on? Has the patient only a small amount of pocket money? Has the patient inadvertently brought in a cheque book, cash dispenser card or credit card? Is it understood that the Health Board cannot be responsible for loss of property? The patient may realise that only essential items should be retained and agree to have unnecessary items sent home and this will lessen anxiety.

The possibility of people being admitted from Accident and Emergency department while they are on holiday and likely to have large sums of money; when they are going to or coming from functions wearing expensive jewellery and clothes has already been mentioned. The patient will naturally be anxious about such possessions and while explaining the why and wherefore of what she is doing, the nurse will be reassuring and lessening anxiety. If the initial nursing assessment reveals any or all, or a combination of the already mentioned circumstances, the admitting nurse has two functions:

- to make a list of the patient's personal possessions and record them in the ward Property Book or whatever it is called, and have the description agreed with the patient if he is capable. If the patient is incapable, it is wise to have them agreed with another person. Only visible facts are recorded about jewellery, for example a gold-coloured ring with a clear stone, not a gold ring with a diamond; a dark brown, full length fur coat, not a natural mink coat
- to commit these personal possessions to safety. This may seem to an inexperienced nurse to be fulfilled by sending them 'home' with the 'accompanying person'. But an experienced nurse knows that great skill is needed to discover the relationship, which may be:
- a family member
- a professional/business acquaintance/ friend
- a peer who was involved in the accident and so on.

If there is any uncertainty, it is safer to have the possessions conveyed safely to a central locked store, accommodating, for example, long dresses on coathangers. Of course if there is an individual wardrobe by the bed it will suffice, so long as it is locked and the key kept in safe custody.

Planning

The document usually associated with this second phase of the process of nursing is the patient's nursing plan. In the older hospitals, the identified 'patient's problems', agreed with him, are likely to be:

- anxiety because he does not have access to a lockable area by the bed for safe-keeping of handbag or wallet, and private mail which may be brought in by visitors even for short-term patients, for example bank statements and credit card accounts. Patients are often away from the ward for long periods in other departments for investigations and so on.
- anxiety because he does not have access to a lockable wardrobe in which to keep day clothes. To be deprived of day clothes is an assault on one's self-image; the person no longer feels independent, confident, able to make decisions and so on. When a patient is up for an increasing number of hours each day in a rehabilitation programme, being dressed in day clothes helps him to identify with his previous daytime life-style.

Although the patient's problems have been clearly identified, they are not amenable to a clinical nursing intervention, so there is no point in writing them on the patient's nursing plan. But a nursing intervention could be to inform management of these requisites so that nurses can apply the principle of nursing — helping patients to avoid loss of personal possessions. The patient's problems are clearly amenable to managerial intervention, but they cannot be solved overnight. Solving them may be constrained by lack of available finance — or the ward may be on the upgrading programme for 3 years hence. However, if the ward staff know this, they can more readily accept the constraint on the quality of nursing carried out meantime.

Implementing

Implementing, the accepted third phase of the process, will depend on whether or not there is a planned nursing intervention to implement.

Thinking about any principle of nursing in process context must help us to understand nursing: the process must be our servant, not our master.

Evaluating

In the early days of using the process, writers who were grappling with the concepts pointed out that evaluating, the fourth phase was the least understood and indeed was frequently omitted, and there was, and still is justification for this. Gradually there seemed to be an increase towards consensus among those gaining more experience of using the process, that evaluating and assessing used the same skills, but evaluating was comparing the current patient status against the status recorded at the initial assessment to discover whether the planned nurse-initiated intervention had achieved the set goal to solve or alleviate the patient's problem. Currently, with even more experience in 'process thinking' we realise that the four phases of the process can be used creatively instead of rigidly. There is an example in the previous chapter (p. 246) and this chapter contains another example, using the definition in the Concise Oxford Dictionary of the word 'evaluate':

- ascertain amount of
- find numerical expression for
- appraise, assess.

It is reasonable for example, for a hospital to collect the number of incidents of loss of patients' personal possessions in each clinical area and to use it as an item in any one of the Quality Assurance programmes which are in use. Can you remember the name of any of them?

APPLYING THE PRINCIPLE

A registered nurse must be capable of:

- implementing the hospital plan related to the safety of patients' personal belongings
- ensuring that conscious patients understand their responsibility for their personal belongings in hospital
- applying the principle — helping patients to avoid loss of personal possessions – in a process of nursing context.

WORKING ASSIGNMENT

Topics for discussion

- the plan in your hospital for the safety of patients' personal belongings
- a patient informs you that some money is missing from the locker drawer
- Mr Jones is ready for discharge and his outdoor clothes are brought to the ward from the central stores. He says that his overcoat is missing.

Writing assignment

- write a short essay on 'Patients' personal possessions in hospital'.

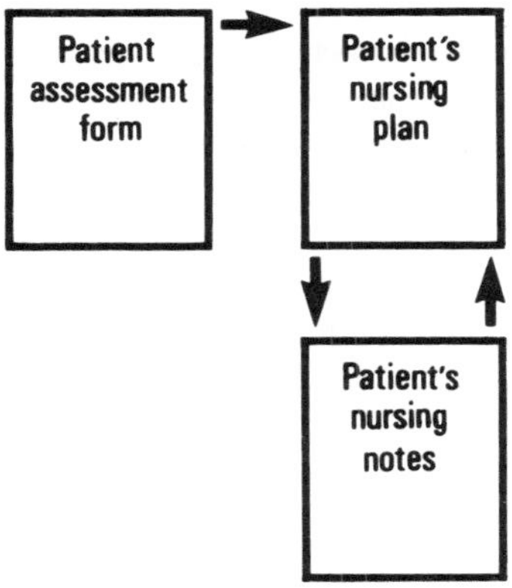

Reading assignment

Background information
Colonisation
Infection
Hospital-acquired infection
Barrier nursing
Handwashing

Community- and hospital-acquired infection and the process of nursing
Plan for assessing and evaluating handwashing

Applying the principle
A registered nurse must be capable of:

Working assignment
Topics for discussion
Writing assignment

20

Helping patients to avoid community- and hospital-acquired infection

READING ASSIGNMENT

Ayliffe G A G, Coates D, Hoffman P N 1984 Chemical disinfection in hospitals. Public Health Laboratory Service

Ayrton N A 1982 Last offices in cases of notifiable disease. The Journal of Infection Control Nursing 19 May: 5–6
The use of cadaver bags in controlling infection.

Ayton M 1985[1] Infection control — a question of balance. Nursing: The Add-On Journal of Clinical Nursing 2 (35) March: 1039– 1040
Contains an illustration of the three main types of hospital-acquired infection. Describes the infection control service.

Ayton M 1985[2] Infection control — protective clothing. Nursing: The Add-On Journal of Clinical Nursing 2 (38) June: 1136, 1138-1339
Discusses the use of gowns and aprons, gloves, masks, goggles, caps, overshoes.

Baker L F 1978 You can get rid of them. Nursing Times 74 (14) April 6: Contact 4–5
Infestation control in hospital.

Brunt M 1978 Bacteriological control in intensive therapy. Nursing Times 74 (16) April 20: 670–672

Burgess N R H, Chetwyn K N 1978 Cockroaches and the hospital environment. Nursing Times 74 (14) April 6: Contact 5–7
Cockroaches can act as a reservoir of pathogenic organisms which can be transmitted to food and utensils.

Casewell M, Phillips I 1977 Hands as a route of transmission for Klebsiella species. British Medical Journal 2 November 19: 1315–1317

Collins B J 1982 Microbial decontamination in hospitals. The Journal of Infection Control Nursing 19 May: 1–4
Describes some of the different methods — cleaning, disinfecting, sterilising, used in controlling infection.

Cowan M, Allen J 1986 Dirty linen. Nursing Times 82 (44) October 29: 36–37
Gives comprehensive guidelines for hospital laundering policies resulting from a study into the use of duvets in one hospital.

Deli-Tucker E, Campbell C 1986 The Friesen concept — a blueprint for care? Nursing Times 82 (6) February 5: 28–30
Each patient's room contains all the requisites for nursing. As they are used they are replaced by technicians' rounds. All the nurses' time is spent in patient contact. The nosocomial infection is 3–4%, compared with the national rate of around 9.0%.

Denton P F 1986 Psychological and physiological effects of isolation. Nursing: The Add-On Journal of Clinical Nursing 3 (3) March: 88, 90–91

Glenister H 1987 The passage of infection. Nursing Times 83 (22) June 3: 68, 71, 73 (The Journal of Infection Control Nursing)
Emptying catheter bags can result in cross-infection. Assesses the problem and looks at ways in which infection can be reduced; effective handwashing being an important contribution.

Grazebrook J 1986 Counting the cost of infection. Nursing Times 82 6 February 5: 24–26
A short history of the Infection Control nurse and how her work can make considerable savings by eliminating ritual practices, as well as making nursing more credible.

Gidley C 1987 Now, wash your hands! Nursing Times 83 (29) July 22: 40–42
Reports a small pilot study assessing nurses' handwashing technique and its appropriateness relative to the task just completed or immediately anticipated.

Griffiths G 1986 Preventive measures. Nursing Times 82 (38) September 17: 92, 95, 97
Describes the role of the Infection Control nurse.

Hawkins C, Taylor B E, Viant A C 1978 Use and abuse of phenolic disinfectants. Nursing Times 74 (14) April 6: Contact 4–5
Table of types of phenolic disinfectants, their strength and reason for use.

Hoffman P 1986 Disinfection in hospitals. Nursing: The Add-On Journal of Clinical Nursing 3 (3) March: 106–108
Gives a useful Table of properties of chemical disinfectants.

Holman R 1979 Our dirty hospitals. Nursing Times 75 (25) June 21: 1035

Larson E, Lusk E 1985 Evaluating handwashing techniques. Journal of Advanced Nursing 10: 547–552
Describes two tools, one for the appropriateness of handwashing, the other to evaluate the technique.

Lawrence M 1984 Patient hand hygiene — a clinical enquiry. Nursing Times 79 22: 24–25

Leonard M 1986 Handling infection. Nursing Times 82 (38) September 17: 81, 82, 84
Compares the effectiveness of an antibacterial soap and an alcoholic hand rub in reducing the transient flora on hands.

Meers P D, Stronge J L 1978 Hospitals...should do the sick no harm. Nursing Times Supplements
Part 1 76 (4) January 24
Part 2 76 (8) February 21
Part 3 76 (12) March 20
Part 4 76 (16) April 17
Part 5 76 (20) May 15
Part 6 76 (25) June 19

Nursing Standard 1985 Nurses told of wedding ring risk. Nursing Standard 381 January 24: 8
The Central Public Health Laboratory working with doctors at a London Hospital found that 20 out of 50 nurses had pathogenic bacteria beneath wedding rings.

Nursing Times 1984[1] Infections in hospital cost £2 billion. Nursing Times 80 (39) September 26: 8

Nursing Times 1984[2] More use should be made of IC nurses. Nursing Times 80 (38) September 19: 7
Describes how use can be made of Infection Control nurses.

Roper N (ed) 1987 Pocket medical dictionary, 14th edn. Churchill Livingstone, Edinburgh, p 35

Roper N, Logan W, Tierney A 1985 The elements of nursing, 2nd edn. Churchill Livingstone, Edinburgh, p 35

Rush D 1987 Infection control in ITU (Intensive Therapy Unit). Nursing: The Add-On Journal of Clinical Nursing 3 (15) March: 552–556
Discusses the microorganisms most commonly found as infecting agents, and patients' compromised immunological state. Infection control and the environment. Procedural measures in I.T.U.

Sedgwick J 1984 Handwashing in hospital wards. Nursing Times 80 (25) : 63–67
Reports a project in which the majority of hands were badly washed, with thumbs showing the greatest failure rate.

Sills G A 1986 Sterilization. Nursing 3 (3) March: 109–110
Discusses heat, gas, radiation, filtration and chemicals, and puts them in a Quality Assurance context.

Speechley V 1986 Intravenous therapy: peripheral central lines. Nursing: The Add-On Journal of Clinical Nursing 3 (3) March: 95–99
An illustration of intrinsic and extrinsic contamination during intravenous therapy.

Ward K 1985 Down the drain. Journal of Infection Control Nursing. Nursing Times 81 (49) December 4: 60–62

Webster M 1986 Control measures. Nursing Times 82 (6) February 5: 26-28
Describes the steps which were taken to combat an outbreak of multiply resistant *Staphylococcus aureus*.

Webster O, Bowell B 1986 Thinking prevention. Nursing Times 82 (23) June 4: 68, 70
Hospital staff must never relax their efforts to keep infection to a minimum. Describes a scoring system which aims to help nurses assess those patients most at risk.

BACKGROUND INFORMATION

Each student of nursing enters the programme with some idea of infection, microorganisms (germs) and infectious disease. Because microorganisms are invisible to the naked eye, things which 'look clean' (including hands) can have many and varied microorganisms on them. Soon after birth microorganisms establish a presence on the skin, in the bowel and respiratory tract, and around the urethral and vaginal orifices and the anus. They are the natural or resident flora and are sometimes referred to as commensals, and are said to 'colonise' the area, where they are not usually pathogenic, but they can become pathogenic if they move to another part of the body.

Colonisation

When the body's defence mechanisms (Roper, Logan & Tierney 1985) are working adequately, 'colonisation' does not become pathogenic, but when man, as host to these parasites, begins to respond to their presence, colonisation ends and 'infection' begins. The concept of colonisation is absolutely basic to understanding the prevention of hospital-acquired infection. Many nursing activities have as their objective preventing the status of colonisation from becoming that of infection.

Microorganisms forming part of the resident flora in the sites mentioned can cause infection if they gain access to another part of the body and this transfer is easily accomplished by hands. It is important therefore for nurses to help patients avoid this, by for instance offering hand-cleansing facilities after defaecation (Lawrence 1984).

As well as a resident flora, the skin can acquire and lose other microorganisms and this concept of a 'transient skin flora' is essential for nurses to understand the rationale of many of the nursing activities discussed in other chapters of this book. It is also important to realise that pathogenic microorganisms may well be part of the transient flora on the skin, especially the hands of both patients and staff in hospital.

Infection

What is infection? Roper (1987) defines it as 'the successful invasion, establishment and growth of microorganisms in the tissues of the host. It may be of an acute or chronic nature.' She goes on to describe hospital-acquired (nosocomial) infection as 'one which occurs in a patient who has been in hospital for at least 72 h and did not have signs and symptoms of such infection on admission.'

Hospital-acquired infection

Hospital-acquired infection is not only a problem in the UK. In 1983, a World Health Organization (WHO) advisory group was set up to collect data from 33 countries; it found that the average prevalence rate was 11.9% (Nursing Times 1984). WHO estimated that the financial cost was around $2 billion a year world wide. Patients over 64 years of age were the most susceptible, followed by babies under one year. The most common site for infection was the urinary tract (p. 257), wounds (p. 257) and the respiratory tract (p. 257). In view of the increased:

- discomfort to the patient
- pain
- length of stay in hospital
- danger to other patients and staff
- avoidable deaths, as well as
- strain on health care systems

the subject of hospital-acquired infection is of major importance in a nursing curriculum, particularly in the microbiology part of it. Items in the Reading Assignment are evidence of the breadth and complexity of the subject, and the references in them will guide students to further reading as they require more information during clinical allocations. In this text, however, only a basic broad overview is given.

The microorganisms on the skin adhere to the cells on the surface and as these are constantly being shed, the clothes and bedding in contact with the skin are impregnated with microorganisms. This is the reason for 'inrolling' the sides/ends of a sheet to the centre before removal (p. 172). Even though domestic duties are designated 'non-nursing', the infection control nurses (p. 92) advise on the methods to be used throughout the hospital and the charge nurse liaises with the domestic supervisor so that the standard of cleanliness in the ward is acceptable to the nurses. Because of the important part played by the ancillary staff in the prevention and control of hospital-acquired infection, it is recommended that in-service educational programmes are arranged for them.

Considering the vast number of microorganisms in and on people, in the atmosphere and on all surfaces, infections in human beings must be considered a relatively rare occurrence. This is because many of the organisms on skin and in the atmosphere are deprived of moisture and as mentioned, humans have a variety of protective mechanisms for dealing with their bacterial population (Meers & Stronge 1980:Part 6).

The subject of infection, its prevention and control are now so complex that many hospitals have appointed specially trained nurses to work in close association with a microbiologist, and together they are responsible for implementing and constantly monitoring the recommendations of the Control of Infection Committee. Many countries have an Infection Control Nurses Association and there are meetings at local, national and international level. *The Journal of Infection Control Nursing* is now published by Macmillan Journals and distributed in the *Nursing Times* several times each year. Readers will gain an adequate base of knowledge about the function of the infection control team, particularly the role of the Infection Control Nurse (ICN), by reading these entries in the Reading Assignment — Grazebrook (1986), Griffiths (1986) and Webster (1986).

The term 'hospital-acquired infection' is more descriptive than the older term 'cross infection' and the current term 'nosocomial infection'. However the 1980 prevalence survey of 43 hospitals in the UK indicated that approximately 20% of hospital patients had infections, and of these approximately 10% were community-acquired, that is were present on admission, and 10% were hospital-acquired. Table 20.1 shows sites and percentages:

Table 20.1 shows sites and percentages:

Site	%
urinary tract	30
wounds	20
respiratory tract	20
other	30
	100

Ayton M (1985) discusses the microorganisms involved. Each hospital should have a prevention of infection policy regarding such things as when and how to use for example disinfectants, antibiotics, decontamination, sterilisation, laundry and equipment, as well as safe clinical procedures. Hoffman (1986) gives guidance about disinfection in hospitals and Sills (1986) about sterilization; while Collins (1982) discusses some of the different reasons for wearing protective clothing and discusses gowns and aprons, gloves, masks, goggles, caps and overshoes.

Students of nursing may not readily appreciate that nurses have a responsibility to prevent *food poisoning* where there is communal feeding. Non-fingering of food and covering drinks and fruit on lockers are all contributions which the nurse can make, together with handwashing (p. 140) before meals for staff and patients. If arrangements are not made to centralise the washing up within the hospital, then the ward kitchen should be supplied with a dishwashing machine or twin sinks so that washed dishes and cutlery can be rinsed in very hot water. When removed they dry quickly; tea towels are then unnecessary. Closed-in, dust-free crockery racks are the safest place for crockery between meals.

The war-time slogan 'Coughs and sneezes spread diseases, trap them in your handkerchief' helped to cut down *respiratory infection* when many people spent the night huddled together in an air raid shelter. Since 50–60% of the population are now known to be nasal carriers of Staphylococci, 'Trap them in a paper handkerchief and throw it into a receptacle which can be closed', ought to be the current slogan, together with 'Ban material handkerchiefs' — for patients and staff in hospital. Plenty of paper tissue dispensers and disposal arrangements throughout the building will help people to observe these maxims. Ideally hands should be washed after nose-blowing and certainly if it is carried out during food preparation.

Barrier nursing

An infectious patient is 'isolated' from the others; *barrier nursing* is the term used to describe this skilled technique. The principle is to retain the infection within the 'barrier' and disinfect everything afterwards. The use of disposable items simplifies the procedure.

Patients with a very low resistance to microorganisms (for example those with agranulocytosis, leukaemia and those undergoing immunosuppressive treatment) are isolated. The principle is to prevent any microorganisms coming in contact with the patient. Everything that goes within the area must be sterile, and an elaborate régime has to be observed. The technique is sometimes referred to as *'reverse barrier nursing'*. Brunt (1978) describes the use of an isolator tent for this purpose.

Handwashing

Several writers state that handwashing is the most important procedure in preventing hospital-acquired infection. Few schools of nursing teach a handwashing technique for use in areas other than the operating theatre, yet after research into nurses' techniques, Taylor (1978) wrote:

> The implications of inadequate techniques are potentially serious, since the areas of the hands most often neglected are those which are most likely to come into contact with patients or materials (Fig. 20.1).

In the second part of the research project the number of handwashes and their quality, as well as the relationship to preceding activity (clean/dirty) was assessed in medical and surgical wards under normal working conditions for 1 hour (Taylor 1978). Table 20.2 shows the number of dirty activities not followed by handwashing. The research report's last paragraph reads:

> It is important that microorganisms in the inanimate and animate environment should be seen in the 'mind's eye'. No amount of sterile supplies, environmental disinfection or ritual procedures will protect the patient from an attendant with contaminated hands. Seventy per cent alcohol, if correctly applied, is an effective hand disinfectant. Its introduction as a routine measure for aseptic techniques should be supported by an intensive teaching programme and well defined indications for its use.

Casewell & Phillips (1977) in their report identify several nursing activities after which the nurses' hands were contaminated (Table 20.3). They wrote:

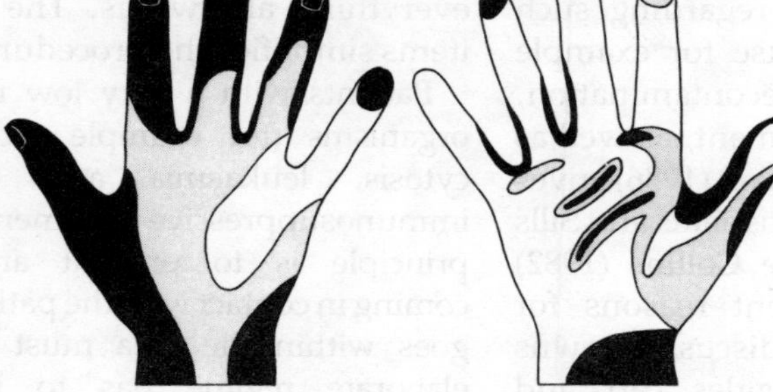

Fig. 20.1 Handwashing. Palm — right. Back — left.
Key: black = most frequently missed areas,
grey = less missed areas (Taylor 1978).

Table 20.2 Handwashes carried out by all grades of staff after clean and dirty activities (Taylor 1978)

	SRN	SEN	Learner	Auxiliary
Number of handwashes	25	25	28	17
Number of nurses performing handwashes	7/8	8/8	8/9	6/6
Number of handwashes after clean activities	13	16	15	9
Number of handwashes after dirty activities	12	9	13	8
Number of dirty activities not followed by handwashing	59%	64%	54%	72%

Table 20.3 Activities which contaminated the hands (Casewell & Phillips 1977)

lifting patients
general nursing
physiotherapy
taking blood pressure and pulse
washing patients
oral temperature
radial pulse
touching shoulder
touching groin
extubation
touching hand
touching tracheostomy

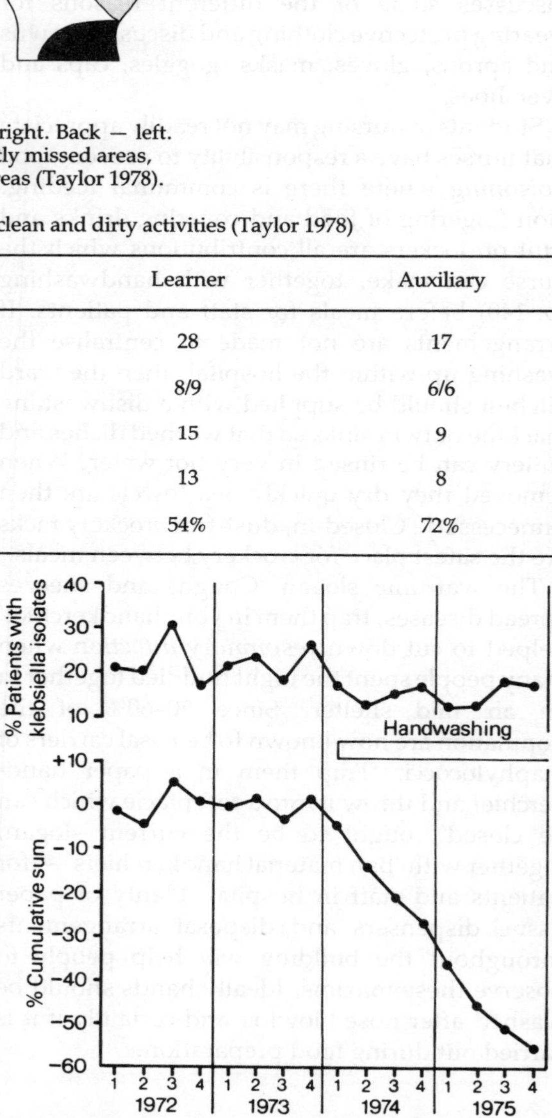

Fig. 20.2 Quarterly percentages of patients colonised or infected with Klebsiellae 1972–1975, and change in cumulative sum of percentages associated with staff handwashing (Casewell & Phillips 1977)

> Furthermore our results show that only slight contact with the patient's skin may be required for the transfer of 100 to 1000 viable Klebsiellae to the nurses' hands. These nurses considered that they had 'clean' hands, and would not normally have washed before attending another patient, unless they were about to undertake an aseptic technique.

Data collected over a 4-year period are demonstrated in Figure 20.2. The reduction in Klebsiella colonisation or infection of newly admitted patients that coincided with increased staff handwashing before moving from one patient to the next is clearly shown. Clorhexidine (4%w/v) hand cleanser was used for hand-washing and it proved to be an easy practical method. The fact that the reduction was sustained over a 2-year period provides perhaps the most convincing evidence that hands are a major route of transmission of hospital-acquired infection.

Although these two research reports are 10 years old, two more recent research projects — Larson & Lusk (1985) and Leonard (1986) — each reported poor technique of the nurses' actual handwashing and inappropriate time of handwashing. There are references in these two reports to the few other projects which were carried out in the early '80s with similar results. All reports stress the inadequacy of teaching about adequate handwashing technique. Here the activity is broken down into component steps:

- remove wrist watch and wedding ring (Nursing Standard 1985)
- hold each hand in a downward position
- place each in turn in the stream so that each palm including the wrist and bulbar eminence of the thumb and the back of the hand is wet
- apply whichever cleansing agent is recommended by the Control of Infection Committee to one palm
- massage the wrist, bulbar thumb eminences, fingers and palms against each other in horizontal movement until all creases are covered
- continue to massage — almost in a figure of eight movement so that the back of each hand including the fingers is adequately cleansed
- with the palmar surfaces of the fingers of one hand massage between the fingers and along the back of the other hand until adequately cleansed
- vice versa
- rinse both hands from the wrists and bulbar thumb eminence downwards, holding in the downward direction
- shake excess moisture from the hands
- dry the hands in the same sequence of movements according to the policy of the Control of Infection team. Where separate linen or paper towels are used, a receptacle with a pedal-operated lid must be provided for used ones.

There is evidence of wedding rings harbouring pathogenic organisms; removing them from the finger and wearing them on a neck chain could be a contribution to prevention of nosocomial infection (Nursing Standard 1985).

COMMUNITY- AND HOSPITAL-ACQUIRED INFECTION AND THE PROCESS OF NURSING

To help students to begin to think in 'process context' about this vast subject, we will start at the beginning, by making a brief survey of how this might be accomplished. The midwife, with the goal of preventing infection, will assess each new mother's understanding and practice of perineal and umbilical cord hygiene, as well as that of bottles, teats and nappies. If the assessment reveals inadequate knowledge and/or practice then the midwife can identify (with the mother) three potential problems:

- the mother's infected perineum
- the baby's infected cord
- infantile diarrhoea and/or vomiting which can be spread by the faecal-oral route, either directly or indirectly.

The plan will contain interventions in the form of teaching sessions; implementation will be recorded, and evaluation will have two dimensions — feedback from the mother about her understanding and practice after the teaching sessions; and whether or not the potential became actual problems. Diarrhoea and/or vomiting could be monitored on a long-term basis.

The health visitor will assess what parents know about, for example immunisation, and the infectious diseases which it can prevent. If their knowledge is deficient or inaccurate, do they have a problem? It might be expedient to state the goal at this point, which could be that they will be able to make an informed decision about whether or not their baby will participate in the immunisation programme. If they agree with this, the health visitor can plan to provide factual information of the many advantages, to be weighed against a few disadvantages. The plan will be implemented and the implementation recorded. As in the previous paragraph, evaluation will have two dimensions, feedback from the parents as to their understanding of the instruction, and the parents feeling comfortable with the choice they have made, and the health visitor feeling comfortable with their choice, particularly if the decision is against immunisation.

The community nurse may have to visit, for example, a patient who has an indwelling catheter and closed urinary drainage for the purpose of taking a monthly specimen of urine for culture of microorganisms because an indwelling catheter carries the potential problem of urinary tract infection. Another of the patient's problems is coming to terms with a changed body image and this may never be accomplished 100%, so a continued expression of interest is part of a high standard of nursing. Nurse will assess the patient's current state of knowledge and practice for achieving the goal of 'no urinary infection'. The criteria used in assessing might include:

- what does he understand about the possibility of urinary tract infection?
- how is the bag emptied?
- how often is the bag emptied?
- are the hands washed before and after emptying?
- how often is the urethral meatal area cleaned?
- how is it cleaned?
- how does the patient prevent the bag being raised above the level of the bladder?
- does he know that the connection of the fluted end of the catheter and drainage tube must remain intact?

Should there be deficits in any of these areas of knowledge and/or practice, the patient's nursing plan will contain interventions such as teaching and/or demonstration to deal with them. Implementation will be recorded on the patient's nursing notes and this may provide summative evidence on the set date for evaluation.

Almost every nursing activity carried out by hospital nurses has a dimension for prevention of hospital-acquired infection. The following list is not exhaustive but it gives an idea of the range of these activities:

- involving use of washbowls (p. 92)
- involving use of bathmats (p. 92)
- use of clinical thermometers (p. 223)
- use of invasive techniques:
  - injections (p. 286)
  - intravenous drips (p. 286)
  - catheterisation (p. 194)
- use of aseptic techniques:
  - wound dressings (p. 269)
  - pressure sores (p. 120)
  - preoperative preparation of skin (p. 309)
  - preoperative shaving (p. 310)

And the most important activity to prevent hospital-acquired infection is handwashing.

Plan for assessing and evaluating handwashing

To finish this chapter here is a suggested plan for assessing and evaluating handwashing:

- absence of wrist watch and wedding ring?
- were the hands held in a downward direction?
- was each, in turn, held under running water?
- was the wrist, palm, back of hand and bulbar eminence adequately wetted?
- were the palms, fingers and bulbar eminences massaged with a cleansing agent using a horizontal movement?
- was a figure of eight movement used to massage the cleansing agent over the back of the hands and fingers?
- were the palmar surfaces of the fingers of one hand used to massage the cleansing agent between the fingers and along the back of the other hand?

- were vice versa movements used?
- was excess moisture shaken from the hands?
- was a safe and efficient procedure used for hand drying?

An additional random objective evaluation could be incubation of laboratory culture plates impregnated with a swab taken from freshly washed hands.

In this chapter colonisation, infection, hospital-acquired infection, barrier nursing and handwashing were discussed before considering the principle — helping patients to avoid community- and hospital-acquired infection — in a process of nursing context. A plan for assessing and evaluating handwashing was suggested.

APPLYING THE PRINCIPLE

A registered nurse must be capable of:

- organising ward work in compliance with the principles of prevention and control of hospital-acquired infection
- organising ward work to prevent food poisoning
- recognising when barrier nursing is necessary
- carrying out and teaching a safe procedure for barrier nursing
- applying the principle — helping patients to avoid community- and hospital-acquired infection — in a process of nursing context.

WORKING ASSIGNMENT

Topics for discussion

- the particular policy for prevention of hospital-acquired infection in your hospital
- the particular method of barrier nursing in your hospital
- the policy in the hospitals to which you are allocated for use of the following — protective clothing: gowns and aprons, gloves, masks, goggles, caps and over-shoes
- the disadvantages of hospital-acquired infection
- does handwashing have to be taught?
- should there be random checks on the standard of each nurse's handwashing technique since it is the most important contribution to 'helping patients to avoid community and hospital-acquired infection?'

Writing assignment

- give the exact routine to be followed in your hospital to render the following articles hazard-free for patients:

  back rests
  bath mats
  baths/outlet
  bed cradles
  bedding
  bedpans
  bedsteads
  commodes and commode pans
  crockery
  cutlery
  denture containers
  lavatories
  mattresses
  pillows
  sanichairs
  sinks/outlet
  thermometers
  tooth cleaning tumblers and bowls
  urinals
  vomit bowls
  washing bowls
- name the requisites for growth and reproduction of bacteria
- name the routes by which bacteria can enter the body
- name the three most common sites involved in hospital-acquired infection
- name the factors concerned in the body's defence against infection
- make a list of factors concerned in the prevention of infection

- define the following (although there are some medical words in the list, they are introduced in a nursing context):

  a carrier
  antibacterial
  antibiotics
  antibodies
  agranulocytosis
  bacteria
  bactericide
  bacteriostatic
  barrier nursing
  body's defence mechanisms
  colonisation
  commensals
  decontamination
  diphtheria
  direct contact
  disinfectants
  disinfection
  fever
  fomites
  fungicide
  fungistatic
  germicidal
  hepatitis
  immunity
  immunosuppressive
  indirect contact
  infection
  ingestion
  inhalation
  inoculation
  leukaemia
  malaria
  measles
  natural flora
  nosocomial infection
  orifice
  parasites
  pasteurisation
  pathogenic
  perineum
  pus
  resident flora
  reverse barrier nursing
  saprophyte
  sepsis
  spore
  sputum
  sterilisation
  subclinical
  susceptibility
  transient flora
  tuberculosis
  typhoid fever
  umbilical cord

- give the exact routine to be followed in your hospital for the disinfection of faeces, sputum and urine.

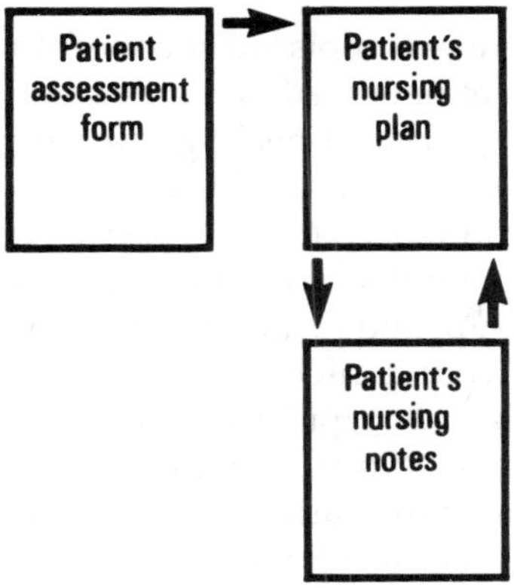

21

Helping patients to avoid hazards related to wounds

READING ASSIGNMENT

Allan D 1977 Complications of T-tube drainage of the common bile duct. Nursing Times 73 (33) August 18: 1270–1271
Function of T-tubes; complications; removal and breakage.

Ayliffe G A J 1978 Screening of hospital staff for *Staphylococcus aureus*. Nursing Times 74 (4) April 6: Contact 6
Gives the reasons why routine nasal swabbing for carriers is unnecessary.

Ayton M 1987 A healing process. Senior Nurse 6 (4) April: 21–23
Wound healing is a delicate process which needs to be understood and nurtured. Outlines the physiological steps involved and discusses the nurse's need to keep up to date.

Ayton M 1985 Wounds that won't heal. Community Outlook November: 16–17, 19
Suggests some ideas for dealing with large chronic wounds in the community.

Bayliss D 1979 New cure for an old problem. Nursing Mirror 149 (7) August 16: 34–36
Synthaderm used on a leg ulcer; dressing has a hydrophilic surface and a hydrophobic backing to create a micro-environment in which epidermal regeneration occurs.

Calmic Medical Division 1985 How wounds heal: a practical guide for nurses. The Calmic Medical Division of The Wellcome Foundation Ltd

Contains multiple choice questions, and some 'case problems' for private study or group discussion.

Cornwall J V (1986) The treatment of leg ulcers. Nursing: The Add-On Journal of Clinical Nursing 3 (6) June: 203–204, 206–208
Describes a classification of ulcers and how they become infected.

David J 1986 Practical Nursing Handbook. Wound management: a comprehensive guide to dressing and healing. Martin Dunitz, London

Draper J 1985 Make the dressing fit the wound. Nursing Times 81 (41) October 9: 32–35
The bias of some ward sisters to certain products used for awkward wounds may hamper the healing process. Argues that knowledge of all available products is necessary to turn a 'hit and miss' process into an exact one. Has a Table of details of some widely used products.

Davis B, Blenkharn I 1987 On the right track. The Journal of Infection Control Nursing. Nursing Times 83 (22) June 3: 64, 66, 68
Sophisticated technical explanation of suction apparatus which was found to be the culprit, but the account of tracking down the source of infection is important basic knowledge.

Dowding C M, Horn S 1986 Scars: formation and effects. Nursing: The Add-On Journal of Clinical Nursing 3 (6) June: 198, 200–202
Patients need as much skilled help in reconstructing their damaged selves as in mending their damaged body tissue. In some countries, scars are a form of beauty and have a social message, for example, that a girl is of marriageable age.

Gould D 1984 Clinical forum. Nursing Mirror 159 (16) October 31: iii–iv
Wound healing depends on the general physiological state of the patient as well as the specific micro-environment of the wound itself. Gives the characteristics of an optimum dressing. Each patient and each wound require individual assessment, planning and treatment.

Ingleston L 1986 Make haste slowly. Nursing Times 82 (37) September 10: 28–30
Describes how an outdated, ritualised wound dressing procedure was replaced successfully after careful trials of new method.

Jaber F 1986 Charting wound healing. Nursing Times 82 (37) September 10: 24–25, 27
Illustrates a wound chart to assist in evaluation of a patient's wounds to ensure systematic follow-up, and to identify incipient or postoperative wound infection.

Johnson A 1984 Towards rapid tissue healing. Nursing Times 80 (48) November 28: 39–43
An understanding of the basic mechanisms of wound healing is fundamental to the planning of care for each individual wound. A Table gives a protocol for the treatment of ulcers using Granuflex Hydroactive dressings, and another gives time of healing.

Johnson A 1986 Cleansing infected wounds. Nursing Times 82 (37) September 10: 30, 32, 34
Describes a small trial (18 patients) to evaluate the efficacy of Debrisan macrogol paste in eliminating pathogens from stasis ulcers. Cost of using this method compared favourably with using topical antibiotics without the risk of resistant microorganisms.

Johnson A 1986 Dressings and rehabilitation. Society for Tissue Viability. Edinburgh Conference Supplement September: 3–5
A case report illustrating the benefit of a new 'odour eating' dressing — Lyofoam C.

Johnson A 1987 Wound healing under the microscope. Community Outlook January: 12–13, 15
An in-depth look at the healing process. A list of dressings to aid natural healing. Wound site must be kept at 37°C; minimal exposure; removing dressings some time before a doctor's round should be discouraged.

Macfie J, Cowell M, Pawsey G, Bancroft J, McMahon M 1979 A liquid alternative to gauze. Nursing Mirror 149 (5) August 2: 30–32
Viscous elastomex poured into open granulating wounds; it sets into a soft pliable 'stent'; removed daily and washed in antiseptic solution; patient baths, after which, stent replaced.

Maggs F A P 1980 Medical uses of charcoal cloth. Nursing Mirror 151 (4) July 24: 45
A dressing for malodorous wounds; air purification; heating blankets.

Robertson J C 1986 Wound healing — the problems. CARE The British Journal of Rehabilitation and Tissue Viability. 1 (1): 4–6
... wounds which can be further damaged by bad dressings and infection. The whole patient has to be considered for the whole 24 hours, as well as the wound, otherwise opportunities for avoiding harm and optimising care may be lost.

Sherman L 1979 A pinch of salt. Nursing Times Community Outlook 75 (45) November 8: 355, 356, 358
Salt has no antibacterial properties other than that some bacteria do not grow in solutions with a high salt content.

Sims R, Fitzgerald V 1986 Wound care in the community. Nursing: The Add-On Journal of Clinical Nursing 3 (6) June: 209–210, 212–213, 215
Useful headings — Assessment and care planning. Wound care products. Disposal of dressings. Patient education. Aspects of wound management. Cleansing. Debridement. Control of wound odour.

Stronge J L, Meers P D 1980 Hospitals ... should do the sick no harm 8 The infection of wounds. Nursing Times 76 (34) August 21: Supplement
A classification of surgical wounds; 24% of hospital-acquired infections are wounds.

Taylor V 1980 Meeting the challenge of fistulas and draining wounds. Nursing 80 (June): 45–51
Turns problems into challenges; assessing the patient with a fistula or draining wound.

Thomas S, Dawes C, Hay P 1980 A critical evaluation of some extensible bandages in current use. Nursing Times 76 (26) June 26: 1123–1126
Cotton crêpe or cotton stretch bandages perform better, and are less expensive than crêpe bandages.

Torrance C 1986 The physiology of wound healing. Nursing: The Add-On Journal of Clinical Nursing 3 (5) May: 162–164, 166, 168
The sequence of events in wound healing are described in four phases which calls for ongoing assessment and changes in the nursing plan.

Vallé-Jones J 1979 Giving a leg-up to 'bad legs'. Nursing Mirror 149 (10) September 6: 43
Trial of a cream, Flamazine, on 10 patients with varicose ulcers; Table shows successful results.

Williams C M 1986 Wound healing: a nutritional perspective. Nursing: The Add-On Journal of Clinical Nursing 3 (7) July: 249–251
Discusses the nutritional physiological consequences of trauma; nutritional support and requirements; the malnourished patient. Gives a Table of some conditions and treatments which may predispose to malnutrition and poor wound healing.

BACKGROUND INFORMATION

The word 'wound' is probably most commonly interpreted by the majority of beginning students of nursing as a 'surgical' wound. Television documentaries may well have contributed to your idea of an 'operation': at the beginning the skin and underlying tissues are incised, and at the end, in most instances, the patient has a 'clean stitched wound'. But a wound can also result from a blow, missile or stab; a 'nonsurgical cut', perhaps from flying glass might be an incised wound with continuous edges; or in the case of other flying debris, it could be a lacerated wound with jagged edges. Other wounds include injury to the skin from:

- chemicals
- cold (frost bite)
- friction (climbers are at risk when using ropes)
- heat
  - — dry heat causing burns
  - — moist heat causing scalds
- pressure (from an overlying plank, girder and so on)
- rays (sunburn, radiotherapy).

Wounds can also be a manifestation in the skin of internal conditions, examples being pressure sores (p. 115); ulcers (Cornwall 1986); and gangrene which has many causes. Applying the principle of 'helping patients to avoid hazards related to wounds' is therefore not the prerogative of the general surgical wards to which you will be allocated, but the principle can be applied to patients in for example:

- Accident and Emergency department
- burns unit (which may cater for patients of all ages, and from distant places in the region)
- children's ward (in a general hospital it is likely to cater for children whatever the medical diagnosis: in a children's hospital it can be medical, surgical, orthopaedic and so on)
- the community
- geriatric ward
- gynaecological ward
- intensive care unit
- medical ward
- orthopaedic ward (which may cater for patients of all ages)
- urology ward.

This list is not exhaustive, it is merely to introduce the idea that clinical experience of a particular kind (in this instance related to wounds) will not only be found in a clinical area bearing a surgical label. As you gain experience as a student, and later as a registered nurse, you will realise that there are many other highly specialised areas where the principle has to be applied.

AVOIDING HAZARDS RELATED TO WOUNDS IN PROCESS CONTEXT

In the last decade there has been an explosion in increased knowledge about wound healing and the number of items in the Reading Assignment, with their many references to journals of several disciplines, are indicative of this. The message is clear from several of them that the focus must be on the patient, not the wound. A nurse and a clinical psychologist (Dowding & Horn 1986) remind us of the meaning of scars and disfigurement, and they discuss adolescence, and sexuality. They quote a research report which shows that those who had previous knowledge of the size of wound to be expected, avoided patient dissatisfaction with technically satisfactory surgery. Other articles show the depth of physiological knowledge required to understand the healing of wounds, but at the same time point out that the 'whole patient' requires to be assessed and planned for (Robertson 1986, Sims & Fitzgerald 1986, Torrance 1986). And it is encouraging that cognisance is being given to the process of nursing. Continuing these themes the four phases of the process will be discussed first in relation to the patient, and then to the wound.

Related to patient

Glancing back at the many different clinical areas in which patients with different sorts of wounds might be found, it will be realised that a text cannot possibly capture the individuality of the patient which provides the base for individualising nursing — the objective in using the process of nursing.

In the Accident and Emergency department, the experienced nurse in a matter of seconds will have 'assessed' the patient by using her clinical judgement, and she will have decided, for example, what has to be done to keep the patient alive, which decision will be followed by appropriate action. In the case of a patient who has an earth-contaminated wound, when he is in a stable condition, he will be asked about tetanus immunisation and the decision made as to whether he needs a tetanus boost or an injection of tetanus antitoxin, and this will be recorded, as the ward nurses need to know so that they can observe (ongoing assessment) for any reaction. The temperature will be measured, the pulse and respiration counted. A rise in temperature will probably not be indicative of infection (the usual cause), but in patients who have suffered tissue injury, it will be due to the release of pyrogens as explained by Gooch (p. 229). Away from the drama of the Accident and Emergency department, there will be patients to be assessed:

- who have been admitted for a surgical operation
- who require specialised investigations before a final decision about surgery

- who already have a wound, including a pressure sore or an ulcer.

Some of these patients may have a medical diagnosis which could interfere with wound healing, examples being:

- one of the many forms of anaemia
- one of the arthritic conditions
- chronic heart failure
- chronic kidney disease
- diabetes
- one of the malabsorption syndromes
- malignancy
- one of the muscular dystrophies.

and there are so many more, but enough has been said to alert the beginning student of nursing to the necessity for assessing the patient's understanding of his 'medical' condition, and the nurse's understanding of the consequences for wound healing.

The general requisites to avoid hazards related to wounds are adequate nutrition and hydration (p. 147); sleep because it facilitates cellular regeneration (p. 59), freedom from pain (p. 62), and information about assessing, planning, implementing and evaluating these is to be found in other parts of this text. Consequently applying the principle 'helping patients to avoid hazards related to wounds', in process context, to a particular patient who is well nourished and hydrated; sleeps satisfactorily and states that he is not experiencing pain, may not require a direct entry on the nursing documents, whereas it is pertinent to record the four phases of the process related to all wounds.

Related to wound

Because of the knowledge explosion related to the healing of wounds, the accepted four phases of the process of nursing have become vitally important in recording the 'history' of each wound. Many factors affect the 'history' such as type of wound, state of wound, discharge from wound, odour of wound discharge and drainage from wounds, so they will be discussed in this order, in the context of assessing, which of course is not a once-only activity, but includes ongoing assessment.

Assessing the wound

Most of the problems identified from assessment data will not be experienced by the patient because they are potential ones, identified by the nurse using her specialist knowledge. Wounds are so individual, only a general scheme can be offered for the nurse to bear in mind when assessing them. However, considerable information about the intricacies of assessing pressure sores (p. 116) is relevant here.

type of wound:
- abrasion (excoriation); superficial layer of skin removed by traumatic friction. Some pressure sores start in this way (p. 115, superficial)
- surgically incised
- non-surgically incised (flying glass, knife wound)
- lacerated (jagged edges)
- pressure sore (decubitus ulcer)
- other ulcers
- gangrene

state of wound:
- is there undue redness?
- is there any swelling? (may be a haematoma)
- is there bruising?

discharge from wound:
- is there any discharge?
- is it serous?
- is it blood-stained serum?
- is there frank blood?
- is there pus?

odour of wound discharge:
- is there any malodour? malodour can cause several patients' problems, for example:
  — the stench is in my nose, and I cannot eat
  — the house stinks and I can't invite friends to visit
  — I cannot visit friends.

Maggs (1980) describes the use of charcoal cloth for malodourous wounds, and Johnson (1986) describes the use of a new 'odour eating' dressing Lyofoam "C". Sims & Fitzgerald (1986) give useful advice in their last paragraph.

Wound drainage: ongoing assessment will provide summative/cumulative evaluation data related to the type and amount of drained fluid. Drainage may be active; the drain is attached to suction apparatus producing a 'closed drainage system'. There is a serious potential problem of suction apparatus acting as a reservoir for hospital-acquired infection. Drainage can be passive, when the drain provides a path of least resistance to the skin and the exudate seeps into a surgical dressing. It is used for as short a time as possible because it provides a route for microorganisms to enter the body.

Planning

If assessing reveals the actual problems from malodour suggested previously, it will result in nursing interventions to overcome them, such as dressing the wound more frequently: timing the dressing so that it is equidistant between meals; increasing ventilation; using air fresheners and so on together with the use of charcoal as mentioned previously to achieve the set goals which might be:

- no odour
- improved appetite
- patient socialising in previous pattern.

Even with a clean stitched wound, infection is a potential problem perceived by the nurse. However spraying it with a soluble acrylic resin minimises the risk; a transparent elastic film is formed which permits the passage of air and water vapour but is impervious to bacteria. The goal will obviously be an uninfected healed wound with minimal scar.

The goal for an infected wound will be to render it uninfected so that the healing process can begin and can end with minimal scar. Johnson (1984) in 'Towards rapid tissue healing' illustrates in a Table the project protocol used for a study of ulcers: if infected follow this regime; if clinically clean follow this régime. The article by Robertson (1986) is at an introductory level. To thoroughly understand the article by Torrance (1986) a considerable knowledge of physiology is required, but on pages 166 and 168 the effects of wound dressings are described and he points out that 'no single dressing will be suitable for all wounds'. Johnson (1987) gives even more detailed and in-depth study of healing. He classifies the new primary dressings designed to aid natural healing as:

- semipermeable adhesive films
- hydrocolloids
- hydrogels
- polysaccharide dextranomers
- polyurethane foams

and each group of dressings can be used for specific purposes. He makes the point that the wound should be kept warm and advises — remove the dressing immediately before inspection, and then redress immediately. As healing is a sequential process, evaluating that one stage is complete and the next beginning, may result in a changed nursing intervention on the patient's plan, yet the goal can remain unchanged.

Selection of the nursing intervention may be affected by availability of resources such as:

- cleansing lotions
- types of dressing
- materials to secure dressings in position

but the intervention must be written unambiguously so that any nurse can carry it out. Nurses may need to 'plan' so that the dressing trolley will be available, for example in wards where team nursing, patient allocation or primary nursing (p. 21) is being practised there may be only one trolley, not necessarily because of lack of money but of storage space.

Implementing

The older nursing texts paid considerable attention to damp dusting to prevent dust dissemination; to the fact that 1 hour should have elapsed after bedmaking before dressings were done. There was to be no smoking and as little talking as possible during a 'dressing round'. The clean wounds were dressed before the infected ones. However after antibiotics were introduced much less attention was paid to these aspects; domestic work became a non-nursing duty. But as strains of microorganisms are becoming resistant to an increasing number of antibiotics — multiply resistant, and the presence of methicillin-resistant Staphylococci is causing great concern — there is an upsurge of interest in preventing dust dissemination in, for example, bedmaking (p. 169).

The individualised planned nursing interventions will be implemented and each time it will be recorded on the patient's nursing notes together with ongoing assessment information re the state of the wound. If in the nurse's professional judgement, knowledge and previous experience she considers that the next nursing intervention should be changed, this will be written on the nursing plan.

Ingleston (1986) describes how an outdated ritualised wound dressing procedure was replaced successfully after careful trials of the new method. Masks are not worn: plastic apron put on at the beginning of dressings. Hands are washed at the beginning and end of the procedure and after removing the soiled dressing. The project tried using an alcoholic hand wipe which was bacteriologically acceptable but it caused skin problems for some nurses. The trolley is washed daily with detergent and only cleaned between dressings if it is physically soiled or contaminated. There will be an exact way in which 'aseptic'/'non-touch' technique is to be used in the hospitals where you work, not only for surgical dressings but also for any invasive technique. It will have been agreed by the Control of Infection Committee and to be accountable, nurses must observe the recommendations of these specialists.

Evaluating the wound

It is customary to interpret the fourth phase of the process of nursing — evaluating — as taking place on a set date, to discover whether or not the set goals have been achieved. The original factual account of the wound will be a starting point. This will be on the assessment form for those who had a wound on admission; and for others it will be on the patient's nursing notes on the day of operation. Thereafter for both sorts of wounds, there is likely to be summative/cumulative information contributing to the 'requested evaluation on a particular date'. From articles in the Reading Assignment, use of the new primary dressings designed to aid natural healing (p. 268) has decreased healing time to a maximum of 50 days in one study (Johnson 1984) from double figures in months. In such trials coloured photographs of the wound provide ongoing and final evaluation. But in their day to day work in the wards, nurses use their increasing knowledge about wound healing; their increasing skill in observing and interpreting subtle changes in the wound: recognising when a change to another dressing will facilitate the next stage of healing, and deciding to act on this recognition, and these are all part of the concept of 'clinical judgement'.

This chapter started by describing various types of wound and considered the variety of clinical allocations in which a student of nursing might gain experience in caring for a patient who has a wound. The principle — helping patients to avoid hazards related to wounds — was then discussed in process of nursing context.

APPLYING THE PRINCIPLE

A registered nurse must be capable of:

- using and teaching a safe technique for wound dressing: in a treatment room, in a ward
- using knowledge about the healing of wounds when dressing wounds
- using knowledge about microbiology when dressing wounds
- writing details of the planned particular wound treatment on the patient's nursing plan so that a nurse on any shift can carry out the individualised treatment
- evaluating and recording progress/deterioration of a particular wound in the patient's nursing notes.

- applying the principle — helping patients to avoid hazards related to wounds — in process context

WORKING ASSIGNMENT

Topics for discussion

- the particular method of doing a dressing in your hospital
- special room for dressings v. doing dressings in the ward
- non-touch technique
- Central Sterile Supplies Department
- the effect on self-image of visible scar on those parts not usually covered by daytime clothes
- the effect on self-image of a scar on those parts usually covered by daytime clothes.
- looking to the future — you are an experienced registered nurse! In your professional judgement a wound requires application of a particular dressing which is not currently provided by the Health Board of which you are an employee. What can you do about it?

Writing assignment

- make a list of the sequence of activities when dressing a wound
- define the following:

  anaemia
  antibiotics
  arthritis
  cellular activity
  clean stitched wound
  debridement
  diabetes
  enzymic activity
  exudate
  gangrene
  haematoma
  incised wound
  lacerated wound
  malabsorption syndrome
  malignancy
  microenvironment
  microvascular
  muscular dystrophies
  pathogens
  pus
  pyrogens
  serous
  tetanus antitoxin
  tetanus immunisation
  topical
  ulcer.

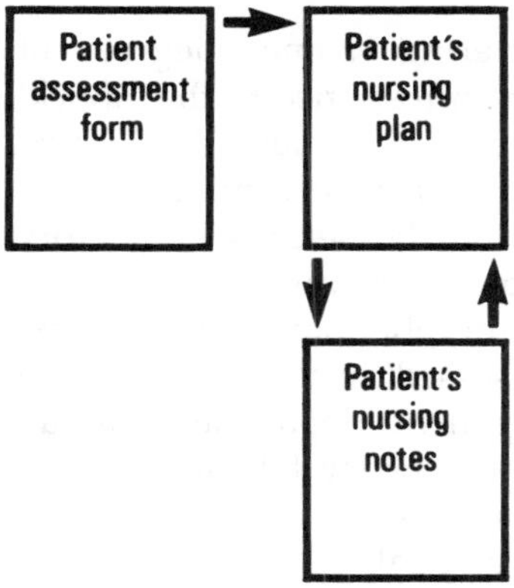

Reading assignment

Background information

The patient in a plaster cast in process of nursing context
Assessing
Planning
Implementing
Evaluating

Applying the principle
A registered nurse must be capable of:

Working assignment
Topics for discussion
Writing assignment

22

Helping patients to avoid hazards associated with plaster casts

READING ASSIGNMENT

Benz J 1986 The adolescent in a spica cast. Orthopaedic Nursing 5 (3) May/June: 22–23

Chilman A, Thomas M 1987 Understanding nursing care, 3rd edn. Churchill Livingstone, Edinburgh, p 56–59
Care of patients in plaster: care of the cast; turning the patient; placing patient on bedpan

Cuddy C M 1986 Caring for the child in a spica cast: a parent's perspective. Orthopaedic Nursing 5 (3) May/June: 17–21

Loder J 1986 The case for combination casts. Nursing Times 82 (45) November 5: 49
Plaster of Paris casts have lost popularity in favour of new expensive casting materials; yet a combination is worth its weight in cost-saving and effectiveness.

Pearce E 1980 A general textbook of nursing. Faber & Faber, London, p 255–256
Application of plaster of Paris; its use as an external splint.

Roper N, Logan W, Tierney A 1985 The elements of nursing, 2nd edn. Churchill Livingstone, Edinburgh, p 36

Shesser L K, Kling T F 1986 Practical considerations in caring for a child in a hip spica cast: an evaluation using parental input. Orthopaedic Nursing 5 (3) May/June: 11–15

Wytch R, Mitchell C 1986 Getting plastered. Nursing Times 82 (36) September 3: 48–50
Gives a list of new splinting materials and

describes their advantages and a few disadvantages.

BACKGROUND INFORMATION

Most beginning students of nursing will be familiar with the fact that plaster casts can be applied to the upper and lower limbs. They may not know that a plaster cast can also be applied to the lower trunk and one lower limb (a single hip spica); to the lower trunk and both lower limbs (a double hip spica), and to the upper trunk and one shoulder (a shoulder spica).

In general, plaster casts to an upper limb leave the fingers and lower portion of the thumb exposed. They are usually applied after a fracture to immobilise the bone ends so that they can heal in 6 to 8 weeks. Similarly plaster casts to a lower limb leave the toes exposed and are usually applied for the same reason, but the bone ends take up to 3 months or longer to heal.

Approximately 30 years ago all casts were made of plaster of Paris (Chilman & Thomas 1987, Loder 1986, Wytch & Mitchell 1986), but the last-named consider that it has poor strength to weight ratio, and a rapid loss of strength in contact with water. They discuss several newer but more expensive agents, while Loder (1986) is in favour of a combination of one of the expensive agents and plaster of Paris which is cheaper. From the information in these two articles it would seem that nurses have a responsibility to discover the drying time of the applied cast; and the time which should elapse before weightbearing on the applied cast is safe.

The application of a plaster cast is rarely a nursing duty; it is usually applied in a plaster room by a highly qualified technician. Patients who have a cast applied to an upper limb for a fracture are often treated as outpatients: they are given a list of instructions for which they sign. It is the nurse's responsibility to check by question and answer, the patient's understanding of these instructions, about which more will be said later.

THE PATIENT IN A PLASTER CAST IN PROCESS OF NURSING CONTEXT

The person requiring application of a plaster cast because of a fracture will be frightened, anxious and probably suffering some degree of physiological change in response to the 'shock' to the nervous system — minimally it might be tremor of the hands which he cannot control, and maximally it could be serious circulatory collapse. Roper, Logan & Tierney (1985) give a succinct account of the phenomenon of shock. The patient to be 'assessed' in a nursing context may be in an outpatient department; in an orthopaedic ward in a general hospital, in a children's ward in a general hospital, or in a special orthopaedic hospital.

Assessing

The objective in collecting information at the initial assessment is to identify problems which the patient is experiencing that are amenable to nurse-initiated intervention. For instance, after a fracture such a patient's problems might be:

- pain
- feeling anxious because a bone is broken
- anxious about how long it will take the bone to heal
- anxious about what he will be able/not be able to do with the plaster in position
- how long he will be away from school/work and so on.

Nurses may learn some of the constraints in carrying out everyday living if a thick bandage is applied to the preferred hand and left on for 24 hours. How does one manage washing and bathing; going to the lavatory? What if sleeves do not accommodate the plaster?

There follows a suggested scheme which can be borne in mind during the initial assessment of a limb to which a cast has been applied; then perhaps hourly for the first 4 hours, and then maybe twice daily as an ongoing assessment tool; or immediately if there is any pain:

- pain : in the enclosed area is reported to the doctor immediately: it may herald plaster sore, pressure sore, ischaemia } serious complications
- pressure : while the cast is damp do not apply any pressure which will dent the plaster

- drying : dry by keeping cast exposed to air; an electric fan or hair dryer can be used
- heat : do not put a hot water bottle in direct contact, as plaster is a good conductor of heat and a burn can result
- blanching : if pressure is applied to a nail or skin, it blanches; normally when released, colour returns in a few seconds: continued blanching is evidence of arterial deficiency
- blueness : either due to bruising of tissues when the digits were held during application of cast; or interference with venous drainage (local cyanosis)
- swelling : same causes as blueness: if it does not respond to raising the limb for several hours, for example using a bed elevator or a protected pillow, it must be reported to the doctor
- motor nerve integrity : ask patient to move fingers and/or toes as appropriate to prove that nerve pathway from brain to muscle is intact
- sensory nerve integrity : pinch digits to discover whether patient can 'feel' the touch
- 'pins and needles' (paraesthesia) : may be symptomatic of nerve compression

Returning to the patient who has a cast applied as an outpatient, and thereafter goes home with written instructions, a useful practical exercise for readers would be to discover the instructions given to outpatients in the hospitals to which they are allocated. Does it say anything about 'preferred hand'? Does it say anything about wetting and soiling of the cast? Are there any suggestions about how everyday living activities might be managed? As a further exercise in 'process thinking' you might consider the fact that the patient knows the state of his fingers on leaving hospital, that is, on initial assessment. As he carries out the instructions, is he carrying out ongoing assessment in the form of 'patient intervention'?

Some actual problems may be identified by using the previously suggested assessment list. But there are many nurse-perceived potential problems which older nurses might well call 'possible complications'. They will only be written on the nursing plan if they manifest as actual problems: they are yet another example of information which nurses require to 'hold in reserve' while carrying out nursing activities. They are listed here; there cannot be an order of priority and they include physical, psychological and social aspects of the problems.

Potential problems:

- stiffness of joints
- weakness of muscles
- lack of nutrients required for bone healing and growth in children; healing after fracture or bone surgery in adults
- inpatients may have a long stay so that young children can have insufficient constructive play activities; older children's education can be disrupted, and adults can be bored which is not conducive to effective healing
- lack of family finance for members travelling to hospital and bringing a gift or even sheer necessities such as soap and shaving cream
- changed body image
- lessened patient self-esteem perhaps because the family is functioning satisfactorily without them
- mental stress, perhaps from feelings of guilt
- physical and psychological problems in passing urine and faeces into sanitary utensil which is difficult to place against a rigid cast
- psychological problem for female patients with a hip spica when they are menstruating.

Planning

The second phase of the process by custom results in setting goals for the patient's actual (and potential) problems; deciding which nursing/patient interventions will be required to achieve the goals. All these will be written on the patient's plan to individualise the nursing which is planned for him.

Because pain is such a valuable indication of something going wrong under the plaster, medical policy may be to avoid strong analgesics. Comforting measures such as 'keep patient fresh and cool', 'apply cold compress to forehead' and distracting activities such as knitting may be written as nursing interventions on the patient's plan. Interventions to prevent plaster sores may include sweeping out particles of plaster and food crumbs, using a soft, long handled brush. Preventing pressure sores (p. 116) will call for ingenuity because of the restrictions imposed by the rigid cast: when a satisfactory solution has been found it should be written on the nursing plan so that nurses on succeeding shifts can benefit from the ingenuity and carry out the 'planned' nursing.

Implementing

Current thinking about implementing, the third phase of the process of nursing, is that as each planned intervention is carried out it is recorded on the patient's nursing notes. But many of the day to day interactions between nurse and patient are not 'planned' in the sense that they are not written on the nursing plan. For example, a nurse might sense that a patient in a plaster cast seems to be preoccupied, and at an appropriate time she offers an opportunity for discussion, during which an actual problem of financial difficulty is identified, and the patient accepts the offer of a visit from a social worker. Looking back at the list of potential problems readers will realise the importance of having this information in reserve, to be used when appropriate. Thinking in 'process context' need not be a rigid interpretation of the four phases: it certainly permits the creative part of nursing which is its art.

Evaluating

Turning to suggested patients' problems which are amenable to nursing intervention (p. 272), evaluation of pain will depend on how it was assessed. If it were written as the patient described it, then the patient's current description of it, or statement of its absence, will be compared with the stated goal which may well be 'not experiencing pain'. Information might be collected about whether or not the comforting measures had improved the pain experience; there may be summative/cumulative information on the patient's nursing notes.

The anxiety related to a broken bone may well have lessened after the nurse explored the patient's knowledge of, and attitude to a broken bone; filling in any discrepancies, and explanation that the cast will keep the bone ends together (in apposition) so that they can heal, should lessen anxiety. Factual information about the approximate time it will take the bone to heal should also contribute to lessened anxiety. Nurses' knowledge about what patients can and cannot do when enclosed in the different casts will be variable. Some may have personal experience and it is worth learning from them, so that the advice given to patients is as comprehensive and realistic as possible. If an anxiety scale was used at the initial assessment, its re-use would provide information as to whether the patient's current anxiety level had increased or decreased and by how much.

In the background information at the beginning of the chapter the various kinds of plaster were discussed. Then the principle — helping patients to avoid hazards associated with plaster casts — was considered in a process of nursing context.

APPLYING THE PRINCIPLE

A registered nurse must be capable of:

- safe and efficient nursing after application of a plaster cast
- recognizing excessive stress in patients who have a plaster cast

- applying the principle — helping patients to avoid hazards associated with plaster casts — in a process of nursing context.

WORKING ASSIGNMENT

Topics for discussion

- change of body image
- psychological trauma after a road traffic accident.

Writing assignment

- state a nurse's responsibilities when a plaster cast is applied to an out-patient
- state the factors about which you would collect information when assessing a patient after the application of a plaster cast
- state potential problems after application of a plaster cast
- state the dietary requirements for new bone formation
- define the following:

active
apposition
congenital
cyanosis
fracture
ischaemia
motor nerves
paraesthesia
passive
plaster sores
pressure sores
sensory nerves
signs
spica
symptoms

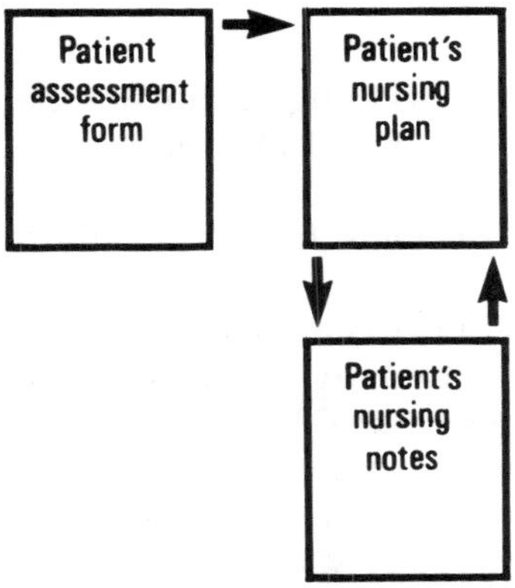

23

Helping patients to avoid hazards related to medications

Reading assignment

Background information
- *Factors which health authorities encourage/discourage*
  - *Most authorities encourage the use of:*
  - *Most authorities discourage the use of:*
  - *Prescription error*
  - *Checking of drugs*
  - *Medicine trolleys*

Routes and methods of giving medications
- *Oral route*
- *Topical applications*
- *Injections*
- *Inhalations*
- *Suppositories*
- *Pessaries*

Medications in a process of nursing context
- *Assessing*
- *Planning*
- *Implementing*
- *Evaluating*

Applying the principle
- *A registered nurse must be capable of:*

Working assignment
- *Topics for discussion*
- *Writing assignment*

READING ASSIGNMENT

Badger C, Regnard C 1986 Pumping in pain relief. Nursing Times 82 (28) July 9: 52, 54
After introduction of a needle subcutaneously or intramuscularly, fine tubing attaches it to an automatic syringe (strapped to the skin) which delivers a consistent volume of a pain relieving drug.

Benson S 1985 A self-medication survey of elderly patients in hospital. British Journal of Occupational Therapy 48 (11) November: 326-328

Bill T 1984 Mental health nursing. Depot drugs in community psychiatry. Nursing Times 80 (3) January 18: 43–46
Study of the effects of Clopixol.

Bleathman C 1985 Pharmacology. Nursing: The Add-On Journal of Clinical Nursing 2 (41) September: 1213, 1215, 1217
Effect of drugs on the elderly.

Bradshaw S 1987 Treating yourself. Nursing Times 83 (6) February 11: 40–41
Elderly people are especially at risk of iatrogenic illness, may be due to poor drug compliance — not understanding what the drugs are for and when they should be taken. Discusses ways in which nurses could improve their practice. References.

Bream S 1985 Teaching the elderly about drugs. Nursing Times 81 (29) July 17: 32–34
Self-medication programmes.

Campbell D 1984 Who carries the drugs can? Nursing Mirror 159 (17) November 7: 31
Drug checking in hospital.

Channer K 1985 Stand up and take your medicine. Nursing Times 81 (28) July 10: 41–42

Clarke G 1983 Pharmaco-kinetics. Nursing Times 79 (49) December 7: 58, 60
Drug absorption rates in different parts of the body.

Clarke-Mahoney J P 1984 Self-medication programme improves compliance. Nursing 14 (12) December: 41
Describes a medication régime after discharge.

Cobb M D 1986 Evaluating medication errors. Journal of Nursing Administration 16 (4) April: 41–44

Cobb P, Eastman M, Hammond M 1984 Cutting down on errors and drugs. Nursing Mirror Community Forum 159 (12) October 3: vi–viii
Evolvement of a system of drug administration in old people's homes. It minimised errors and decreased the number of prescriptions. References.

Cohen M R 1985 Drug-induced anaphylaxis. Nursing 15 2 February: 43
An adverse reaction can occur in many tissues throughout body.

Collins B J, Robinson M G, Spence B K, Hunter J, Nelson J K 1983 Safety of reusing disposable plastic insulin syringes. Lancet: 559–560

Cox J, O'Malley K 1986 Problems of drug treatment in the elderly. Journal of the Royal Society of Health 106 (2) April: 46–68

David J 1987 Injection equipment. Nursing: The Add-On Journal of Clinical Nursing 3 (19): 727–729
Uses the headings — syringes, needles, useful extras and disposal.

De Mont A 1984 Medicine chest laxatives. Community Outlook Nursing Times 80 (6) February 8: 48–49

Devlin R 1985 Home comfort. Nursing Times 81 (36) September 4: 19– 20
Nurses caring for the terminally ill administering pain-killing drugs.

Donovan A 1985 Counteracting side-effects. Nursing Mirror 161 (14) October 2: 38–39
Clinical trial of a drug (Nabilone) used to treat cancer.

Downie G and others 1984 Drug administration. Safer than plastic cups. Health and Social Service Journal 94 March 29: 376
Wiegand system in home for the elderly in Aberdeen.

Fielo S, Rizzolo M A 1985 The effects of age on pharmacokinetics. Geriatric Nursing 6 (6) November/December: 328–331

Gaunder B N, Winkle D 1984 Anaphylaxis. Managing and preventing a true emergency. Nursing Practitioner 9 (5) May: 17–20

Gibb S 1985 The yellow one is my water pill. Nursing Times 81 (9) February 27: 29–30
A self-medication programme to overcome confusion on discharge.

Glasper A, Ireland L 1987 Drugs: children are different. Senior Nurse 6 (4) April: 5
Many paediatric nurses have misgivings about the UKCC's new guidelines on drug administration.

Glasper A, Oliver R W 1984 A simple guide to infant drug calculations. Nursing: The Add-On Journal of Clinical Nursing 2 (22) February: 649–650

Goodinson S M 1986 Fundamentals of drug action. Nursing: The Add-On Journal of Clinical Nursing 3 (10) October: 386–390
Contains a detailed Table of parenteral routes for giving drugs.

Goodman C 1985 Cytotoxic drugs: their handling and use. Nursing Times 81 (47) November 20: 36–38
A project to answer the question — are nurses fully aware of the hazards involved in administering cytotoxic drugs? The known local reactions are described. References.

Harper D C 1984 Application of Orem's theoretical constructs to selfcare medication behaviours in the elderly. Advances in Nursing Science 6 (3) April: 29–46

Holmes S 1984 Chemotherapy and the gastrointestinal tract. Nursing Times 80 (8) February 22: 28–31

Hopkins S 1983 Minihep darts. Nursing Mirror 157 (24) December 14: 31
New system for subcutaneous injection of heparin.

Hopkins S J 1977 The law and the misuse of

drugs. Nursing Mirror 144 (20) May 19: 25–26
The Misuse of Drugs Act (1973): the responsibility for the safe custody of Controlled Drugs rests on the nurse in charge of the ward; a doctor has no right of access to ward stocks.

Hosking J 1985 Knowledge and practice. Nursing Mirror 160 (5) January 30: ii–vi
Research supplement.

Johnson M 1987 Drugs and discipline. Senior Nurse 6 (2) February: 14-16
Questions the use of formal disciplinary procedures for drug errors.

Jones B 1984 How drugs act. Nursing Mirror 158 (19) May 9: 17–19

Journal of District Nursing 1986 Drug reactions: sensitivity and allergy to drugs. Journal of District Nursing 5 (1) July: 18

Journal of District Nursing 1985 Drug reactions: that worn out feeling. Journal of District Nursing 4 (1) July : 24
Drug reactions.

Kallas K D 1984 Establishing a self-administered medication programme. Journal of Nursing Administration 14 (11) November: 38–42

Kofoed L L 1986 OTC drugs: a third of the elderly are at risk. Geriatric Medicine 16 (2) February: 37–38, 41–42
Describes over-the-counter medications.

Lamy P P 1986 Drug interactions and the elderly. Journal of Gerontological Nursing 12 (2) February: 36–37

Mackenzie J 1984 The ward pharmacist and the nurse — a Scottish view. Nursing Times 80 (22) May 30: 61–63
Discusses pharmacist as member of ward team.

Macquire J, Preston J and Pinches D 1987 Two pink and one blue ... Nursing Times 82 (2) January 14: 32–33
Reports a nursing study of self-medication in elderly people. Explains establishment of a tablet-taking régime in hospital before discharge.

McMillan E 1984 Patient compliance with antihypertensive drug therapy. Nursing: The Add-On Journal of Clinical Nursing 2 (26) June: 761–764
Discusses factors influencing compliance, reasons for non-compliance and the nurse's role in education. Contains a plan of education.

McMillan E 1984 Oxygen therapy. Nursing: The Add-On Journal of Clinical Nursing 2 (28) August: 822–825.
An illustrated up-to-date account of equipment via which oxygen can be given to the patient.

Monahan F D 1984 When swallowing pills is difficult. Geriatric Nursing 5 (2) March/April: 88-89

Morris B 1984 Prescription for disaster. Senior Nurse 1 (8) August: 21–22
Role of the community psychiatric nurse (CPN) in prescribing and administering drugs to the elderly.

Nicholson H 1986 The success of the syringe driver. Nursing Times 82(28) July 9: 49–51
Describes use of a syringe driver to control pain in advanced cancer.

Nisbet F 1986 Taking the tablets. Nursing Times 82 (11) Community Outlook June: 20–21
Describes how to help the elderly people sort out their drug regime.

Parke D V 1985 Adverse effects of drugs — their causes and prevention. Journal of the Royal Society of Health 105 (2) April: 39– 46

Parkinson E 1984 Stop thieves in the ward. Nursing Times 80 (17) April 25: 61–62
The author, a security adviser, includes a section 'Security of drugs'. No references.

Punton S 1985 Burford Nursing Development Unit Newsletter Self-medication. Nursing Times 81 (43) October 23: 45

Raynor D K 1985 Labels on medicines: do patients understand them? Self Health 7 (June): 11–12

Ritchie P J, Greenburgh G E 1985 Guidelines for the administration of medication in day care centres. Journal of Community Health Nursing 2 (3): 145–149

Rivers P 1986 Towards safer drug administration. Geriatric Nursing 6 3 May/June: 25–26
A system for use in residential care homes.

Roper N (ed) 1987 Appendix 4 Drugs. Pocket medical dictionary, 14th edn. Churchill Livingstone, Edinburgh, p 314–358
Explains drugs and the law; The Misuse of Drugs Act 1971; The Medicines Act 1968; drug measurement; weight; volume; concentration; body height and surface area.

Contains a list of approved and proprietary (brand) names of drugs.
Rowland T 1985 Darting in with heparin. Nursing Mirror 160 January 23: 34–35
New method of subcutaneous administration of heparin.
Royal College of Nursing 1980 Drug administration — a nursing responsibility. Royal College of Nursing, London, p 1–10
In hospital; community; Controlled Drugs; The Medicines Act 1968; acute allergic reaction.
Seaman D 1984 Managing a syringe driver. Journal of District Nursing 3 (2) August: 6
Smith R E, Birrell J 1986 Compliance: a shared responsibility. The Professional Nurse 1 (11) August: 302–303
Gives three hypothetical situations in which the nurse involved may influence the likelihood of compliance. Nurses are encouraged to consider non-compliance not only as a patient behaviour, but as a shared responsibility. One reference.
Smith S 1984/85 How drugs act.

1. How drugs are absorbed and reach their destination. Nursing Times 80 (48) November 28: 24–27
2. Elimination and cumulation of drugs. (44) December 5: 44–46
3. Side-effects. (50) December 12: 46–47
4. Intolerance, idiosyncrasy and hypersensitivity. (51) December 19:34–36
5. Overdoses and poisoning. 1985 81 (1) January 2: 29–31
6. Drugs at different ages. (2) January 9: 37–39
7. Vitamins. (3) January 16: 35–37
8. Antibacterial and antiviral agents. (4) January 23: 34–36
9. Describes how the most commonly prescribed analgesics work. (5) January 30: 36–37
10. Drugs and sleep-hypnotics. (6) February 6: 36–37

Smith S 1987 Drugs and the heart. Nursing Times 83 (21) May 27: 24– 26
Smith S 1987 Drugs in angina and myocardial infarction. Nursing Times 83 (22) June 3: 52–54
Smith S 1987 Diuretic agents. Nursing Times 83 (23) June 10: 53–55
Smith S 1987 Drugs and the parasympathetic nervous system. Nursing Times 83 (24) June 17: 36–38
Smith S 1987 Drugs and the eye. Nursing Times 83 (25) June 24: 48– 50
Smith S 1987 Drugs and the gastrointestinal tract. Nursing Times 83 (26) July 1: 50–52
Speechley V 1984 Administration of cytotoxic drugs. Nursing Mirror 158 January 11: 22–24
Spencer R, Alexander D 1986 Counselling clients regarding over the counter drug use. Journal of Community Health Nursing 3 (1): 3–9
Thomas S 1979 Medicines: care and administration. Nursing Mirror 148 (15) April 12: 28–30
Hospital stocks; scheduled poisons; storage rules; nurses' responsibilities; administration methods; injections.
UK Central Council 1986 Administration of medicines: an advisory paper. UKCC London.
Vickerman L 1984 Involuntary medication: your patient advocacy role is on the line. Canadian Nurse 80 (5) May: 32-34
Psychiatric patients' right to refuse medication.
Williams A 1984 Medicine management. Nursing Mirror. Community Forum 159 (12) October 3: i–viii
Describes and illustrates some practical aids to help patients with problems. No references.
Williamson J 1985 Beyond the limits. Nursing Times 81 (13) March 27: 18–19
Includes the government's official limited drug list.

Drug abuse and drug abusers

Caroselli-Karinja M, Zboray S D 1986 The impaired nurse. Journal of Psychosocial Nursing and Mental Health Services 24 (6) June: 14, 16–19
Description and discussion of nurse addicts.
Child-Clarke A, Cotterell D 1984 Occasional Paper An 11-year follow-up of drug clinic attenders. Nursing Times 80 (50) December 12: 52–53
Dobson M 1984 Mental health nursing.

Responding to problem drug users. Nursing Times 80 (47) November 21: 57–58

Gay M 1986 Drug and solvent abuse in adolescents. Nursing Times 82 (5) January 29: 34–35

Ghodse H and others 1986 A comparison of drug-related problems in London accident and emergency departments. British Journal of Psychiatry 148 June: 658–662
The report of a survey carried out between 1975 and 1982.

Green P L 1984 The impaired nurse: chemical dependency. Journal of Emergency Nursing 10 (1) February: 23–26
Drug or alcohol abuse.

MacLennan A 1986 Taken over by heroin. Nursing Times 82 (7) February 12: 45–47

Merker L and others 1985 Assessing narcotic addiction in neonates.
Paediatric nursing 11 (3) May/June: 177–181

Orr R 1984 The cost of blessed tranquillity. Nursing Times 80 (36) September 5: 48–50
Discusses addiction to benzodiazepines.

Phillips K 1986 Neonatal drug addicts. Nursing Times 82 (12) March 19: 36–38

Rickard T 1984 Drug dependence. Nursing: The Add-On Journal of Clinical Nursing 2 (24) April: 710–713

Robertson J R and others 1986 Epidemic of AIDS related virus infection among intravenous drug abusers. British Medical Journal 292 February 22: 527–530

BACKGROUND INFORMATION

Overprescribing of drugs has become a serious and expensive problem for the health service. It can result in patients being prescribed several drugs (polypharmacy) and it can also result in the 'medicalisation' of emotional and social problems. Nurses have an important role to play in supporting and counselling patients who are in a low mood, and in helping them to understand that dispiritedness (p. 82) does not usually respond to medication. They also have a role in educating the public not only about the merits, but also about the disadvantages of analgesics, antibiotics, antidepressants, laxatives, sedatives and tranquillisers.

Various surveys have shown that a substantial proportion of the population indulge in excessive self-medication, that is, the taking of medicines available without a doctor's prescription, 'over the counter' medications (Kofoed 1986, Spencer & Alexander 1986). Remedies for headache, indigestion, constipation, muscular discomfort, coughs and colds come into this category.

Other surveys have shown that only 50% of drugs prescribed by general practitioners are taken by their patients. Various reasons are given such as when the patient feels better he ceases to take the pills. Other reasons given for not completing a course of drugs are that after a few doses the patient does not feel any better, or that the pills do not agree with him. These deviations from a prescribed programme, whether they are due to non-comprehension or non-compliance of the patient are a frequent cause of admission and re-admission to hospital. They also result in 'left-over' tablets in the home which are a danger.

To help patients to avoid hazards associated with medications there are stringent rules and regulations enforced by the government; it has published a 'Guide to the Misuse of Drugs Act 1971, and to certain Regulations made under the Act'. Hopkins (1977), interprets the Act for use by nurses and doctors (Roper 1987). Of course the precautions have to be carried out by all staff employed in the manufacturing, testing, buying, selling, and storing of drugs. As a precaution, most Health Boards issue a booklet of instructions about the care and use of drugs, lotions and poisons to be observed by their staff. The statutory nursing body, the United Kingdom Central Council (UKCC) published an advisory paper on the administration of medicine (1986).

The usual system is for each ward to hold a supply of the commonly used drugs, which are directly ordered by the ward and supplied by the pharmacy. Sometimes the last doses of tablets or medicine were put into an open vessel while the container went to the pharmacy for replenishment. To avoid this dangerous practice many wards have two 'stock' bottles permitting one to be used while the other is being replenished. Another method of overcoming the problem is for the pharmacy to conduct a 'topping up' service.

Because of the many dangers inherent within the traditional system, an increasing number of hospitals have introduced an individual patient dispensing service that is, instead of a patient being given a tablet from a stock bottle, the bottle is labelled with the patient's name.

Nurses are beginning to be more comfortable with discussion about whether or not able patients in hospital could be responsible for their self-medication. The majority of the population are elderly and may well have no one to help them with their drug régime when they go home. There is now ample documentation of patients' admission and readmission to hospital, the main cause being faulty taking of prescribed medicines. To avoid this it would seem to be necessary for nurses to teach patients and to assess and evaluate their ability to be independent in taking their medicines. Several articles in the Reading Assignment describe ways in which this has been dealt with: they are identifiable from the title or the annotation.

In America some hospitals have installed an automatic drug dispenser in the wards. The machine dispenses the drug after sending a coded message to a central tape-recorded, card punch, or computer, where a complete record is kept of what drugs have been issued and to which patient. It is claimed that the use of these machines has eliminated any error in dispensing and in addition, practically eliminated the theft of drugs which is an increasing hazard with the modern tendency towards more widespread use of, and addiction to, drugs.

Several items in the Reading Assignment under the heading *Drug abuse and drug abusers* give adequate information about this very important subject. Two of the items remind us that nurses are not immune from abusing drugs and alcohol (Green 1984, Caroselli-Karinja & Zboray 1986).

Factors which health authorities encourage/ discourage

There are generalised instructions pertaining to the writing of prescriptions; the packaging of prescriptions and checking of the drug into the patient, and they are obviously necessary — Raynor (1985) entitles her article 'Labels on medicines: do patients understand them?'

Most authorities encourage the use of:

- legible handwriting for prescriptions
- printing for prescriptions — where hand-writing is difficult to read
- words written in full
- arabic numerals
- the doctor's prescription as a check during the administration of drugs
- two stock bottles for each ward or department
- screw tops for bottles
- return to the pharmacy of discoloured solutions, disfigured tablets, unlabelled or illegibly labelled bottles, bottles labelled with a patient's name after discontinuance of the medicine, drugs unused on their date of expiry
- identification and instruction on the containing part of the vessel
- a second person checking the drug into the patient as well as withdrawal of the drug from its labelled container where checking is necessary.

Most authorities discourage the use of:

- Latin abbreviations
- Roman numerals
- ward medicine lists
- checking of drugs into a syringe but not into a patient
- checking of tablets into a spoon or container and not into the patient
- putting tablets or the last dose of medicine into an open vessel while the container goes to be refilled
- corks as they are difficult to sterilize
- discoloured solutions
- disfigured tablets
- unlabelled or illegibly labelled bottles
- any substance with an expiry date in the past

- an excessive number of medications for any one patient
- identification and instruction on the lid of any container
- the giving of drugs, labelled with one patient's name, to any other patient.

These are examples of precautions to be taken by members of a multidisciplinary team to help patients to avoid hazards related to medications.

Prescription error

In case of prescription error, the Law recognizes the person of greater experience as being more responsible, for example, an inexperiencd houseman prescribes too large a dose; an experienced nurse gives the dose; the Law does not expect blind obedience from a nurse.

Checking of drugs

Hospitals vary as to which drugs need to be checked and who has to do the checking. The strictly legal requisites are the minimum, that is the 'Controlled Drugs' should, when given, be witnessed by a second person. In order to give better protection to patients, many hospitals have more stringent rules and require Scheduled drugs as well as Controlled Drugs to be checked. Most hospitals designate the status of the checker. It is important that a student of nursing can differentiate between hospital and legal responsibilities with regard to drugs, lotions and poisons (Royal College of Nursing 1980, Campbell 1984).

Medicine trolleys

In the past when task allocation ruled (p. 21), nurses spent a lot of time lifting the necessary items for doing a ward medicine round on to an ordinary trolley, and putting them back into the locked medicine cupboard, at least three, and often four times a day.

Industry, ever ready to help nurses to give medicines safely, marketed 'medicine trolleys' which, over the years have become more functional, and most health authorities provide this equipment for the wards.

The suggested routine when using the trolley illustrated in Figure 23.1 is that all the patients' medication cards are loaded into one holder at the beginning of the round. Previously identification of ambulant patients presented a problem; however it is now customary for all patients to wear an identification bracelet (p. 246) which has solved the problem for nurses new to the ward. At each bed or chairside, the patient's card is extracted and propped up on the inside lid while carrying out instructions. The drug, dose and time are recorded on the card, together with the signature of the giver: in 'process context' this is documenting the implementation of the planned delegated nursing intervention. Whereas an 'implementation' is usually recorded on the patient's nursing notes, it is different for medicines. The signed medication card is then put in the other holder.

Another specially designed medicine trolley is illustrated in Figure 23.2. At the rear left side is a lock-up Controlled Drugs and Schedule Section. Patients' medicine charts are in a slotted holder attached to the 'lid'. Racks in front contain clean

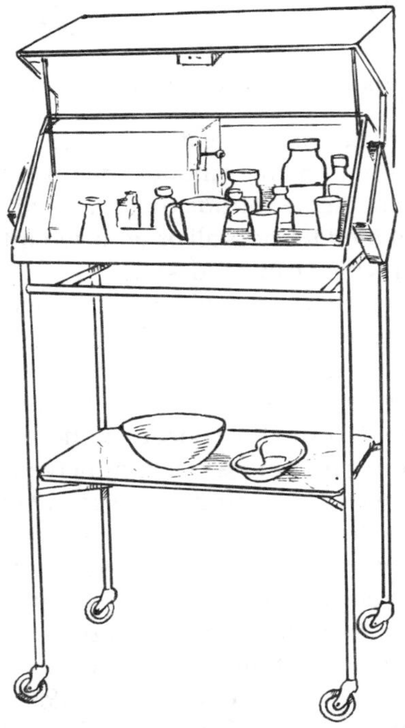

Fig. 23.1 Medicine trolley with card holders fixed at each side of the cabinet

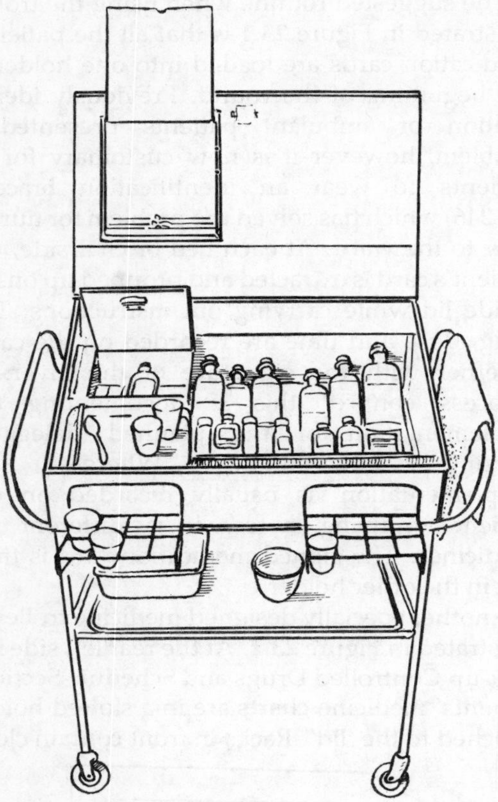

Fig. 23.2 Medicine trolley: racks in front contain clean glasses

glasses. A tray underneath takes used glasses. Large castors ensure smooth, silent wheeling. Between medicine rounds these 'locked' trolleys can be chained to the wall or wheeled into a wall cupboard which can be locked.

However, there are two tendencies which may change the need for, or the design of, medicine trolleys. One is the move towards team nursing (p. 21), or patient allocation (p. 21), or primary nursing (p. 21) and the concept of these methods of organising nursing is not conducive to that of the 'ward medicine round'. The second tendency is towards teaching patients self-medication to enable them to manage their medication régime safely after discharge from hospital. The references show how this concept is being put into practice in different ways and in different circumstances (Clarke-Mahoney 1984, Kallas 1984, Benson 1985, Bream 1985, Gibb 1985, Punton 1985).

It may be that medicine trolleys will give way to a medicine cabinet on the wall by each bed, opened by a combination number, and serviced by the pharmacy. It would seem to be an asset which would help nurses to achieve their objective of carrying out 'individualised nursing' in relation to medications, about which more will be said later.

ROUTES AND METHODS OF GIVING MEDICATIONS

'Giving medicines' is only part of the medication scenario and nurses administer drugs by several other routes and each of these involves participating in several methods. They will be discussed under the headings — oral route, topical applications, injections, inhalations, suppositories, and pessaries before ending the chapter by considering medications in process context.

Oral route

The route of giving medication in which nurses most frequently participate is the oral one, and the tablet or capsule is swallowed by the patient, usually with a drink of water. Monahan (1984) offers advice which can be used for patients who find swallowing pills difficult.

The majority of prescriptions written by a general practitioner state that the medicine has to be taken after meals. Many lay people believe that medicines are less irritant when taken 'on a full stomach'. 'Medicine rounds' therefore need to be considered in relation to meal times: they are still being carried out, even in some of those areas which are participating in 'patient allocation' (p. 21), usually to comply with the Health Authority's policy of drug checking. Many tablets release the medicament slowly, so that its absorption by the gastrointestinal mucosa is gradual and the intended action lasts throughout the 24 hours. The instruction with an increasing number of drugs is to 'take 1 hour before meals'. Some people believe that it is harmful to take medicines 'on an empty stomach' — more will be said about this later. Special arrangements will need to be made in the ward for these 'before meal' medications. Some drugs which are absorbed from the oral mucosa have to be sucked and consequently nurses need to teach patients about this method of absorption.

Suggestion is so powerful that it has cured a person taking only coloured water, with the belief that is was something special. Encouraging the patients towards optimism is an important part of their therapy. The patients are glad of reinforcement along the road. 'These red pills will soon have your blood up to normal' conveys the necessary optimism. 'A few more pills to make you rattle' is likely to make the patient query the wisdom of all his medications. It is not in the nurse's province to tell the patient the name of the drug being taken. This is wise and necessary when the drug is habit forming. It is the nurse's duty to give an explanation of what the drug is expected to do, for example, 'Doctor wants you to take these tablets to soothe your nerves, but he doesn't want you to be sleepy during the day. If you do feel sleepy during the day, will you please tell me, so that we can adjust the dose?' People who are taking antihistamines should be warned of the possible side effect of daytime sleepiness. They should be advised against driving, cycling, and so on.

Addiction can result from continued use of barbiturates. Their action is potentiated in the presence of alcohol, but patients do not know this unless they are told. The classic example is the old lady who, having taken her sleeping pill, has a nightcap from the 'special' bottle in her locker. She is difficult to rouse in the morning and when roused, her confusion appears to be inexplicable. For the same reason patients taking tranquillisers need to be advised not to take alcohol. Patients taking monoamine oxidase inhibitors should understand that their action is potentiated by barbiturates and alcohol. They are also advised to abstain from cheese, Marmite, Bovril and broad beans because they can produce a hypertensive attack. They are asked to refrain from any drug not ordered by their doctors.

Some patients with high blood pressure (hypertension) are treated with antihypertensive drugs that can cause mental depression and the nurse must recognize this development. Such patients should be advised to rise slowly from the lying to the sitting position to avoid fainting from a sudden fall in blood pressure due to sudden change of posture. Constipation may be troublesome, and the ambulant patient's co-operation is necessary so that this can be reported and dealt with. Patients on sulpha drugs and antibiotics must understand that such substances can be harmful unless taken as instructed. Patients taking belladonna in any form, for example, preoperative medication or antispasmodics, need to be advised about the side-effect of a dry mouth. Patients taking iron or bismuth should be advised about passing dark-coloured stools, so that they are relieved of anxiety. Patients on anticoagulant drugs are advised to shave with special care as their blood-clotting mechanism is reduced. Patients taking antimalarial drugs are advised to stop the tablets if there is any blurring of sight.

Because of the diversity of shapes and sizes of spoons in a household, a 5 ml plastic one is provided with each bottle of liquid medicine.

Topical applications

The word 'topical' describes application of such substances as anaesthetics, powders, ointments, lotions and creams to the skin or mucous membranes and they have a local effect. A recent result of pharmacological research and modern technology has produced drugs impregnated into a special 'patch' which, when applied to the skin, releases the drug gradually so that it is absorbed to maintain its effective level in the blood stream throughout 24 hours.

Injections

The majority of adults in Britain today have some knowledge about injections and the nurse can discover this as she assesses people before giving injections. People's attitude and level of anxiety may well reflect the circumstances which prevailed at their previous experience of having an injection. Not all injections are given in hospital; for example health visitors carry out immunization programmes in health clinics; community nurses give injections in patients' own homes, or in a clinical room in a building from which GPs practise; occupational health nurses may well give injections to minimise a worker's time away from work should he otherwise have to attend his GP's surgery. Of course some people such as those who have diabetes learn to inject themselves, and many drug abusers choose this method for introducing the drug. Because of the anxiety about drug abusers sharing needles, with the consequent risk of spreading Aids, some Health Authorities are providing them with disposable syringes which have an attached needle; and these units are now prescribable for diabetic people.

Patients, wherever they are in the health care system, requiring injections, become dependent on the staff:

- to provide a reliable service of sterile syringes and needles whether or not of the disposable variety
- to store the drugs under conditions which maintain their potency
- to give the right medically prescribed drug, in the right dose, at the right time, to the right patient by the appropriate route, using a skilful, reliable technique.

The various routes include intradermal, intramuscular and subcutaneous. *In the last two instances, the needle can be left in situ and fixed by fine tubing to a syringe driver which injects the drug continuously to give a constant level in the blood stream to, for instance keep the patient free from pain (Badger & Regnard 1986).* Some specialist nurses, particularly in oncology departments, learn to give cytotoxic drugs by the intravenous route. The doctor places the needle in position when a drug has to be introduced epidurally, but before and during the procedure, the midwife or nurse provides both physical and psychological support for the patient, and thereafter closely supervises the drug flow. Drugs are sometimes introduced intrathecally, when the nurse's role is similar to that in the previous sentence, except that the whole dose is given at one injection. Whichever route is used, the skin is pierced, therefore theoretically it is deprived of one of its functions — to act as a barrier to infection. Considering the large number of injections which are given, only a relatively small number result in infection. In the process of assimilating a knowledge base required for nurses to make professional decisions about safe practice for each injection, the reader should realise that some of the concepts discussed in other chapters of this text are appropriate here; they are:

- hygienic handwashing (p. 258)
- resident microorganisms on the skin (p. 255)
- transient microorganisms on the skin (p. 255)
- virulence/pathogenicity of microorganisms (p. 308)
- immunological status of the injected person (p. 257)

People who give themselves therapeutic subcutaneous injections at home, for example those who have diabetes, are advised on research-based knowledge (Collins et al 1983) to return the disposable syringe with its sheathed needle attached, to its packet after injection, and store it in a domestic refrigerator at +4°C. Those without a fridge use a glass syringe which is immersed in 70% industrial methylated spirit, and disposable needles which are safely discarded after each use. Such people are taught that their hands and the injection site must be clean; the injection site should not be cleansed with alcohol because of its drying and hardening effect on the skin, and because the risk of an abscess following subcutaneous injection is negligible. One has to remember that the number of microorganisms in the home environment is likely to be less than in a hospital, and the organisms much less likely to be pathogenic.

However, it may well be the policy that inpatients who require subcutaneous injections should have the skin-site disinfected, because of the possibility of transient pathogenic microorganisms and should such patients have been in for some time their immunological system may not be functioning maximally, and their skin may have been colonised by pathogenic microorganisms. It is advised that a perfunctory wipe with a swab dipped in alcohol will not adequately remove or kill microorganisms on the skin. In situations where disinfection is required, the alcohol should be well rubbed into the skin and allowed to dry.

Skin disinfection policy for intramuscular and intravenous injections is usually agreed by the infection control committee for each district and applies to all health premises as well as hospitals. The student of nursing should be familiar with and carry out the policy agreed for the district in which she is working.

Sterile syringes and needles, usually disposable, are supplied by the CSSD (Central Sterile Supplies Department). They may be separate and after use the needle point can be put through the nozzle of the syringe; they may be the all-in-one variety with the needle protected by a sheath so that after use the sheath can be replaced to avoid 'needle stick' (pricking) injuries to any members of staff. The used syringes and needles are then put in a special receptacle for 'sharps' and the health authority's policy for dealing with the receptacles must be strictly adhered to. The greatest danger of 'needle stick' injury which has been recognised for over 15 years is the transmission of hepatitis B. Over the past few years an additional danger is infection with the virus causing AIDS (Acquired Immune Deficiency Syndrome), recently re-named HIV (Human Immunodeficiency Virus).

The majority of drugs are dispensed in single dose containers as manufacturing firms try to overcome the problem of legibility of writing on such small glass ampoules. The liquid in the phial is sterile thus minimising the hazard of infection. Figure 23.3 illustrates withdrawal of fluid from a single dose container. All staff members should take precautions against accident from broken glass.

To help those diabetics who have difficulty injecting themselves, Hypoguards are available (Fig. 23.5). They consist of a needle holder and sleeve which can be attached to a hypodermic syringe. It is claimed that injection can be given painlessly. A nurse may need to teach a patient to use one of these to give his own injections. The same firm, Hypoguard Ltd, has used modern technology to produce a click/count syringe for blind, and partially sighted diabetics.

It is unfortunate that 'into the buttock' is used to describe one of the sites for intramuscular injection. The common conception of the buttock is of the lower, prominent, fatty portion (Fig. 23.6).

Fat causes delay in absorption of the drug. The skin of the lower area is more likely to be infected with microorganisms from the bowel which increase the risk of abscess formation. The sciatic nerve traverses this region. All authorities are agreed that only the upper, outer quadrant of the buttock (Fig. 23.7) is suitable for intramuscular injection.

The belly of the deltoid muscle (Fig. 23.8) is

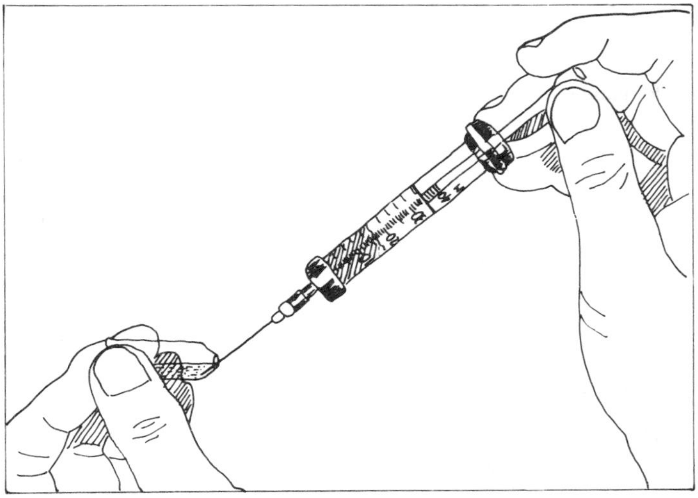

Fig. 23.3 Drawing up fluid from a single dose container

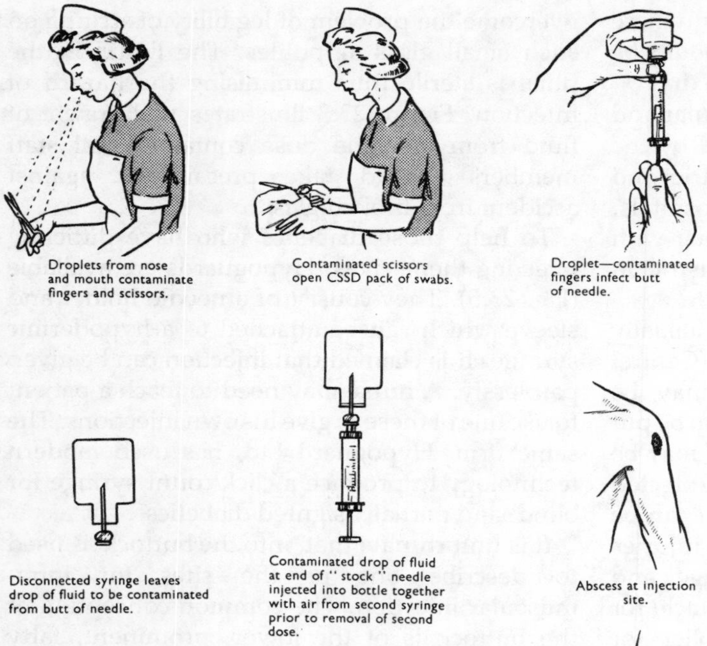

Droplets from nose and mouth contaminate fingers and scissors.
Contaminated scissors open CSSD pack of swabs.
Droplet—contaminated fingers infect butt of needle.
Disconnected syringe leaves drop of fluid to be contaminated from butt of needle.
Contaminated drop of fluid at end of " stock " needle injected into bottle together with air from second syringe prior to removal of second dose.
Abscess at injection site.

Fig. 23.4 Withdrawing fluid from a multidose container

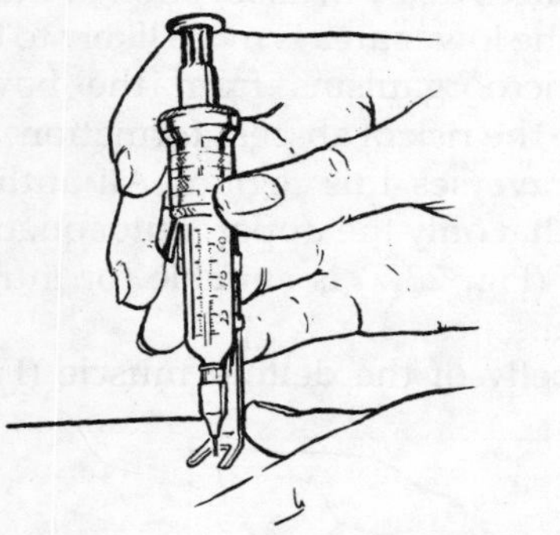

Fig. 23.5 A hypoguard useful for patients injecting themselves

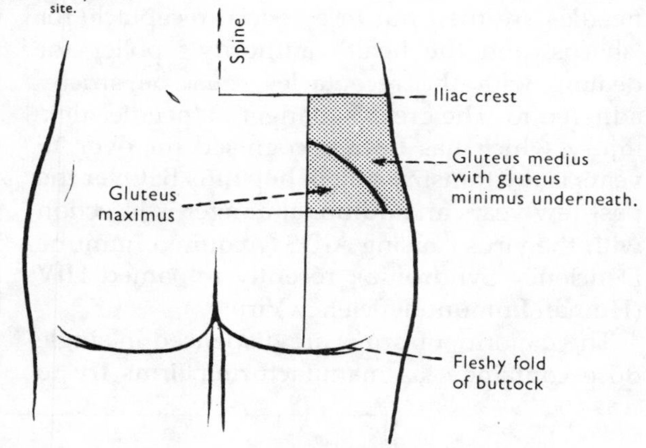

Fig. 23.7 Upper, outer quadrant of buttock

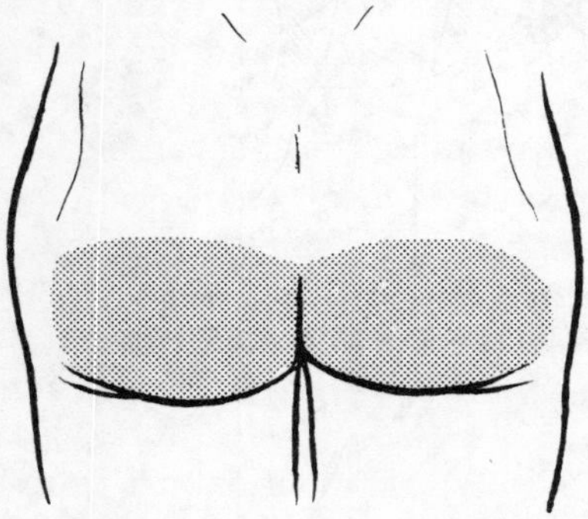

Fig. 23.6 Common conception of the buttock

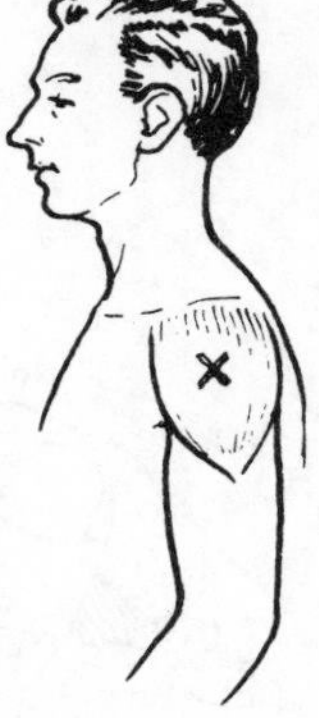

Fig. 23.8 Belly of deltoid muscle

pierced by entering the lateral aspect of the upper third of upper arm.

The belly of the lateral muscle (vastus lateralis) making up the quadriceps muscle is pierced by entering the lateral-medial aspect of the middle third of the thigh. The belly of the middle muscle (rectus femoris) is pierced by entering the anterolateral aspect of the middle third of the thigh (Fig. 23.9).

Iron is sometimes given by intramuscular injection. The thick, dark liquid tends to leak along the needle track and stain the skin producing an area like a bruise. To prevent this it is recommended that the skin is drawn well over to one side, the needle inserted, the drug given, the needle half withdrawn, pressure on the flesh released and the needle completely withdrawn. This is said to produce an angulation in the tract, past which the fluid is less likely to leak.

The precautions which a nurse must take to prevent herself becoming sensitized to an antibiotic include the following points. Antibiotic powder in a sealed container keeps at ordinary room temperature for long periods. As soon as it is dissolved in sterile, distilled water it starts to decompose. Wherever possible the powder should be freshly prepared. Should there by any *solution* left over, it should be stored in the refrigerator for a maximum of

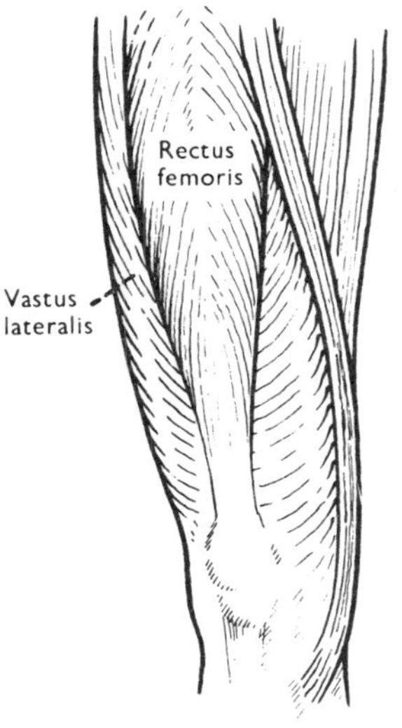

Fig. 23.9 Belly of lateral and middle position of quadriceps muscles

24 hours. Thereafter it should be put into a plastic bag for disposal to prevent sensitivity in anyone handling it. Any antibiotics stored temporarily in the refrigerator must be removed half an hour before use. Some of the antibiotic *suspensions* are difficult to give, especially in cold weather. They are inclined to block the needle. The patient should be prepared first so that the suspension is in the syringe for the minimum length of time. The nurse assesses by question and answer that the patient understands the procedure. Rolling the container in the palms of the hands tends to make the suspension thinner. It is then well shaken. It is best to use a wide-bore needle and exert a steady, strong pressure on the piston.

The rules for checking with the prescription, having some medicaments checked by a second person, identifying the patient (p. 246), and recording the giving of medicaments are the same for injections as for oral medication (p. 283). In some hospitals the route is recorded, for example oral penicillin, IM penicillin; oral paraldehyde, IM paraldehyde; IV atropine. In some hospitals the site used for intramuscular injection is recorded with each dose, so that the patient is protected from the hazard of having consecutive injections in the same site.

Inhalations

Some people when afflicted with the common cold get relief from nasal blockage by using decongestant sprays or inhalants which are available at the chemists. Others get relief from smearing the inside of the nose with Mentholatum or Vick and inhaling the vapour therefrom. Many lay people know that relief for respiratory infections can be gained from inhaling steam. Most people know that Friar's balsam or menthol crystals can be added to the water providing the steam. Few households possess a Nelson's inhaler but most have a jug or basin which can be used for this purpose. Many households keep a bottle of smelling salts in the emergency cupboard for use when anyone feels faint. Some asthmatics and their relatives and friends know about inhaling bronchodilator drugs in spray form. Most people know from films and television that oxygen can be given by various sorts of masks and that a person can be put in an oxygen tent. Some people have heard of hyperbaric oxygen.

Inhalations may be ordered for the following purposes:

- to relieve upper respiratory infection, e.g. rhinitis, coryza, sinusitis, pharyngitis
- to decongest the nasal mucosa, e.g. pocket inhalers obtainable from a chemist
- to treat some nasal conditions post-operatively
- to relieve lower respiratory infections, e.g. laryngitis, tracheitis, bronchitis
- to render sputum less tenacious, e.g. Alevaire or other mucolytic agents administered in aerosol form
- to render sputum less foul-smelling, e.g. creosote inhalations for patients with bronchiectasis
- to warm and moisten the air when a patient has a tracheostomy
- to dilate the bronchi, e.g. ephedrine in asthma
- to improve circulation of blood to the heart, e.g. ampoule of amyl nitrite
- to relieve hiccoughs
- to supply oxygen
- to stimulate the respiratory centre, e.g. carbon dioxide
- to produce anaesthesia.

Inhalation of steam

Whether a Nelson's inhaler (Fig. 23.10) or a jug with a narrow top (Fig. 23.11) is used the patient must understand that the loosened secretions need to be evacuated to gain full benefit from the treatment. From the upper respiratory tract this is achieved by blowing the nose but there is one exception; after some nasal operations the patient is discouraged from blowing the nose and any secretion drains on to a pad secured to the upper lip; it is changed at frequent intervals. With infection of the lower respiratory tract the patient is encouraged to cough and expectorate after steam inhalation. Graduated waxed sputum cartons are often used for patients with bronchiectasis. The amount of sputum evacuated daily is recorded on a graph. The nurse may need to give these patients their steam inhalation just before the physiotherapist's visit, so that the patient gets the greatest benefit from the treatment.

Patients can be advised to use an astringent lotion to close the pores which are opened with steam from a jug inhalation. Cold water is astringent to the skin. The eyes should not be exposed to the vapour from a medicament.

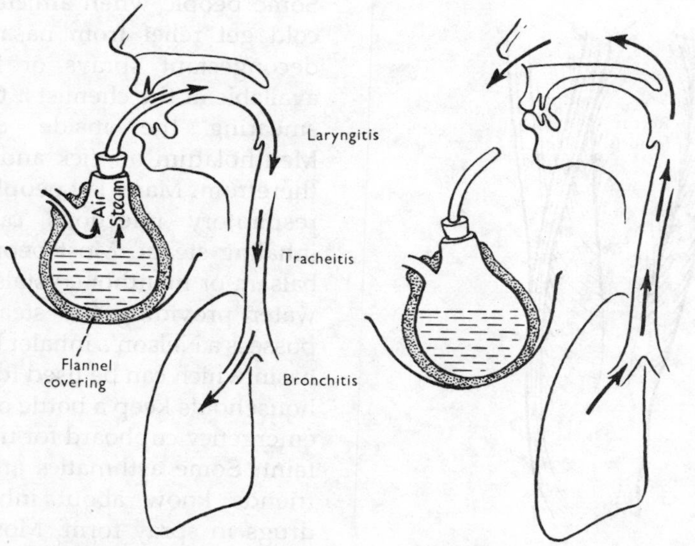

Fig. 23.10 Breathing in from Nelson's inhaler; exhaling through nose

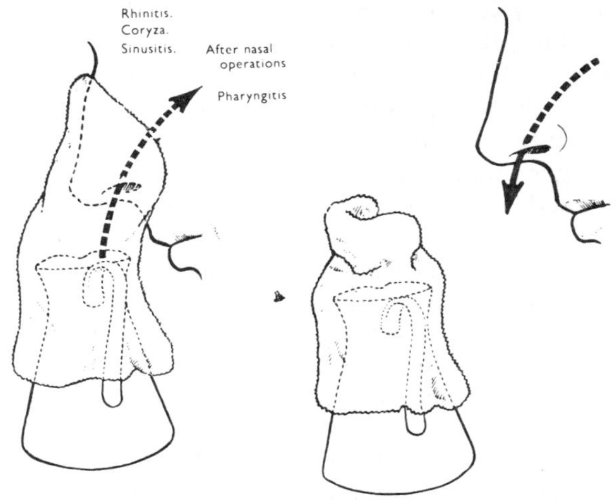

Fig. 23.11 Inhaling and exhaling through nose, using a jug inhaler

A swab soaked in methylated spirit and held in a long-handled forcep is useful for removing Friar's balsam from the inside of a Nelson's inhaler or a jug with a narrow top.

When steam is produced from a kettle, the spout of which is introduced into a steam tent, water can bubble out of the spout if the kettle is overfull. Accident from this cause is less likely if a special long-spouted kettle is used. In some hospitals one nurse is made responsible for putting 1 pint of water into the kettle each half hour and signing her name and the time and amount of water (and medicament, if any) added; a pad and pencil by the kettle is useful for such recordings.

Where steam is unsuitable, apparatus is available for humidification of atmosphere using cold water. The Croupette and Humidair types are like oxygen tents, but the Croupaire (Fig. 23.12) has no enclosing canopy. The minute particles of water are sprayed on to the patient from a distance of 60–90 cm. Inhalation of this cool, soothing vapour is said to loosen bronchial secretion, ease breathing and prevent thirst and dryness of the mouth. The fineness of the spray prevents damping of the bedclothes. The risk of burning from touching a boiling kettle or scalding is eliminated.

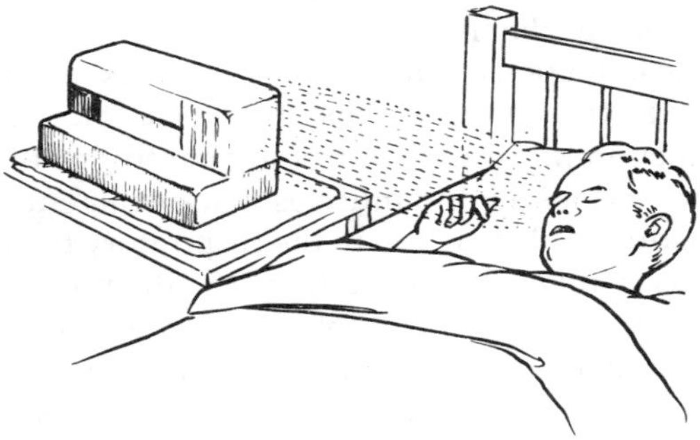

Fig. 23.12 Croupaire on locker

Oxygenation → Deoxygenation cycle

Administration of oxygen (O_2) is an important

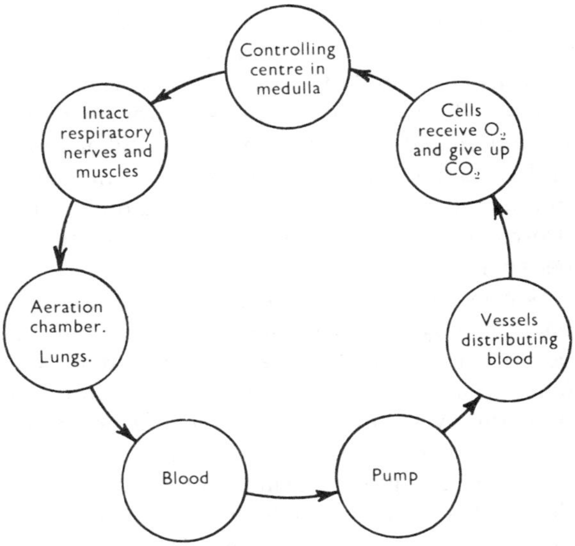

Fig. 23.13 Oxygen — deoxygenation cycle

nursing activity. To facilitate understanding of the rationale for this procedure, the student of nursing needs to be familiar with the oxygen deoxygenation cycle in man; its complexity is portrayed in Figure 23.13. Interference at any point can result in hypoxia, generalized or local, for which warmed, moistened oxygen may be necessary.

The *controlling centre in the medulla* is normally stimulated when there is simultaneous excess of carbon dioxide (CO_2) and lack of oxygen in the blood. The centre can fail to function properly in the presence of some toxins, chemicals and electric shock.

Tetanus, poliomyelitis, bulbar paralysis, diphtheria and muscle relaxant drugs can interfere with the *respiratory nerves and muscles*.

Hypoxia can result from *lack of oxygen in the air entering the lungs*, for example, at high altitudes. Hypoxia can result from lack of air entering the lungs. This may be due to dysfunctioning of the controlling centre, or the respiratory nerves and muscles. Lack of air entry can be due to obstruction in the respiratory tract, such as a relaxed tongue (Fig. 15.10), plug of mucus or vomit, clot of blood, foreign body, membrane as in diphtheria, muscular spasm as in asthma, or the presence of a tumour. Lack of air entry can be due to external pressure on the respiratory tract as in strangulation, hanging, enlarged glands including the thyroid, tumour, pneumothorax, haemothorax and hydrothorax.

Lack of exchange of gases in the lung can be due to faulty diffusing membrane as in bronchiectasis, pneumonia, atelectasis, emphysema, tuberculosis and pneumoconiosis. The presence of fluid may interfere with gas exchange, for example, after drowning, or in the presence of pulmonary oedema.

Severe lack of blood as in anaemia and after haemorrhage, and the haemoconcentration that occurs as part of the 'shock' syndrome (circulatory inadequacy p. 311) can interfere with the cycle. In carbon monoxide poisoning the haemoglobin combines with this gas to form carboxyhaemoglobin, a stable compound, which does not readily dissociate; haemoglobin is thus 'locked up' and not available for oxygen transportation.

The heart can suffer from congenital abnormality or become abnormal as the result of disease. The heart can succumb to acute or chronic (congestive) failure and it can be rendered less effective by myocardial infarction.

The vessels distributing blood can be affected by atherosclerosis, thrombosis, embolism, vasoconstriction or vasodilation, giving rise to local or generalized hypoxia according to site, for example, coronary thrombosis and pulmonary embolism can result in generalized hypoxia; vasoconstriction as in Raynaud's disease causes local hypoxia. Vasodilation in the 'shock' syndrome (circulatory inadequacy) gives rise to generalized hypoxia.

The cells in the body can suffer from metabolic upset which can interfere with their use of oxygen and release of carbon dioxide, thus upsetting these balances in the blood.

An understanding of the way in which oxygen is absorbed and transported in the body is necessary for the nurse to help patients with decreased oxygen. Oxygen is essential for the production of energy to keep the body warm and to initiate the many chemical processes going on within it. The energy cycle is the ATP = ADP cycle. ATP (adenosine triphosphate) is present in every cell in the body. It is continually being broken down to release its stored energy; at this point it becomes ADP (adenosine diphosphate) which is continually being converted back into ATP by energy released from the breakdown of food. One can use the analogy of a car battery which releases energy to start the engine and is recharged during the run. If ATP is not continually regenerated, metabolism is impossible and death ensues. Oxygen is necessary for the reactions which maintain the supply of ATP. Lack of oxygen in the tissues leads to a deviation from the normal metabolic pathway, resulting in the production of lactic acid. This metabolic acidosis combined with respiratory acidosis stops metabolism. ATP ceases to be regenerated — there is no source of energy left — death ensues.

Administration of oxygen

Oxygen can both kill and cure. The doctor's

prescription for oxygen includes the apparatus via which it is to be given, the rate of flow; if this rate of flow has to be changed, at what time, and to what rate it has to be changed, and the duration of the inhalation. The nurse's responsibilities include being familiar with and able to use the apparatus available with safety to all concerned. The nurse must understand the prescription and carry it out faithfully. This means being with the patient until he loses his fear, then frequent supervision to see that the apparatus is in situ and working efficiently. The patient will not be prepared for the blood estimations which are often necessary during this treatment. He may well complain (if he has sufficient breath) that he came to have his breathing, not his blood seen to, if a suitable explanation is not given and understood. Conversation needs to be arranged so that minimal contribution from the patient will assure the nurse that the patient understands. Such patients need dietary considerations (p. 145). Into the bargain they may be afflicted with coughing (p. 209). The breathless patient is discussed on page 206. The temperature will be recorded in the axilla.

Apparatus via which oxygen can be administered includes face masks. The type of mask usually depends on availability rather than on which one would be most appropriate for the particular person requiring oxygen. The design usually permits air to be drawn into the mask to dilute the oxygen, in most instances by varying a valve setting. For acute conditions a concentration of oxygen of about 50% is desirable. McMillan (1984) gives an illustrated up-to-date account of equipment via which oxygen can be delivered to the patient.

Application of a mask to the face is suggestive of smothering. A person needing oyxgen is already 'short of breath'. The oncoming stream of oxygen needs gradual introduction until the patient becomes used to it, before the mask is finally fixed in position. A similar situation arises when a healthy person runs against a high wind which rushes into his open mouth creating an alarming feeling. The fact that the patient cannot talk while wearing a mask may create anxiety. He needs an alternative means of communication which should be written in the nursing plan; it could be a bell for attracting attention, or a pad and pencil for conversation. He must not be ignored. The staff must learn the art of communicating with him under these restricted conditions; observation and accurate interpretation of non-verbal cues is of paramount importance. The face invariably becomes hot and sweaty when wearing a mask. The patient is refreshed for taking nourishment by sponging with cool water before meals. An astringent such as eau-de-cologne or after-shave lotion may help him to feel cooler. Prevention of dry lips and a dirty mouth call for the staff's attention. The mask can be dried at mealtimes.

Delivering oxygen via nasal cannulae is less confining for the patient. There is no association with smothering as with a mask. The patient is free to speak, eat and have his mouth and lips attended to without interruption of oxygen flow. Anaesthetic spray or ointment makes introduction and positioning of the cannulae more bearable until the patient gets used to them. If the patient is asked to stretch and tighten his upper lip over his upper teeth the entrance to the canals along the floor of the nose are more easily seen. The cannulae are passed into these canals for 8cm so that they reach the nasopharynx. The apparatus can rest over the pinna and the weight of the tube can be supported by a safety pin attached to the pillow in such a manner that it does not constrict the tube. After discussion with the patient the fine adjustment valve on the cylinder head is turned very slowly and gradually until the prescribed rate of oxygen flow is established.

Where there is a piped oxygen supply to the wards, turning the control tap releases the gas into a glass bobbin flow meter, which registers the rate of flow in litres per minute. Antistatic rubber tubing is attached to the oxygen outlet pipe from the flow meter to deliver the oxygen to the humidifier (or nebulizer) if one is used, and then another piece of tubing is attached to the humidifier and the prescribed apparatus via which oxygen is delivered to the patient.

Where there is no piped oxygen supply, each ward is supplied with an easily, quietly transportable cylinder stand, a humidifer which often fits into a bracket on the stand, a cylinder key and a cylinder head. The hospital authorities are responsible for storing cylinders flat in a cold, dust-free room. The porter transports them from this store, on a trolley to the ward. The cylinder may be strapped to the trolley to prevent accident. Oxygen cylinders are black with a white shoulder. They have oxygen stencilled in black on the white shoulder. At one end there is a metal mount with a threaded central depression to receive the cylinder head. Projecting at right angles from this metal mount is the main tap with arrows pointing in the direction of turn for 'on' and 'off'. The ward cylinder key opens this main tap momentarily to blow away any grit or dust, which by friction could ignite in a stream of oxygen. This is best done outside the ward as it can be noisy. If the cylinder head has not been used for some time a blast of oxygen on its threaded base will blow away grit or dust. It is recommended that a duster is not used for this purpose. The threaded base is put into the threaded central depression in the cylinder and the winged nut screwed down securely (Fig. 23.14). The main tap is now fully opened with the key and the pressure gauge will register 'full'.

Opening the fine adjustment valve releases oxygen through the reducing valve (which does not need adjustment) and is turned until the necessary number of litres per minute are indicated on the flow meter. Tubing attached to the flow meter conducts oxygen to the humidifier (or nebulizer). Another piece of tubing leads from the humidifier to the patient and is connected to the prescribed delivery apparatus.

Patients with chronic pulmonary disease who are having oxygen therapy need to be observed carefully for any increase in pulse rate, showing that the heart is trying to compensate for lack of oxygen in the blood; any change in mental state, e.g. confusion, disorientation, euphoria or any change in the level of consciousness (p. 65) which indicate that the brain is not receiving sufficient oxygen. Absence of cyanosis and a change in respiration to shallow breathing may indicate that too much oxygen has been given. The respiratory centre in these patients has

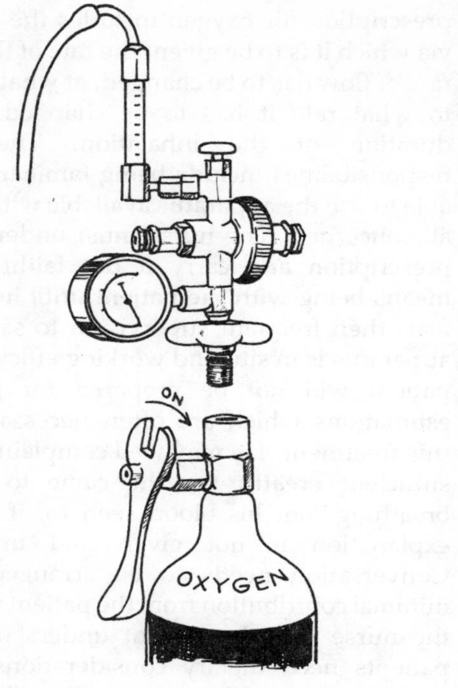

Fig. 23.14 Oxygen cylinder with ward key and cylinder head

become insensitive to the carbon dioxide in the blood and relies on complex hypoxic stimuli from cells in the aorta and carotid bodies for respiration. In other words, such patients depend on a slight degree of hypoxia in order that they can function best with their disability. Above a certain level of CO_2 in the blood, the patient is dependent for breathing stimulus, on the carotid bodies which function during oxygen lack. If we give such patients too much oxygen these carotid bodies fail to keep the patient breathing. Apparatus which delivers low oxygen concentration, such as the Venturi mask, is needed for such patients. The doctor is dependent on the nurse's skill and integrity in carrying out his oxygen prescription and on her intelligent observation of the patient which is recorded in the nursing notes, and reported to the doctor should there be any gross change in the patient's condition.

Many authorities state that effective humidification needs to be incorporated in any system of oxygen administration. Other people think that bubbling oxygen through water does not result in adequate humidification and that an

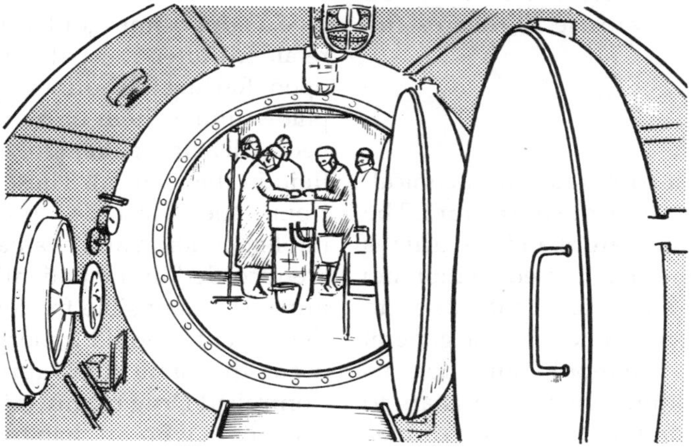

Fig. 23.15 Hyperbaric oxygen chamber in which surgery can be performed

efficient nebulizer should be used.

In America a machine which removes nitrogen from the air has been patented. It is claimed that it raises the oxygen in room air to at least 45%. It avoids the inconvenience of and possible psychological reaction to wearing a mask or being enclosed in a tent. It leaves the patient free to move about the room.

Of recent years hyperbaric oxygen chambers have been used for an increasing number of conditions. The early ones are cylindrical metal tanks into which oxygen under pressure can be pumped. Some accommodate the patient, nurse and equipment. Others are large enough for surgery to be performed in them (Fig. 23.15). The most recent ones resemble a bed (Fig. 23.16). Some units which specialise in pressurized oxygen treatment use flame-proof clothing for patients and staff to reduce the risk of fire.

Measures to reduce the hazards associated with oxygen therapy

- an oxygen cylinder is never put near a source of heat, for example a radiator
- the cylinder is opened to remove grit and dust outside the ward
- any grit or dust on the cylinder head is removed with a blast of oxygen
- hammering is avoided for fear of sparks
- the ward key is attached to the cylinder stand
- grease is not applied to mechanical parts

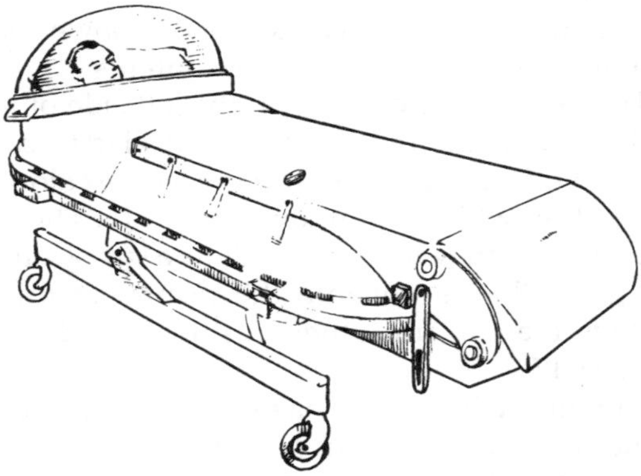

Fig. 23.16 Hyperbaric oxygen chamber in which patient can be nursed as in a bed

- empty cylinders are clearly marked
- an adequate supply of oxygen is kept in each ward and is tested daily
- apparatus for administration is ready to use in emergency
- the cylinder stand must be easy and quiet to move
- smoking is not permitted in the vicinity of oxygen apparatus
- alcohol or oil is not used on patients receiving oxygen
- mechanical toys, push bells, electric heating pads or lights are not put in an oxygen tent
- bedmaking, hair combing and movement of clothing and bedclothes is done carefully to avoid spark from static electricity

- every member of staff must know the location of, and how to use, the nearest fire extinguisher.

Suppositories

Medicaments can be incorporated in a conical, gelatinous base for insertion into the rectum. The base melts at body temperature and the drug is liberated. It may: soothe an inflamed membrane; relieve local pain such as that due to haemorrhoids; be absorbed to have a general effect, for example, aminophylline for its respiratory effect in asthma which is resistant to adrenaline; have a diuretic effect in cardiac oedema; draw fluid from surrounding tissues to lubricate dried faeces thereby enabling evacuation; have a direct effect on the bowel wall producing evacuation of bowel contents.

The descending colon is on the left side of the abdomen. In the region of the left iliac fossa it makes an S-shaped bend to connect the colon to the rectum which is a midline structure. The left lateral position will therefore allow a suppository (or fluid) that is put into the rectum to travel further than if any other position is adopted (Fig. 23.17).

Patients who have haemorrhoids of long standing may be used to self-insertion of a suppository to give relief from pain. Most other people's concept of the back passage is of excretion — and not very nice at that. Those patients requiring insertion of a suppository need instruction as to what is expected of them during the procedure and what result is expected from the procedure before they can minimise their anxiety level and co-operate. It is best to give a suppository for local effect, (or fluid to be retained) after the patient has had his bowels open. Raising the buttocks by putting a protected pillow under them or by raising the foot of the bed, will help a patient to retain a suppository (or fluid in the rectum). These treatments are given from the doctor's prescription and the implementation and evaluation of the treatment are recorded in the patient's nursing notes. The nurse is responsible for correct identification of the patient. Should a morphine suppository be used, the same rules apply as when giving a Controlled Drug by any other route.

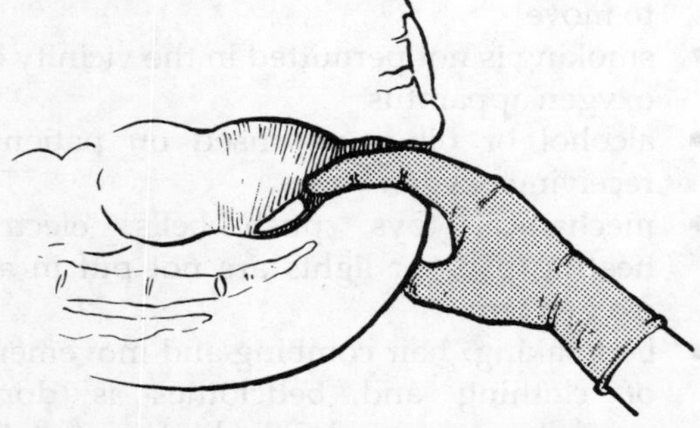

Fig. 23.17 Left lateral position for insertion of a suppository, or introduction of fluid into the rectum

Patients who are habitually constipated may benefit from instruction about diet and exercise. On the other hand nurses may find such patients very knowledgeable about the condition. This is yet another example of how important it is to ask patients what they know about a condition such as constipation.

Pessaries

Drugs can be introduced into the vagina for their local effect. A medicated pessary is similar to a suppository. It may contain Flagyl to kill the *Trichomonas vaginalis* which causes vaginitis, nystatin to kill the organism which causes thrush, stilboestrol to produce lactic acid in the postmenopausal vagina or sulphonamide or antibiotics to sterilize the vagina prior to operation. Some women are in the habit of inserting spermicidal pessaries.

Most pessaries are ordered daily and inserted at night before the patient goes to sleep (Fig. 23.18). The patient is best advised to wear sanitary protection as there may be a drip from the vagina as the upright position is assumed in the morning because there is no sphincter on the vagina. In hospital, patients may have insertion more frequently than daily. Treatment should be arranged so that the patient lies recumbent for 2 hours after insertion, which should be after she has visited the lavatory or used the commode. Such treatment is given from doctor's prescription and the implementation and evaluation are recorded in a patient's nursing notes.

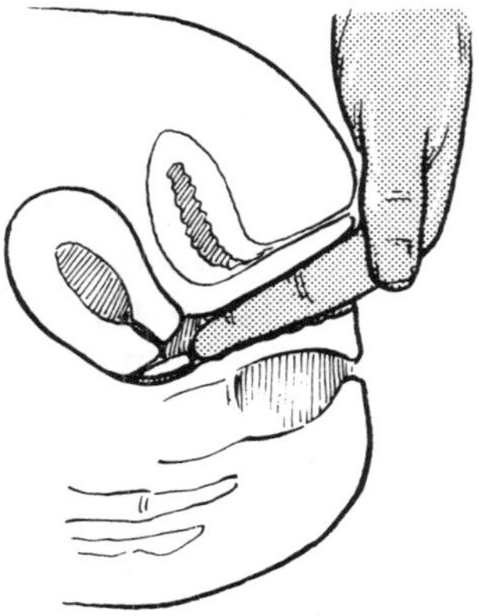

Fig. 23.18 Recumbent position for insertion of pessary into the posterior vaginal fornix

The routes and methods of giving medications are obviously an important part of nursing. To recapitulate — it has been discussed under the headings:

- oral route
- topical applications
- injections
- inhalations
- suppositories and
- pessaries.

An attempt will now be made to consider the wide ranging subject of medications in the context of 'process thinking'.

MEDICATIONS IN A PROCESS OF NURSING CONTEXT

The objective in using the process is to individualise nursing, which surely is its art. The foregoing text shows clearly that the art of nursing is of paramount importance. However, attempting to discuss medications in a process context does help us to clarify our thinking about the cognitive aspects of the nursing activities and interventions necessarily related to medications. They need to be supported by background information about the drugs, their absorption, intended action and any known side-effects, a subject increasingly being called pharmacokinetics. Equally, knowledge from the social sciences is required, together with great sensitivity and skill in therapeutic relationships to help the patient gain maximum benefit from the medication.

Assessing

The accepted first phase of the process, assessing, is associated with the initial assessment interview, information from which is recorded on some type of assessment form. It is usual to enquire whether or not the patient is taking any medicine or tablets. If so, does he know the name? What colour are they? Why is he taking them? How long has he been taking them? How often does he take them? At what time of day are they taken? Have they been brought into hospital? Have they been taken as prescribed, relating to both dose and times per day? What is done if a dose is 'missed'? For example a person who has to take a drug three times a day may go out in the morning, meet a friend unexpectedly, have lunch, and arrive back at 16.00 h. Answers to some of these suggested prompts may alert the nurse to the patient's inadequate understanding of the disease and the medications. It would be inappropriate to arrange a teaching session so early in the patient's stay because the tablets may be changed and so on. But the nurse, having perceived a potential problem of 'non-compliance because of inadequate knowledge', could record this: the nursing intervention 'teach patient about medications' would be written on the nursing plan at a later date. This demonstrates that information on the assessment form can be useful throughout the patient's stay. Or if it is the custom to put potential problems on the nursing plan, in this instance, there will not be an immediate nursing intervention. The nurse will also get some idea of the patient's attitude to medications and his beliefs about whether or not they are 'doing him any good'.

For those patients who are not taking any medication, the nurse, using information collected from other sources before the initial assessment will bear in mind whether or not the patient is likely to need medication during the stay. Those admitted for surgery will minimally have a premedication before going to the operating theatre. Should the patient rate himself as a poor sleeper, the nurse may elicit that in spite of this, he does not believe in taking sleeping pills.

Considering the different sorts of medications and the routes by which they may be administered, collecting information about the patient's knowledge, attitudes and beliefs may be needed at any time during the patient's stay, for example if a suppository or a pessary is prescribed, or if the patient requires to be rehydrated via an intravenous drip.

Planning

Planning, the second phase of the process, is associated with the patient's nursing plan. Examination of the collected information and discussion with the patient will help to identify any problems which he might be experiencing in relation to medications. Poor sight can cause anxiety about reading the label correctly; disabled hands can find opening containers difficult; the tablet may be too large for comfortable swallowing and so on. Of course many patients will not have a problem, either on admission or during their stay. How-ever, the number of articles in the Reading Assignment which mention non-compliance regarding drug taking after discharge, or indeed in those who have never been in hospital, shows that nurses do have a responsibility to teach patients about their drugs, how to identify the different ones, what each one is expected to achieve, and about contacting their GP should anything untoward happen. Maybe lack of teaching (to avoid noncompliance) has occurred because of too rigid an interpretation of the process of nursing, for example that a nursing intervention is selected to solve or alleviate a patient's problem. As practice in 'process thinking', it was suggested earlier that the possibility of non-compliance could be thought of as a potential problem. Bradshaw (1987) discusses ways in which nurses can improve their practice and McMillan (1984) discusses factors influencing compliance, reasons for non-compliance and the nurse's role in education, giving a plan for same.

Implementing

Several points about this third phase of the process, implementing, have already been made. The subject of this chapter — helping patients to avoid hazards related to medications — is so wide-ranging that a list is going to be presented of the possible nursing interventions arising from the doctor's prescription for medication, which includes:

- application of ointment to the skin
- application of a drug patch to the skin
- giving medicines
- giving injections
  - — intradermal
  - — intramuscular } syringe drive
  - — subcutaneous } syringe drive
  - — intravenous
- participating in injections
  - — intrathecal
  - — epidural
- giving steam inhalations
- administering nebulisers
- giving oxygen via
  - — a variety of masks
  - — nasal catheters
  - — a tent
- administering hyperbaric oxygen
- inserting a suppository
- giving enemeta
- inserting a pessary.

Any of the preceding prescriptions will be recorded on the patient's medication Kardex which, where appropriate, the nurse signs as she 'implements' the planned prescription. However, the nurse's responsibiity does not end with the signature. The doctor has an objective/goal when prescribing medications. For example, antihypertensive drugs lower a raised blood pressure; but how low? It will depend on age of patient for one thing. If it goes too low he may have problems of a different kind. The medication Kardex caters only for implementing its instructions — giving the medication. The patient's plan should therefore contain the nursing interventions arising from the medical prescription, agreed by both nurse and doctor, which are to be implemented, for example in this instance: 'take blood pressure before giving medication'. This implementation will be recorded on the blood pressure chart and there will be immediate evaluation as the levels are compared with the previous recording. The nursing intervention on the patient's plan may continue, 'if diastolic pressure below ... withhold dose and inform charge nurse'. The fact that the dose is not given will be recorded on the patient's nursing notes.

The intervention on the nursing plan for a patient having an intravenous infusion may be 'change dressing at IV site'. Each nurse therefore implements this according to her knowledge and expertise, and the patient may well be aware that the arm is much more comfortable after being dressed by Nurse X than Nurse Y.

Evaluating

Where time-related goals have been set, on the appointed day, the assessment data and the patient's nursing notes will be inspected to see whether or not there is any summative/cumulative evaluation data. In the interest of minimising paper work it is important to realise that different 'implementations' are written on different charts — the medication Kardex and blood pressure chart have already been referred to. There may be an intake and output chart if the patient is being stabilised on a diuretic, and of course the temperature, pulse and respiration chart if, for example, antibiotics or antipyretics are prescribed.

Inspecting the medication Kardex may reveal that a medication error occurred — strength of dose, volume of dose, number of tablets and so on (Cobb 1986) and an opportunity to discuss this is given in the Topics for discussion (p. 300). A simple guide to infant drug calculation is given by Glasper & Oliver (1984).

The fact that potential problems have not become actual ones is an important factor in evaluation. For example, no scalding from steam inhalation; no explosion or fire from using oxygen; no sepsis at injection site; no instances of non-compliance.

If teaching drug regimes is broken down into tiny steps, they will provide criteria for evaluation, for example:

- patient recognises different tablets
- knows what each is for
- knows when to take each of them
- knows what untoward signs or symptoms should be reported to the doctor.

The length of this chapter is indicative of the important role which nurses can enact in achieving with patients, outcomes that are safe and maximally therapeutic in relation to medications. The various routes and methods of giving medications were discussed at the beginning of the chapter before considering the principle — helping patients to avoid hazards related to medications — in a process of nursing context.

APPLYING THE PRINCIPLE

A registered nurse must be capable of:

- ordering, storing and using Controlled Drugs and Scheduled drugs
- conducting a safe self-medication programme in the ward
- instructing and supervising staff so that they learn a reliable method for giving medicine
- carrying out a reliable policy for the giving of injections
- instructing and supervising staff members so that they learn a reliable policy for the giving of injections
- giving steam treatment with safety and maximum benefit to the patient
- instructing and supervising staff in the administration of steam
- giving oxygen with safety and maximum benefit to the patient
- instructing and supervising staff in the administration of oxygen
- using the fire extinguisher; seeing that all staff know where it is and how to use it
- giving of a suppository to be retained
- giving of a suppository to produce evacuation of the bowel
- giving of fluid which has to be retained by the rectum

- giving of fluid which has to be returned from the rectum.
- inserting a pessary into the posterior vaginal fornix accompanied by suitable conversation with the patient
- ascertaining a patient's knowledge about self-insertion of pessaries, correcting any misinformation and supplying any needed information.
- applying the principle — helping patients to avoid hazards related to medications — in a process of nursing context.

WORKING ASSIGNMENT

Topics for discussion

- the particular method of giving medicines in your hospital
- self-medication — at home, and in hospital
- when a person leaves the chemist's counter having exchanged a National Health Service prescription for drugs, to whom do they belong?
- the advantages and disadvantages of ward day rooms
- identification of patient prior to medication
- different cultural attitudes to medicines
- a patient's right to refuse medication
- a nurse commits a prescription error — should it be reported?
- the policy for disposal of 'sharps' to be carried out by staff members in the employment of the health board in your area
- sensitisation of staff to antibiotics
- diseases transmitted by blood
- administration of oxygen
- carbon dioxide narcosis
- steam inhalations
- the enema v. the suppository
- disposable enemata
- pessaries

Writing assignment

- why must medicine (in a powder) never be put in milk for a child?
- what are the rules for the storage of drugs and lotions in your hospital?
- what are the rules for giving medicines in your hospital?
- define the following words which have been introduced in a nursing context:

addiction
adrenaline
AIDS
allergy
analgesic
anaphylactic
antacid
anthelmintic
antibiotics
anticoagulant
antidepressants
antiemetic
antihistamine
antipyretic
antisecretory
antispasmodic
atropine
barbiturates
belladonna
benzodiazepines
bismuth
bradycardia
bronchodilator
cachet
capsule
carminative
chemotherapy
chlorpromazine
clinical trial
Controlled Drugs
coramine
cytotoxic
depot drugs
depression
diuretic
emetic
expectorant
hallucinogens
hepatitis B
HIV
hyoscine
hypersensitivity

hypertension
hypnotic
hypotension
hypotensive
iatrogenic
idiosyncrasy
Imferon
insulin
intolerance
laxative
linctus
liniment
mixture
monoamine oxidase inhibitors
morphine
mucilage
narcotic
non-comprehension
non-compliance
opium
over the counter drugs
papaveretum
paracetamol
paraldehyde
parenteral
patient's advocate
penicillin
pessary
pharmacokinetics
pill
Scheduled drugs
sedative
sensitivity
side-effects
stimulants
streptomycin
sublingual
suppository
tablet
tachycardia
tincture
tinnitus
tranquilliser
trimester
vasoconstrictor
vasodilator
vitamin B_{12}

- state the reasons for giving drugs by injection
- state the advantages of the intramuscular over the hypodermic (subcutaneous) route for giving drugs
- state the method for giving the different injections in your hospital
- draw diagrams to illustrate the sites used for intramuscular injections
- define the following:

hygienic hand disinfection
immunological status
intra-articular
intradermal
intramuscular
intrathecal
intravenous
pathogenicity
resident microorganisms on the skin
subcutaneous
therapeutic
transient microorganisms on the skin
virulence of microorganisms

- state the reasons for which intermittent steam inhalations may be ordered
- what medicaments can be used in conjunction with a steam inhalation?
- how would you instruct a patient about to have a jug inhalation for sinusitis?
- how would you instruct a patient about to have a Nelson's inhaler for tracheitis?
- give the first-aid treatment for burns and scalds
- how would you recognize a cylinder containing oxygen?
- state some conditions for which oxygen may be administered
- what rules are observed in your hospital with regard to the administration of oxygen?
- where is the fire extinguisher in the ward in which you are working?
- define the following:

acute
Alevaire
amyl nitrite
anaemia
anoxaemia
anoxia
asthma

atelectasis
atherosclerosis
bronchiectasis
bronchitis
bulbar paralysis
carboxyhaemoglobin
chronic
coma
confusion
congestive heart failure
coryza
cyanosis
disorientation
dysfunction
dyspnoea
emphysema
ephedrine
euphoria
haemoconcentration
haemorrhage
haemothorax
hydrothorax
hypoxia
isoprenaline
laryngitis
mucolytic
muscle relaxant
myocardial infarction
pharyngitis
pneumoconiosis
pneumonia
pneumothorax
poliomyelitis
pulmonary oedema
Raynaud's disease
retrolental fibroplasia
rhinorrhoea
shock
sinusitis
tetanus
tracheitis
tracheostomy
tuberculosis
tumour

- name the medicaments given by suppository in your hospital
- name the fluids given rectally to be retained in your hospital
- describe your conversation with a patient before introducing a suppository or fluid intended to produce evacuation of the bowel
- describe your conversation with a patient before introducing a suppository or fluid to be retained in the rectum
- define the following:

adrenaline
aminophylline
diuretic
Flagyl
haemorrhoids
hygroscopic
menopause
nystatin
oedema
pessary
spermicidal
stilboestrol
suppository
thrush
Trichomonas vaginalis
vaginitis

- describe your conversation with an outpatient who needed daily insertion of a medicated pessary.

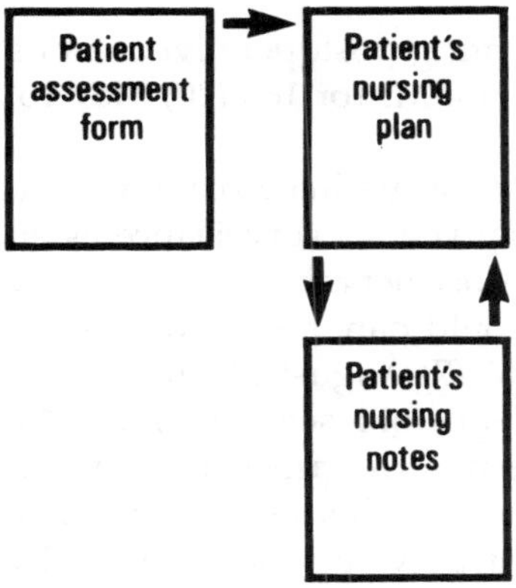

Reading assignment

Background information
Informed consent
Routes of admission

Surgical patients and the process of nursing
Assessing the surgical patient
Planning
Implementing
Evaluating

Applying the principle
A registered nurse must be capable of:

Working assignment
Topics for discussion
Writing assignment

24

Helping patients to reduce the hazards associated with operations

READING ASSIGNMENT

Ayton M 1985 Infection control — a question of balance. Nursing 2 (35)35 March: 1039–1040

Bond S 1980 Shave it…or save it? Nursing Times 76 (9) February 28: 362–363
Pre-operative shaving in minor gynaecological surgery and obstetrics: shaving can be harmful: why does shaving persist?

Boore J 1978 Prescription for recovery. Royal College of Nursing, London
Research monograph.

Coates V 1984 Inadequate intake in hospital. Nursing Mirror 158 (5) February 1: 21–22

Cowan V 1987 Documentation. Nursing 3 (14) February: 527–529
Discusses several intricacies of informed consent.

Date J 1984 Sterile pursuit. Nursing Mirror 159 (23) December 19: 14
Normal bathing pre-operatively for skin cleanliness; careful disinfection of operation site with isopropyl alcohol or povidone-iodine immediately before the incision. Not removing hair produces the lowest infection rate.

Hamilton Smith S 1972 Nil by mouth. Royal College of Nursing, London
Research shows varying interpretation of nursing order 'Fast for anaesthetic'.

Hayward J 1975 Information — a prescription against pain. Royal College of Nursing, London
Research monograph.

Gooch J 1984 The other side of surgery. Macmillan, London

Hunt M 1987 The process of translating research findings into nursing practice. Journal of Advanced Nursing 12 101–110
Pre-operative fasting.

Kennett A 1986 Informed consent: a patient's right? The Professional Nurse 2 (3) December: 75–77

Leeson L 1985 Pain and the postoperative patient. Nursing: The Add-On Journal of Clinical Nursing 2 (43) November: 1259–1290
What is pain? Discusses non-invasive methods of acute pain control.

Leonard M 1984 At the surgical site. Nursing Mirror 159 (16) October 31: (Wound management supplement)

Medical Defence Union 1970 Consent to treatment. Medical Defence Union, London

Melia K 1986 Dangerous territory. Nursing Times 82 (21) May 21: 27

Moir-Bussy B R 1986 The surgical wound. Nursing 3 3 March: 92–94
Gives the classification of clean; clean-contaminated, and contaminated.

O'Brien D K 1986 Postoperative wound infections. Nursing 3 (5) May: 178, 180–182.
The risks of postoperative wound infection are rarely discussed with the patient prior to surgery, but such risks are very real. An infection control nursing officer discusses the risks in detail.

Pettersson E 1986 A cut above the rest? The Journal of Infection Control Nursing 3: March 5: 68, 70
Looks at how electric hair clippers have proved to be a popular method of removing hair.

Pyne R 1986 Tell me honestly. Nursing Times 82 (21) May 21: 25–26
The concept of informed consent.

RCN, the Association of Theatre Nurses, and the medical insurance organisations. 1987 Theatre safeguards. Royal College of Nursing, London (Booklet).

Saxey S 1986 The nurse's response to post-operative pain. Nursing: The Add-On Journal of Clinical Nursing 3 (10) October: 377–381
Reports a study of nurses' knowledge of analgesic nursing interventions. References.

Smith K 1985 Preventing postoperative venous thrombosis. Nursing Mirror 160 (20) May 15: 29–30
Describes a study using graduated compression stockings and daily venous surveillance as an alternative to low-dose heparin.

Summers R 1984 Should patients be told more? Nursing Mirror 159 (7) August 29: 16–20
Medical hospital doctors seem to hide the truth from patients. Describes an investigation to discover whether appropriate information might prevent worry caused by this veil of secrecy.

Tait A 1986 When the doctor doesn't always know best. Senior Nurse 5 (2) August: 19–21

Tweedle D 1978 How the metabolism reacts to injury: tissue repair. Nursing Mirror 147 (21) November 23: 34–38 August: 19–21

UKCC 1984 Code of professional conduct for the nurse, midwife and health visitor. London

Wells R 1986 The great conspiracy. Nursing Times 82 (21) May: 22–25

Winfield W 1986 Too close a shave? Journal of Infection Control Nursing 31 March 5: 64, 67-68
How safe is preoperative shaving? In a study into the different methods of shaving, razor shaving caused the most discomfort to patients.

Wright S 1985 Patient's page: Conspiracy of silence. Nursing Mirror 160 (20) May 15: 47–48
A very clear account of what the postoperative period meant to an intelligent and articulate patient after a vaginal hysterectomy.

BACKGROUND INFORMATION

Most laymen's concept of the operating theatre is tinged with drama and mystery. Most people's concept of having an anaesthetic is of having a mask put over the face. In many people this engenders a feeling of repulsion. Anything that is put over the face tends to have an unpleasant association with smothering. Some people have the idea that all one's secrets are spoken while under the influence of an anaesthetic. Some people have a deep-rooted fear of not waking up from an anaesthetic; from the number who make a will before entry to hospital it is evident that they have faced the possibility of death. Most people have experienced bleeding from a cut in the flesh and they may have an unspoken fear that one could bleed to death during an operation.

Many lay people read in the daily press of the occasional misadventure of an instrument or a swab left in the abdominal cavity at operation, of the wrong patient or the wrong side being operated on. The Theatre safeguards' booklet (RCN 1987) advises on how to avoid such occurrences. Every ex-patient becomes an ambassador for good or ill; his account of his sojourn in hospital, having an anaesthetic and undergoing an operation may influence other people's attitude to these things.

Coming from this complex background it is usual to arrange for most surgical patients to be admitted 24 hours before the operation. This allows for the establishment of mutual understanding and trust between the patient and the surgical team. Obese patients for elective surgery are usually asked to reduce their weight before admission. Smokers are similarly asked to refrain from smoking for at least 1 week before admission.

Drugs such as antidepressants, antihypertensives, cortisone, diuretics, oral contraceptives and phenobarbitone can cause a reaction to the anaesthetic. In some areas the patients are asked to bring to hospital any pills and/or medicines which they are currently taking so that they can be checked. In other areas the patient's general practitioner is sent a form before the proposed day of admission so that he can fill in the names of the drugs which the patient is taking; there is a stamped addressed envelope and the response has been good. Oral contraceptives may not be covered by this method as some women get them from the Family Planning Clinic, so it is important to check this at the initial assessment of the patient.

Informed consent

In the past it has been customary for the nursing staff to get the patient to sign the 'consent form' as part of the admission routine. The Medical Defence Union (1970) recommends consent forms which include a signed declaration by the medical practitioner that he has explained the nature and purpose of the operation to the patient. The booklet explains:

> To be an effective answer to a claim for assault, the consent must have been fully and freely given. The patient should therefore be told in non-technical language, the nature and purpose of the operation. This should be done by a medical practitioner. If an inadequate or misleading explanation is given, the apparent consent obtained may be held to be ineffective.

Wells (1986), a nurse, contends that this is:

> solely intended to protect the surgeon and the hospital, and not the patient. Many consent forms contain phrases such as 'and any other procedures which may become necessary during the operation'.

Certainly this allows the surgeon to implement necessary life-saving procedures should anything untoward occur during the operation. However there are instances when a patient has wakened to find that for instance a colostomy or a mastectomy has been what the surgeon considered 'necessary during the operation'. Members of a better educated public are beginning to realise that there are alternative operations which can be performed for particular conditions. As an example, in many instances of breast cancer, the breast can be preserved, resulting in less psychiatric disturbance and preservation of body image (Wells 1986). Not all patients are informed of this alternative and therefore routinely undergo mastectomy. The concept of 'informed concept' as propagated by the medical profession mentioned previously will increasingly be subjected to pressure from members of the general public. Pyne (1986), Director of Professional Conduct, the United Kingdom Central Council (UKCC) for Nursing, Midwifery and Health Visiting, tells of nurses who contact him on behalf of patients who are 'told little of the surgery for which their consent is sought, or of being told the benefits of a particular operation, but nothing about possible complications, adverse effects and impact on daily living'. Pyne goes on to say that:

> To develop a positive system which takes the patient into partnership requires interprofessional discussion and cooperation, particularly between the medical and nursing professions ... the UKCC ... hoped to engage in official discussions with another statutory body with a view to the preparation of a joint statement or advisory document on the issue of informed consent.

On the other hand Melia (1986) after discussing the routine consent for surgery, explains that even when the legal position is adhered to and the doctor has fulfilled his obligations, there remain ethical considerations for nurses. These arise when patients, after signing the form, say they do not understand the course of action to which they have agreed. She concludes that

> consent to medical treatment is not an area in which nurses can ever truly be held responsible. It would perhaps be not only prudent but also morally sound to recognise this fact and leave doctor's business to doctors.

There is no doubt that the concept of informed consent will develop further and the role of the registered nurse will be clarified. Students reading this text should understand that when they become registered nurses, they have a responsibility to update their knowledge by continuing to read at least some of the nursing journals.

The Royal College of Nursing and the National Council of Nurses of the United Kingdom (RCN) is often told that there is difficulty in the working situation because medical practitioners still delegate to nurses the duty of obtaining consent and giving the explanation to the patient. In view of problems which might arise if there is any legal action concerning the operation it is unwise for nurses to accept this duty. Should the patient ask for a further explanation from the nurse, this should be referred to the medical practitioner who first talked to the patient. It is most important that any doubts (Wells 1986) expressed by the patient about the operation should be reported to the surgeon and the anaesthetist so that they can decide whether or not to proceed. Where members of the nursing profession have any difficulty concerning consent to treatment, they should seek advice from the RCN Labour Relations Department.

Anyone over 16 can now give consent to surgical, medical or dental treatment even in face of objections by parents or guardians.

Occasionally one meets a patient, who, because of his beliefs, refuses life-saving treatment. This an adult is entitled to do, but it poses a problem when a parent refuses such measures for a child. After time was lost while an emergency session of a juvenile court was convened to override the refusal of the parents to consent to a life-saving transfusion for their baby, the then Ministry of Health (1967) advised:

> Hospital authorities should therefore rely on the clinical judgement of the consultants concerned after full discussion with the parents. If in such a case the consultant obtains a written supporting opinion from a colleague that the patient's life is in danger if operation or transfusion is withheld, and an acknowledgement (preferably in writing) from the parent or guardian that despite the explanation of the danger he refuses consent, then the consultant would run little risk in a court of law if he acts with due professional competence and according to his own professional conscience, and operates on the child or gives a transfusion.

Routes of admission

Patients admitted for elective surgery have already been mentioned (p. 305), and the usual interpretation is that it will be to a general surgical ward. These are increasingly rare, usually because of the surgeon's particular interests. In the interest of financial economy some hospitals have a one-day surgical ward — the patient is given the necessary information, both verbal and written as an outpatient and attends the day ward on the appointed day and is collected by a relative in the late afternoon. There are also 5-day surgical wards — Monday morning admission, Friday afternoon discharge. Both these short stay systems depend on co-operation and good communication with the community nursing services. Highly specialised surgical wards are to be found in many cities, such as a burns unit, cardiac surgery, cardio-vascular surgery, plastic surgery, ophthalmic surgery; ear, nose and throat surgery. So patients for elective surgery can be found in wards with a variety of clinical labels. And nurses are expected to be able to apply 'process thinking' to the nursing which is planned for patients with such different medical diagnoses.

However, many patients arrive in the various types of surgical ward as an 'emergency' from the Accident and Emergency department; or they may have gone straight to the operating theatre from that department, to be transferred to the ward after surgery. Absolutely minimal nursing assessment will have been possible, and will not be possible in the ward until the patient's condition permits. This was discussed on page 90. Bearing such diverse routes of admission in mind an attempt will now be made to consider surgical patients in a process of nursing context.

SURGICAL PATIENTS AND THE PROCESS OF NURSING

The main purpose in using the process is to individualise nursing, and this surely depends on the patient's individuality, shaped by his experience of living, up to the time of entry to hospital for surgery. This can be at any stage of living — infant, child, adolescent, adult or elderly. As can be seen from the previous text, the stay can be as short as one day, or several days or weeks, or months; the example given for a longer stay was a patient in a hip spica (p. 273). It would seem that:

- if we are to progress beyond the torrent of abuse about excessive paperwork imposed by implementation of the process of nursing
- if we are to use the process as our servant and not our master in helping us to understand the complexities of 'nursing'
- if we are to provide an equivalent standard of nursing to short, as well as long stay patients,

then we need to become skilled in 'process thinking' so that it guides our clinical nursing. This text has demonstrated that every aspect of nurse/patient interaction cannot possibly be documented, but ipso facto we have to acquire the skill of recognising the essentials which must be documented in as succinct and precise terms as possible.

Assessing the surgical patient

The document associated with assessing (usually interpreted as the initial interview) is variously called patient's assessment form, nursing history or patient profile. It usually requests the nurse to discover what the patient understands about the reason for admission. In the context of this chapter it is for surgery: the following questions do not need to be asked; they are to be borne in mind to guide the nurse as to relevant information required. Question form is used to encourage an enquiring mind:

- has there been any previous experience of surgery? self or other?
- what does the patient know about the operation for which he has been admitted?
- what is the patient's perception of the wound resulting from the operation? (p. 266)
- what is the patient's perception of infection? A wound exposed to bedclothes which 'look' clean may be ignored. Co-operation is needed postoperatively in not touching the wound
- what does he understand about drainage from the wound, if appropriate (p. 268)?
- if the operation involves the small or large intestine, what does he know about 'germs' which normally live there and do no harm? — if they invade the wound, they can become pathogenic and cause infection there – not necessarily due to poor surgical technique: it is one of the risks of intestinal surgery.
- does he know that he will have to use, for instance:
  a bedpan
  crutches
  feeding cup
  a straw for drinking?
  anxiety may be lessened by using these preoperatively
- what does he know about preventive activities which he will need to implement, such as:
  coughing
  breathing
  leg exercises?
  again, starting these preoperatively will reduce the 'strangeness' postoperatively
- is there any suggestion of:
  allergy
  sensitivity
  predisposition to bleeding?
  If these are mentioned as being present in some other member of the family,

questions may need to be asked about these matters without alarming the patient. If relevant, information should be recorded on the assessment form.

- what does he know about being 'fasted'? From the jesting that goes on in the ward when the 'Nil by mouth' card is hung on the bed, it may well be that it is common knowledge. However some ex-patients tell tales of having felt famished before an afternoon operation. Malnutrition can delay wound healing (p. 147)
- what does the patient know about preparation of the operation site?
  - will it be covered before operation?
  - will there be a preoperative bath?
  - will the area be rendered free from hair?
  - how will this be achieved?
- what does the patient know about wearing special clothing for theatre?
  it is customary to wear a theatre gown, cap and socks/boots
- does the patient realise that dentures (or any other prosthesis) cannot be worn in the theatre?
- what does the patient know about 'having an anaesthetic'?
- what does the patient expect will happen on the day of operation?
- will there be any bowel preparation such as an enema or suppository? when?
- what does the patient expect about possible discomfort, soreness, pain after the operation?
- has he any idea of the length of stay?
  people worry about things like being away from the family, from work, from their favourite hobby: the annual holiday may be planned and he may be wondering if he will be well enough to keep to the plan
  the very fact that the nurse is willing to put the patient's operation into the context of his life is reassuring.

This focused conversation will probably not need to be recorded, and will not give rise to a specific nursing intervention on the patient's nursing plan. Yet it is an essential nursing activity. There is now sufficient research evidence (Hayward 1975, Boore 1978) that patients who are adequately informed preoperatively are less anxious, which in turn decreases postoperative pain, vomiting and complications, thereby minimising the patients' stay in hospital. This surely must be advantageous for patients, as the longer they stay, the more likely they are to become colonised with 'hospital microorganisms', some of which are resistant to antibiotics. Although Hayward's work was published 12 years ago and Boore's 9 years ago, an account of an investigation (Summers) published in 1984 revealed that only 30% of nurses had heard of Hayward's or Boore's research.

The areas of knowledge to reduce anxiety, suggested by Hayward (1975), are:

- recognition of staff
- length of time to be spent in hospital
- knowledge of operation
- preoperative preparation
- anaesthesia
- postoperative care
- medication
- exercises
- ambulation.

These areas should be borne in mind during the initial assessment and it is important for nurses to remember that assessing is a two-way process; the patient should be given opportunity to express ideas and ask questions.

Planning

The second phase of the process, planning, in the context of 'helping patients to avoid hazards associated with operations', relates to potential problems.

Wound infection is an ever present possibility, so the nursing plan may carry an instruction for a preoperative bath approximately 1 hour prior to the scheduled time of operation. In some wards it is customary to add a bactericidal lotion to the bath water, but Dale (1984) discusses briefly the research reports on this subject and they show no significant difference in wound infection rates because of the addition. Although bathing can improve morale by removing those substances which accumulate on the skin surface

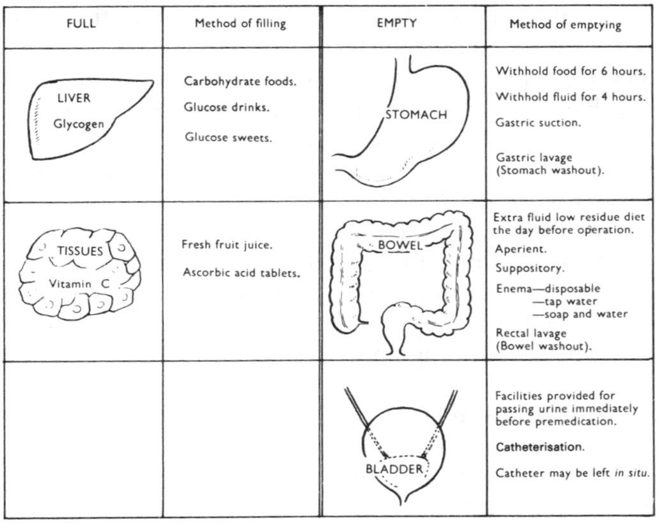

FULL
Method of filling
EMPTY
Method of emptying
LIVER
Glycogen
Carbohydrate foods.
Glucose drinks.
Glucose sweets.
STOMACH
Withhold food for 6 hours.
Withhold fluid for 4 hours.
Gastric suction.
Gastric lavage
(Stomach washout).
TISSUES
Vitamin C
Fresh fruit juice.
Ascorbic acid tablets.
BOWEL
Extra fluid low residue diet the day before operation.
Aperient.
Suppository.
Enema—disposable
—tap water
—soap and water
Rectal lavage
(Bowel washout).
BLADDER
Facilities provided for passing urine immediately before premedication.
Catheterisation.
Catheter may be left *in situ*.

Fig. 24.1 Some preoperative measures

before they decompose and cause an unpleasant odour, it cannot be relied on to remove all bacteria. The site is therefore cleaned with a bactericidal solution immediately before incision. Leonard (1984) quotes an American study in which bacterial colonies on the skin of volunteers were counted before and after the application of the disinfectant used in the operating theatre. The average predisinfection count was 133.3 colonies per cm^2, reducing to 8.2 after disinfection. Most people's defence mechanisms can cope with this reduced number so that infection does not intervene. The donning of clean clothes, and returning from theatre to a freshly made bed with clean linen, both have the rationale of helping to prevent wound infection. The questionable contribution of shaving will be discussed later. Should the wound require to be dressed, the nursing plan will carry the intervention which has to be implemented using an aseptic technique.

Respiratory infection is also a potential problem for the patient undergoing surgery. The nursing plan will have an instruction to give the premedication injection 1 hour before operation to lessen secretion from the upper respiratory tract membrane. The anaesthetic gas is likely to be less irritant to a drier mucous membrane. It is to prevent respiratory obstruction, which can lead to infection, that the plan will request removal of dentures, especially a dental plate with only a few teeth attached. Aspiration pneumonia can occur if food is regurgitated up the oesophagus to be inhaled. It is for this reason that a preventive nursing intervention will be written on the nursing plan to withhold food for 6 hours and fluid for 4 hours (Fig. 24.1). The diversity of practice in preoperative fasting is given by Hamilton Smith (1972) in a research monograph. Hunt (1987 p. 106) reports a replication of this study — with strikingly similar results. She explains in detail how the multidisciplinary team developed the policy, and faced such problems as changing the time of theatre lists; changing the order of the theatre lists. Kitchen and domestic staff had to make a contribution by providing early morning breakfasts. Some nursing staff at ward level had great difficulty in accepting the change — after all it is much easier to hang 'Nil by mouth' notices on the beds of all patients having an operation the next day!

However, considering the evidence of malnutrition in surgical patients (Tweedle 1978, Coates 1984), it would be desirable for nurses in other hospitals to initiate multidisciplinary investigation to identify problems and systems which require to be changed so that preoperative fasting will be a research-based activity. When this is so, tales of ex-patients saying that they suffered 'hunger pains' before afternoon surgery will belong to the past.

Another potential problem is deep vein thrombosis (DVT) and the planned preventive nursing intervention will be supervising deep breathing and leg exercises hourly (p. 203,215). There may be a delegated intervention if the surgeon prescribes the wearing of support hose, or even pneumatic stockings during the operation. And some surgeons prescribe a course of small dose heparin, an anticoagulant given by injection.

Discussion of potential problems related to having an operation would not be complete without considering discomfort, soreness and pain. When one considers 'cutting the flesh', and handling the tissues, before stitching it up again, there will minimally be discomfort and soreness. Even acknowledging this will comfort the patient; ignoring it may well make the patient feel that the nurse does not care. The fact that the surgeon usually prescribes pain relieving drugs to be given 'as necessary' means that judging when it is necessary is a nursing skill.

Saxey (1986) found in her research that nurses under-used the 'as necessary' medical prescription, and their knowledge of narcotics and analgesics varied, and in some instances was deficient. Pain is discussed in Chapter 4, but a reminder here, pain is what the patient says it is. It is a subjective experience and it is not the business of nurses to imply that the patient cannot be experiencing that much pain; or to compare patients. Each patient's pain experience is individual, and regular use of a painometer (p. 52) after operation would be desirable. When nurse and patient work together it should be possible to keep the patient free from pain, by implementing the planned interventions.

Implementing

Implementing, the third phase of the process, is associated with the patient's nursing notes in the documentation system used in this book. Implementing has already been mentioned in this chapter, and this serves to show the circularity of the four phases. As each planned nursing intervention is implemented it will be recorded. Some of the interventions will be prescribed on the medication Kardex, and each time the prescription is implemented, the nurse's signature on the Kardex should be sufficient without writing on the patient's nursing notes, unless of course something untoward has happened such as the patient having a reaction to an antibiotic. However a system needs to be worked out for recording administration of pain relieving drugs and their effect as evaluated by use of a painometer. To recapitulate, the planned nursing interventions to be implemented are likely to be:

- preoperative bath
- special theatre clothes
- bed made up with clean linen
- premedication
- removal of prostheses
- pre-anaesthetic fasting
- supervising deep breathing and foot exercises
- pain relief programme
- aseptic dressing of wound.

The surgeon may request a hair-free operation site. In order to help patients to reduce the hazards associated with this request, nurses should be familiar with the research into hair removal. For many years shaving was, and still is, the method most commonly used (O'Brien 1986). However, scanning electron micrographs have shown that every skin shave causes epidermal damage (Moir-Bussy 1986). She goes on to say that 'If a shave is performed it should be carried out immediately prior to surgery to reduce colonization of these damaged areas which may lead to wound infection'. O'Brien (1986) elucidates 'colonization' and says it is with potentially pathogenic 'hospital microorganisms'. It has to be remembered that some of these are now antibiotic resistant. If the surgeon insists on shaving, knowledge from research indicates that it is preferable to:

- use a disposable razor, and foam rather than soap, or
- an electric razor with a removable head which can be disinfected.

There are alternative methods of removing hair from the skin. It can be cut off with scissors, the blades of which have rounded ends to avoid nicking the skin. Pettersson (1986) describes how to assemble and use electric hair clippers for pre-operative hair removal. As they are non-traumatic to the skin, hair can be removed the day before surgery which can help to shed the workload if several patients are on the operating list. Data were not collected regarding post-operative wound infection.

Winfield (1986) reports a study in which the use of a disposable razor was compared with a depilatory cream, using several criteria as well as wound infection; these included patient satisfaction, medical staff satisfaction, cost and nurse's time spent/saved in the two different procedures. She says 'Present evidence indicates that the infection rate with no shaving would not be different than using a cream' and she gives the references for the two studies supporting the statement.

Other 'unwritten' plans are implemented.

The beds of patients having operations are placed near sister's desk or the nurses' station to facilitate the frequent assessments (pp. 311 to 314) which have to be made and recorded. The principle of such grouping of patients is the same as that of intensive care units, but elaborate monitoring and other special equipment is available only in the units.

The position of, and respiratory care necessary for, an anaesthetized patient is given on page 210. Early ambulation is discussed on page 155. Early ambulation is not a licence for the patient to be up and about all day. Getting out on the commode five or six times is ample ambulation on the first postoperative day for a patient who has had a straightforward appendicectomy. Walking a short distance to and from the lavatory once or twice is sufficient increase of ambulation for the second day. From then on, the rate of increase of activity should fit each individual patient. Clear written instruction in the nursing plan is necessary so that the eager patient cannot play one nurse off against another by saying that he has permission to stay up all day. The patients should understand that gentle early ambulation does not mean that they can stop doing their breathing and leg exercises at least six times daily. Pulmonary embolism is a postoperative hazard.

Those who are apprehensive about getting up so early after operation need time to establish confidence in the fact that their wound comes to no harm, and that they feel better for the gentle, unhurried exercise. It is easy for nurses to think that all patients should respond in the same way to having a clean-stitched wound. A few months in the wards should be sufficient to convince any nurse that this just is not true. There are a myriad of ways in which people can respond to a given situation, which is what makes nursing so interesting.

Postoperative assessment of patient

Assessment	Rationale	Nursing Intervention
Temperature of skin —		
Below normal	Circulatory inadequacy (Shock)	Complete rest. Adequate bedclothes. Extra warmth only applied if prescribed by doctor. Head of bed lowered to an angle of 5°.
Above normal	Upset of temperature regulating centre	Blanket can be removed as extra blood should not be out in the skin vessels, but should be conserved for vital organs.
	Infection	Observe patient for other signs, e.g. pulse of normal volume, but increased in rate; increased respiration rate; moist respiration suggestive of respiratory infection.

Assessment	Rationale	Nursing Intervention
Colour of skin —		
Ashen grey	Circulatory inadequacy (Shock)	As for below normal temperature.
Waxen pallor	Haemorrhage External Internal	Inspect dressing. Apply sterile pad and firm pressure over existing dressing. Notify doctor. Observe for other signs and symptoms of haemorrhage, i.e. subnormal temperature, pulse increasing in rate, decreasing in volume, sighing respirations, restlessness. Notify doctor.
Blue (Cyanosis)	Shortage of oxygen May be due to:	
	1. Failing circulation	As for below normal temperature. Oxygen via mask at the rate prescribed by the surgeon for emergencies. Notify doctor. Have ready injection tray and heart stimulant.
	2. Failing respiration	As for below normal temperature.
	(a) From interference with respiratory centre	Notify doctor. Have ready O_2 and CO_2 for inhalation, injection tray and respiratory stimulant drugs.
	(b) Prolonged action of curare preventing full excursion of respiratory muscles.	Notify doctor. Have injection tray ready. If there is sufficient chest movement to benefit from O_2 this is given by mask. Manual compression of rib cage (Fig.15.24). Mouth to nose breathing (Fig.15.15). Expired air resuscitation with a special tube (Fig.15.16). Use of inflating bellows (Figs15.18–15.20).
	(c) Blockage of respiratory tract by: (i) Plug of mucus (ii) Plug of vomit (iii) Plug of blood	Preventive position (Fig.15.9). Use metal spatula or wooden wedge to prise teeth apart; insert gag, open same. With swab clipped on to long-handled forceps clear back of throat. If colour fails to improve, use suction (Figs.15.21&15.22).
	(iv) Flaccid tongue on posterior pharyngeal wall (Fig. 15.9)	Hold the jaw forward (Fig. 15.10). If colour fails to improve, open mouth as above, draw tongue forward manually or by forceps (Figs15.10–15.14).
Humidity of skin —		
Clamminess	Circulatory inadequacy (Shock)	Take temperature using low-reading thermometer if necessary. If subnormal act according to the surgeon's prescription for this emergency. Usually environmental warmth, i.e. atmosphere and clothing are increased to bring body to normal temperature when it will immediately evaporate the sweat arriving on the skin. Other external warmth, e.g. hot water bottle, electric blanket is seldom applied. Cool tissues need less oxygen.
	Haemorrhage	Take temperature, using low-reading thermometer if necessary. If subnormal look for signs and symptoms of bleeding, given above. Notify doctor.
	Infection	Take temperature. If raised look for other signs of infection as given in Above normal temperature of the skin.

Assessment	Rationale	Nursing Intervention
Pulse —		
Slow and bounding	Early stages of circulatory inadequacy (Shock)	As for Below normal temperature.
Increasing in rate, decreasing in volume	Late stages of circulatory failure (Shock) Haemorrhage	Notify doctor. Have transfusion trolley and injection tray ready. Drugs and fluid replacement will probably be necessary.
Irregular	Ventricular fibrillation	Notify doctor immediately. Send for resuscitation trolley. Defibrillator may have to be used.
Absent	Cardiac arrest	Place patient on floor or board. Start external cardiac massage and expired air resuscitation within 3 minutes. Notify doctor immediately. Send for resuscitation trolley.
Blood pressure —		
Raised	Probably present before operation. Increases operative risk. Anxiety and restlessness can cause cerebral haemorrhage	Discover what patient is anxious about. Help him to cope with anxiety. Give hypotensive drugs as prescribed. Prevent restlessness by nursing measures and judicious use of prescribed sedatives and analgesics.
Lowered	Circulatory inadequacy (Shock)	As for Below normal temperature. Come to an arrangement with doctor as to the level at which he wants to be notified about the falling blood pressure. Observe urinary output as kidneys are unable to secrete when there is low blood pressure. Doctor may ask for a catheter to be left in the bladder and released hourly, urine measured. Have injection tray and transfusion trolley ready.
Respiration —		
Shallow and increased in rate	Circulatory inadequacy (Shock)	As in *Colour of skin —* 2. Failing respiration (b) Prolonged action of curare, etc. p. 312
	Respiratory failure	As in Failing respiration, (a) and (b)
Sighing	Haemorrhage	As in Haemorrhage, External and Internal
Dyspnoea	Respiratory obstruction	As in Failing respiration, (c)
Stertorous and bubbling	Pooling of secretions at back of throat	As in Failing respiration, (c)
Rapid and moist	Infection	Take temperature and pulse. If raised, notify doctor immediately.
Smell of acetone	Metabolic upset Fat incompletely metabolised	Test urine for acetone. Give glucose by mouth, unless patient vomiting, when tray or trolley should be ready for doctor to give glucose intravenously.
Apathy	Circulatory inadequacy (Shock)	As for Below normal temperature. Spare patient any activity until treatment has had time to effect improvement.
Restlessness	Pain	Pain can only be felt when patient has recovered consciousness. Judicious use of prescribed analgesics.
	Haemorrhage	As given above.

Assessment	Rationale	Nursing Intervention
Level of consciousness —		
Response to ordinary voice	Consciousness fully regained	If at all sleepy, patient encouraged to go off to sleep again to get the best advantage from the anaesthetic and premedication. If fully awake patient will appreciate replacement of dentures. Refreshment by sponging hands and face, exchanging theatre for personal clothes, a mouth wash followed by a sip of water may induce further sleep.
Response to loud voice	Consciousness sufficiently regained for coughing and swallowing reflexes to be safe	As above.
Response to touch	Consciousness not sufficiently regained for coughing and swallowing reflexes to be safe	Patient needs constant or frequent observation.
Response to pain (Can be produced by pinching flesh between two finger nails)	Coughing and swallowing reflexes absent	The air tube must be kept patent by all measures already mentioned.
Time of return to consciousness —		In some hospitals it is customary to record this in the patient's nursing notes.
Dressing —		
Damp yellowish patch on outer bandage	Serous oozing	On top of existing dressing and bandage apply sterile wool and another bandage. Continue to inspect at intervals. When oozing has ceased, dressing taken down. Wound redressed with aseptic technique.
Damp blood-stained patch on outer bandage	Blood-stained serous oozing	As above. There may be a drainage tube to attend to.
Frank blood	Haemorrhage	As for haemorrhage.
Inspected to see that it completely covers wound	A clean-stitched wound exposed to patient's clothing and bedclothes will probably become infected	Use of adhesive occlusive dressings or sprays wherever possible.

Evaluating

Evaluating, the fourth phase of the process, necessarily addresses itself to whether or not the potential problems became actual ones. Recordings of the myriad implementations and observations related to a patient having an operation will provide summative and cumulative information on the date set for evaluation. Specific wound infections are a traumatic experience for the patient. They take up extra nursing time: they are not only expensive to treat, but also involve the cost of extra days in hospital. The same can be said of respiratory infection. And should deep vein thrombosis supervene, it is not only one potential problem which has become an actual one, but in its actuality it creates a potential problem of pulmonary embolism! A date will not be set for evaluating the pain control programme because there will be immediate evaluation as the score on the painometer is compared with the last recorded score.

In this chapter the complex concept of informed consent has been discussed, together with the various routes by which patients arrive for surgery. The principle — helping patients to reduce the hazards associated with operations — was considered in a process of nursing context.

APPLYING THE PRINCIPLE

A registered nurse must be capable of:

- giving a patient adequate psychological and physical preparation for surgery
- performing gastric suction and lavage
- administering medicines, injections, infusions
- inserting a suppository, giving an enema and rectal lavage
- catheterising a patient
- taking and recording blood pressure
- assessing the patient postoperatively, interpreting the observations and taking action accordingly
- taking measures to prevent postoperative potential problems from becoming actual ones. Should they become actual ones, recognising them early so that efficient treatment can be started
- dressing a wound with aseptic technique
- knowing and recognising wound complications
- teaching and supervising staff in the acquisition of the aforementioned skills
- having equipment such as oxygen and suction ready to be used in emergency, seeing that all staff know the location of this equipment
- coming to an arrangement with the surgical staff about the treatment to be instituted in emergency by nursing staff pending the doctor's arrival, for example, for cold, clammy skin; rate at which oxygen is to be given; organisation for cardiac massage and expired air resuscitation. Communicating to all staff the exact procedure to be followed.
- applying the principle — helping patients to reduce the hazards associated with operations — in a process of nursing context

WORKING ASSIGNMENT

Topics for discussion

- handwashing
- informed consent
- hair removal from skin as a preventive preoperative nursing activity
- preoperative preparation of a patient for surgery
- postoperative nursing
- postoperative potential problems
- complications of a wound
- making a will as a 'preoperative' activity
- if you had an operation and suffered cardiac arrest, would you want the staff to institute resuscitation?
- your 50-year-old husband has been an invalid for 10 years with progressive multiple sclerosis. He is in hospital for surgery and develops a severe chest infection. He collapses. Would you want the staff to institute resuscitation?

Writing assignment

- for how long before an anaesthetic is food and fluid withheld? Why?
- what factors are important in the preparation of a patient for surgery?
- what observations would you make of the postoperative patient?
- if this patient had an airway in situ, when would you remove it?
- what would you do with it?
- if a postoperative patient went blue, to what might it be due?
- what measures would you take if a patient went blue?
- what is the technical name for this blueness?
- in what position would you place an anaesthetised patient? Why?
- when would you give him a pillow?
- when would you give him a drink?
- why is the bladder and rectum emptied before an anaesthetic?
- what precautions can be taken to ensure that the correct patient is operated on?
- what precautions can be taken to ensure that the correct side is operated on?
- what precautions can be taken to ensure that the correct digit is operated on?
- name the fingers as advocated by the Medical Defence Union
- name the toes as advocated by the Medical Defence Union

Finale

Nursing skills span a lifetime. Midwives care for the needs of pregnant women, are present at the birth of each baby, and care for the mother and baby during the puerperium. A nurse with health visiting skills keeps the family under surveillance until the child is ready for school. A nurse may well be attached to the school medical service and have surveillance of the child's health until he leaves school. Complications can arise at childbirth, and the mother and/or the baby can die, so that all that has been said about the skills of caring for the dying and the grieving will be needed in such an event. Some children are born with congenital abnormalities and need special care throughout their lives. Those who are born blind or deaf may be physically healthy and they will attend special schools for those with their particular handicap. Accident, illness that is predominantly mental or predominantly physical can happen to any person at any time, and such people are usually cared for in hospital, at least in the initial stages. Some unfortunately have a prolonged stay, but the aim as portrayed in this book is to organise the community resources so that as few as possible are cared for as long stay patients. Nursing skills are needed when caring for people at work, when travelling, in the armed forces, suffering accident or disaster. Up to press, the public's image of a nurse has been of a hospital nurse. This will undergo change in the coming years as more and more people are supported in the community. Then as never before, hospital experience will be but an incident in a person's life.

If this fourth edition of *Principles of Nursing* helps nurses to practise process thinking in their daily work related to people in any of the aforementioned groups, then the time and effort allocated to it will have been worth while. Also, if the patients' stay in hospital is achieved without loss of dignity, and patients are returned to their maximum function in the community, or they are helped to a peaceful death, then the nurses' function will have been fulfilled.

Index